Pelvic Yoga Therapy for the Whole Woman

of related interest

Yoga and Science in Pain Care
Treating the Person in Pain
Edited by Neil Pearson, Shelly Prosko and Marlysa Sullivan
Foreword by Timothy McCall
ISBN 978 1 84819 397 0
eISBN 978 0 85701 354 5

Yoga Therapy for Digestive Health
Charlotte Watts
ISBN 978 1 84819 354 3
eISBN 978 0 85701 312 5

Yoga Therapy for Fear
Treating Anxiety, Depression and Rage with the Vagus Nerve and Other Techniques
Beth Spindler
ISBN 978 1 84819 374 1
eISBN 978 0 85701 331 6

Yoga Therapy for Insomnia and Sleep Recovery
An Integrated Approach to Supporting Healthy Sleep and Sustaining Energy All Day
Lisa Sanfilippo
ISBN 978 1 84819 391 8
eISBN 978 0 85701 348 4

PELVIC YOGA THERAPY for the WHOLE WOMAN

A Professional Guide

CHERI DOSTAL RYBA

Foreword by Shelly Prosko

Illustrated by Evelyn Rosario Andry

SINGING DRAGON
LONDON AND PHILADELPHIA

First published in Great Britain in 2022 by Singing Dragon,
an imprint of Jessica Kingsley Publishers
An imprint of Hodder & Stoughton Ltd
An Hachette UK Company

1

Disclaimer: The information contained in this book is not intended to replace the services of trained medical professionals or to be a substitute for medical advice. The complementary therapy described in this book may not be suitable for everyone to follow. You are advised to consult a doctor before embarking on any complementary therapy program and on any matters relating to your health, and in particular on any matters that may require diagnosis or medical attention.

A CIP catalogue record for this title is available from the
British Library and the Library of Congress

ISBN 978 1 78775 664 9
eISBN 978 1 78775 665 6

Printed and bound in Great Britain by CPI Group

Jessica Kingsley Publishers' policy is to use papers that are natural, renewable and recyclable products and made from wood grown in sustainable forests. The logging and manufacturing processes are expected to conform to the environmental regulations of the country of origin.

Jessica Kingsley Publishers
Carmelite House
50 Victoria Embankment
London EC4Y 0DZ

www.singingdragon.com

To my mother, for encouraging me to teach.

To my daughters, for joyful play and big feelings.

To everyone bravely exploring embodiment.

Contents

PART 4: HOW DO WE SOURCE INSPIRATION AND SUSTAIN ACTION?

Acknowledgments

First, I bow to all who have received these teachings and expanded my understanding, compassion, and skill. As my students, you've been some of the best teachers. Thank you for sharing stories and celebrating victories with me.

To Laura Kupperman, for the sweet surprise of connecting me with Singing Dragon. Thank you for instigating this project! Immense gratitude to my editor, Claire, for meeting me each step of the way with enthusiasm.

To Shelly Prosko, for embracing the full spectrum of rigorous, technical accuracy, pelvic-floor jokes, compassion, personal healing – you've enriched my life and this book with your presence.

For the beautiful illustrations and heartwarming friendship – thank you, Eve.

To this crew for candor and providing loving feedback on drafts: Kristin, Julie, Emily, D. Chasse, Lisa, Linda, and Kelsey. I feel so grateful for close sisterhood and the broader community that holds me in positive regard. You know who you are.

To Leila Stuart, for your friendship, frank advice, and generous mentorship. I treasure you.

To Donna Farhi – thank you for sharing your craft. I'm honored to have observed closely as a student and assistant teacher.

To all my teachers, including: Eric Franklin; Scott Anderson; Sandra Helpsmeet, for suggesting I travel to New Zealand and sharing in practice; Susan Gingrasso, distinguished dance educator and my first client in 2003.

To past, current, and future yoga therapists in training with AlcheMe Yoga Therapy, Orange County, CA, for choosing this path. Thank you, Katie, Tess, and Megan for the joy of leading and teaching beside you as co-directors.

To my dad for his entrepreneurial tenacity and my mom for nurturing, painting, praying – I found my way into work I love. To my mother-in-law for praise and presence.

Jason, my love, for participating in "research" and supporting my ambition. The way we partner in the dance of householding, parenting, and marriage makes me proud. To my girls – may you be safe and protected, happy and free. I hope you contribute boldly to a kinder, more embodied world. Thank you for choosing us.

To my body, for the gift of exuberant life.

To nature for her solace, beauty, adventure, and rhythm.

Lastly, to peers and colleagues sharing the vision of pelvic vitality. We do this work together to liberate past and future generations. Thank you for bringing this book to life in your communities.

Foreword

"Have you lost sensation in the area of your perineum, genitals, or anus, or have you had any significant problems controlling or emptying your bowel or bladder?" As a physiotherapist, this is the question I was trained to ask each patient who presented with low back pain. I hoped the person would say no, otherwise it meant a red flag for cauda equina syndrome, a neurological condition that would require immediate medical attention.

That was the extent of our pelvic health training in physiotherapy a few decades ago, in addition to a few minutes of education on the importance of addressing modifications for positions during sexual intercourse for those with back pain, which was offered in the form of a pamphlet that was passed around in class briefly. Thankfully we have come a long way since then in the area of pelvic health and rehabilitation.

During the first decade of my clinical practice, research surrounding pelvic-floor health issues was growing and being translated into physiotherapy practice as a specialty area of pelvic-floor rehabilitation through professional continuing education courses. As I gained knowledge, skills, and experience, my clinical practice evolved to include helping an increasing number of people struggling with a variety of pelvic-floor issues. I am grateful to the pioneers who I have learned from and who have paved the way for us to continue to explore this path: the many researchers, educators, clinical instructors, and clinicians. However, like many specialties, the lens zooms in sharply and often does not zoom back out, resulting in a myopic view of the person and their situation. As Carolyn Vandyken, one of our pioneers in pelvic-floor rehabilitation, states, "We must put the pelvic floor back in the body."

In addition to addressing the pelvic floor within the context of the rest of the body, we also need to extend beyond a postural-structural-biomechanical model and address the whole person and all of their layers of existence within the context of their environment, community, and their relationships. Due to growing and compelling evidence that can no longer be ignored, the modern-day healthcare paradigm is slowly, steadily, and thankfully shifting toward integrating a more biopsychosocial (BPS) approach in many areas of care, including pelvic healthcare. However, attempts at implementing a BPS approach often fall short, perhaps because we are immersed in a reductionistic way of thinking (the belief that individual parts simply make up the whole). If the BPS model is to be used to its fullest potential, it must be applied in a dynamic, interdependent way, in line with the complexity of the human experience.

Pelvic Yoga Therapy for the Whole Woman is a timely and much-needed contribution to conventional pelvic rehabilitation and wellness care as it offers a nuanced and compassionate exploration and understanding of the whole person and their suffering. Yoga therapy uses an accessible biopsychosocial-spiritual framework, supports person-centered care, promotes sustainable self-care and self-efficacy, and nurtures the essential and impactful therapeutic alliance; all of which are vital components of pelvic healthcare. Yoga therapy includes a salutogenic approach, focusing on the factors that help the person progress towards what they value as health and wellbeing rather than focusing on fixing pathologies. The principles and practices of yoga teach us that any aspect of an individual's existence can be changed by any other aspect of their existence, therefore influencing the person's experience and healing journey.

Cheri successfully captures and translates the extensive scope of yoga therapy in the following pages, including the essence of yoga as an inward journey of self-discovery.

I first met Cheri at the Symposium on Yoga Therapy and Research several years ago when she was attending my presentation on yoga therapy and incontinence. I recall her steadfast and kind attentiveness, welcoming and warm smile, and a genuine curiosity that was admirable. Cheri's inquiries during and after the session were a testament to her in-depth and nuanced understanding of the topic, her vast background knowledge and experience, and her immense passion and curiosity that drove her desire to learn more and gain deeper insight in order to best serve her students and clients. Cheri and I consistently met throughout her writing process for this book. It was remarkable to observe her patience, persistence, and ability to clearly explain complex concepts. She skillfully blends current evidence with her knowledge, skills, and experience she has gained over the years as a yoga therapist, dancer, and movement and dance educator, with her ongoing studies in pelvic health. She creatively integrates her novel ideas, assessments, and practices with what she has learned from various teachers, her clients, and her personal experiences. She courageously and playfully shares her own personal stories that the reader will find impactful.

I especially appreciate the embodied experiences Cheri eloquently describes and offers as we make our way through each chapter. The book is a gentle, loving, and compassionate exploration and invitation to embrace an embodied understanding of pelvic yoga therapy, with an abundance of guided self-experiential practices that the therapist can enjoy and learn from, and also offer their clients. This can be one of the most powerful ways to cultivate the emergence of embodied wisdom that supports quality whole person care.

The time is ripe for this book, as a growing number of healthcare professionals are seeking to integrate yoga and a biopsychosocial-spiritual approach to pelvic care, and a growing number of yoga professionals are eager to learn more about pelvic health and using yoga therapeutically.

I am confident that this book will reach and impact a wide audience and serve its purpose as a guide for yoga and healthcare professionals in pelvic health and rehabilitation in this moment in time and in years to come.

Shelly Prosko, PT, C-IAYT
Physiotherapist, yoga therapist, educator
www.physioyoga.ca

Introduction

One question I've investigated for most of my life asks, "How is it that adversity for some people leads to growth, a strengthened commitment to vital health, and meaningful connection, while for others a similar event or conditions breed disconnection, despair, disease?" How do we take what happens to us and turn it into gold? I believe compassionate self-awareness, a curiosity about ourselves, could be a key ingredient – relationship plays another vital role. Yoga therapy prompts discovery of this deep well of knowing, self-actualization, and connection. Leaving no stone left unturned in our lived experiences, yoga makes the unconscious conscious.

I'll keep my story brief here, as my personal experiences have been woven into the text organically. While I had taken up interest in the pelvis several years prior, motherhood galvanized my desire to debunk body myths, raise the standard of care for pelvic health, hold women's stories, and leave a bigger impact on our world through embodiment teachings and writing.

I've found that putting my proverbial pelvic-health flag in the sand has opened dialogue with girlfriends, family members, and even new acquaintances on social media and strangers at the park while our children played. Creating awareness about pelvic health can create an open-door policy where "TMI" (too much information) no longer exists. I adore the moment when a woman boldly asks a question or discloses private details for the very first time and feels seen, heard, and respected. This courageous vulnerability and compassion that we welcome in ourselves and others, and which normalizes this entire conversation, I believe is at the center of our role as yoga therapists specializing in pelvic care. May we welcome our students with grace and skillful presence.

My intentions around language

This is a book about the pelvic floor, but you may have noticed how the word "floor" is absent from the title. This is intentional. The term can be found in these pages like a remnant of our collective understanding, as it is still widely used and accepted. As you'll find, however, many other images and words may better describe the pelvic tissues and their dynamic function – my favorites being a dome, trampoline, and jellyfish. I invite you to expand your understanding from a flat plane of muscles sitting at the bottom of your pelvis and bring awareness to the volume and contours, relationships, and metaphors that will arise from your own exploration.

I hemmed and hawed for months about whether to keep the word "woman" in the title of this book. We have plentiful research showing pelvic-floor dysfunction impacts far more women than men. I've supported hundreds of clients, most of whom have been women. After completing an eye-opening training on transgender-inclusive language for pelvic health, the title felt potentially exclusionary. I wondered how I might better serve and include people with different identities, experiences, and anatomy than the "typical" cisgender woman.

Most of us were socialized to understand gender as a strict binary. In reality, gender identity and anatomy cover a continuum. Even within cisgender groups, we need to be careful not to make assumptions, as there's a range of possible experience *and* biology represented. It may feel polarizing, confusing, and difficult to move through such topics. We're at a time societally that requires discernment, compassion, and great nuance.

Much of what you'll learn in this book can be adapted to suit the needs of clients with male biology or genitals, as the skeletal and muscular structures function similarly to some degree. Transgender individuals also deserve to feel their needs are understood and can be met appropriately.

Work together with your student to identify language that fits their needs and preferences. Take responsibility to get educated about gender identity and gender-affirming treatment.

I sat with all these considerations and settled into a "yes – and" approach. You'll see I use both gendered language (woman, she) and gender-neutral language (they, their, person, student) to attempt to show that we can adapt our language according to audience. As you read, substitute neutral or gendered terms as you see fit.

Mothering two small children amidst writing this book – during a global pandemic – afforded little space or social contact. I would have liked to included clients as models for diversity. I chose to take sample photographs of myself in each posture and hire an artist. It felt important to use hand-drawn images to bring a soft, human touch to these pages – enjoy the illustrations!

Lastly, my writing style is largely tethered to the way I speak when teaching movement (minus the abundant sound effects). I believe firmly that learning anatomy experientially and the attention we invest in personal embodiment gives us the presence to impact our students more deeply than information alone can. Explore the contents of this book as a student first, making it an intellectual *and* somatic experience. Then move into critical reasoning and applications as you consider your role as a yoga, fitness, or healthcare professional.

How this book is organized

The first principle to honor when providing yoga therapy (and healthcare) is to do no harm. As yoga professionals, we seek to provide a safe and consensual, experiential and embodied, trauma-informed approach. This is true regardless of one's specialty, and becomes even more essential to pelvic care as we respect the prevalence of trauma and abuse. In Part 1, we'll cover the ethical, philosophical, and physiological frameworks that guide our delivery of the transformative potential of yoga therapy.

So often, students ask me, "What should I feel when I do this pose?" and "Is this right?" Getting it right doesn't exist – there isn't "one way" to do a posture, or one correct outcome of a practice. Guiding a student well means drawing out their direct experience – identifying what they feel and where their blind spots might be, and offering suggestions that we trust will point them toward their desired outcome. We cannot feel what they feel, nor can we be with them every moment. We can equip and empower our students to meet their own needs with increasing skill.

Just like studying individual pelvic-floor muscles (PFM) extracted from their relationship to the whole body, the act of dissection creates separation where none exists. My understanding of the human body expanded exponentially with one deep week of study with the brilliant Gil Hedley. Donning my nurse scrubs and white lab coat, we began and ended each day in the cadaver lab in circle. His palpable reverence for learning allowed everyone in the room to become investigators, backed by the spiritual significance of receiving the gift of studying together in community, and entering into another's human form by conscious choice and deliberate action.

Our body remains after we die, and tells stories of the life we lived. I marveled at seeing an uncircumcised penis for the first time. We also deducted another donor had been a mother by the shape of her cervix, and that she had not yet crossed the threshold of menopause – a tampon had been left intact by those who had prepared her body. We traverse intimate terrain as pelvic yoga therapists.

It may be useful to reflect on what judgments, sensations, or emotions came up for you when envisioning me in the dissection lab handling the genitals of cadavers. We may feel a similar response wash over us during a session; we can practice observing our discomfort rather than allowing it to overwhelm our focus on the student. If we squirm, grimace, or become tense from believing urine, stool, discharge, or masturbation is too taboo to talk about, we'll be hard pressed to have an effective, heart-to-heart exchange with a client entrusting us with their secrets. These topics come up readily when working with clients experiencing pelvic-health issues, and we all have layers of shame to unravel before we can welcome these conversations and sensations with equanimity.

In Part 2, we'll zoom in to study the pelvis itself in detail, developing what I call X-ray vision, and explore the use of breath and sound. We'll examine how postural relationships can hinder or help one's pelvic function, gather insights about pelvic conditions, and name the varied functions of happy pelvic muscles. Ultimately, our work is always about the whole person in front of us. May this section create a map and compass in your mind, to better assess and guide students toward wholeness.

Our task may be to become more competent and skillful in pelvic matters, yet so profoundly neutral in our presence that we can serve as a vessel for prana to move through us. Holding space is an active state; rather than a state of "doing," however, I believe it's a state of "being." If we impose, fix, or jump to an assumed agenda in response to a student's suffering, we end up clouding our capacity to see them as intricate, inherently whole people. First, we witness. From this state of open perception, the way forward emerges.

In yoga therapy, this constitutes our formal intake and assessment process, which opens Part 3 of this book. You'll then find restorative practices supported by developmental patterns and somatic inquiry, as well as a selection of asana adaptations for pelvic health. Being supports doing, and "doing less" is a common theme I see when training yoga teachers and yoga therapists as they learn to curate more potent, personalized "yoga medicine." We march against the societal drumbeat of "more is better," too, when we invite our students to find a more sustainable pace of life that supports growth and healing.

We can be highly skilled professionals, yet if we fail to inspire and support our students in integrating yoga therapy into their lives, they won't receive its benefit. We'll conclude, in Part 4, with a discussion around bolstering a student's intent and consistency with program adherence strategies. Then we'll elevate the individual's commitment through connection and community support.

If we get to share life with someone as their yoga therapist, let's recognize it as truly sacred. We get to witness our student's ever-growing confidence, help them navigate new concerns and inevitable setbacks, and celebrate new triumphs. The yoga-therapy practice evolves as they do, yet the commitment and relationship carries through as a constant connection to source.

Welcome, dear reader, to the adventure that
awaits in these pages and within you.

PART 1

WHY YOGA THERAPY FOR PELVIC HEALTH?

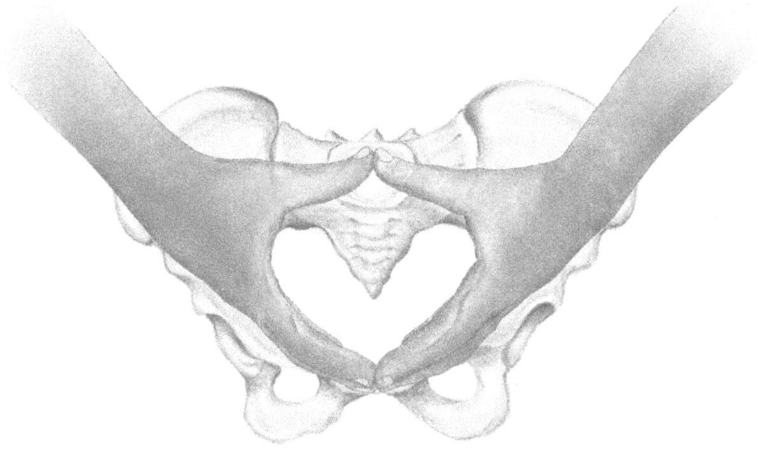

CHAPTER 1

The Role of a Yoga Therapist

Intended to expand the biomedical approach, not replace it, a biopsychosocial paradigm (Wade and Halligan 2017) may reflect the quality of care many consumers have come to understand they deserve. A holistic, collaborative, person-centered approach respects the complexity and lived experience of people with pelvic concerns. The future of healthcare embraces *and integrates* a biopsychosocial-spiritual (BPSS) model (Saad, de Medeiros, Mosini 2017).

Yoga therapy provides distinct methods for the assessment and care of these powerful aspects of the student's experience (McCall, Satish, Tiwari 2016, pp.31–46). Their beliefs and values, mental-emotional patterns, and social relationships, and how connected they feel to a sense of purpose, all hold clues and keys to healing as much as their physical symptoms and medical history. May this book equip you to deliver true holistic care to the students who come to work with you.

In this chapter, we'll explore the definition and scope of yoga therapy, the advantages of a yoga therapist's approach, and the limits of our scope. We'll also clarify how a clinical pelvic therapist and yoga therapist can collaborate to deliver interdisciplinary care. Lastly, informed consent and community care are presented as essential tenets for offering safe and effective pelvic yoga therapy.

Defining yoga therapy and our scope of practice

Quality yoga instruction focuses on customizing and adapting the practice to suit the individual's needs and the season of life they find themselves in – a sort of call and response song in which the student reports what they feel or how they're challenged, and we respond with modifications or refinements to their practice. Wise teachers know how to draw out a student's own insights, develop their kinesthetic skill and discernment, and utilize all the various aspects of yoga practice from asana to pranayama to the ethical observances. Some might ask, "What's the difference between yoga instruction and yoga therapy?"

Crossing the threshold from yoga teacher to yoga therapist entails rigorous training and well-defined therapeutic processes. One hallmark distinguishing yoga therapy is conducting a thorough intake and assessment (Kepner *et al.* 2014). The International Association of Yoga Therapists (IAYT) has worked diligently to standardize the field and provide comprehensive, ethical guidelines for how we train and certify yoga therapists, how we operate our businesses, and how to respect the boundaries of our scope of practice (Kepner 2015, pp.548–560). The role of yoga professionals does not include providing a diagnosis. In fact, our students will likely continue their medical or clinical pelvic care as prescribed while concurrently implementing their yoga-therapy practice.

Author and activist, Matthew Remski, believes "A scope of practice both *limits* the power of the teacher or therapist, and *shares* it with the student" (Remski 2019, p.286). Yoga therapy is a collaborative, co-regulating process in which the responsibility and power is shared between teacher and student. Oversight from an organizing body like the IAYT provides a clearly defined scope, as well as accountability for us as yoga professionals. Thus, students may come to yoga therapy more informed about the quality and types of care they can expect.

The panchamaya model of the five koshas serves as one of the primary models of assessment for yoga therapists (Sovik and Bhavanani 2016, pp.17–29), which we'll cover in detail in the next chapter. This model demonstrates how the interconnected sheaths or layers of each person function as the gem through which the light of prana, or life force energy, filters. A rare and exquisite way of viewing the individual's many facets of self, this model differentiates yoga therapy from a conventional, biomedical model of care. It gives us a container to discern at each level where there's potential for greater awareness, function, and integration, bringing all parts of the whole into consideration for our assessment and therapeutic application of the teachings of yoga. As yoga therapists, we polish this gem as we practice holistically, and share its beauty with each student.

While certain advantages of yoga therapy identified next may also exist within clinical environments, especially in private, out-of-pocket clinics for example, they are fundamental within the role of yoga therapy. Let's examine how yoga therapy can excel in supporting women with pelvic concerns.

Quality and longevity of relationship

Many yoga therapists work in an entrepreneurial, private-practice capacity. Operating outside of the Health Insurance Portability and Accountability Act (HIPPA) requirements and clinical environments, and therefore mostly free from insurance coding protocols, we set the length of each session, frequency of meetings, and longevity of relationship. Whereas a patient might receive a 20-minute office visit in a clinical setting, they likely receive sessions of a full hour, and sometimes longer, with a yoga therapist. Physical therapy, for example, may also have insurance-dictated expectations on the number of billable sessions available to a patient. Clinicians may feel limited by these policies – at times, a driving force for pelvic-floor specialists to make their own entrepreneurial leap in the interest of their patients and career sustainability. Thankfully, there's typically no overarching protocol that dictates when someone is to be "discharged" from yoga therapy – the work continues to unfold with dynamic consent between teacher and student.

We play a unique, often nonclinical role that affords us more time and creative license to witness each client, hear their stories and concerns, and follow our critical reasoning and intuition when developing a plan for their practice. As stated in *The Heart of Yoga*, "Yoga is not fixed. Yoga is creation" (Desikachar 1999, p.xxvi).

Powerful medicine, yoga's efficacy slowly grows as the practitioner maintains the behaviors instilled through a yoga-therapy practice over a duration of time (McCall 2019, p.10). Its strengths may better suit prevention and health maintenance, whereas allopathic medicine, thank goodness, exists for the acute and complex scenarios in which we may find ourselves. While medicine can save lives, yoga seeks to extend and enrich the quality of our lifespan.

As yoga professionals, we can establish business practices that honor this desire for quality and longevity of relationship with our students. This has been a guiding principle in my work for years, and I've found that remaining in touch even well after a working relationship has ended nourishes both my business and the student's continued self-reflection. A small but thoughtful email or a holiday card can reignite one's devotion for practice, and at times help a student return to the safe haven of a group class or resume private sessions for another season of discovery. What better way to serve than to provide continuity – to bear witness to one's life?

We continually reassess, identify progress, and celebrate milestones. The longer an imbalance has existed, or the more complex the variables involved, the more gradual the process of recovery may be for that student. The deeper our rapport runs with a student, the more we see root-cause material and their essential nature rise to the surface over time. Of course, with the right spark of inspiration and the skillful selection and delivery of practices, we may also celebrate more rapid results. By developing a heart-to-heart relationship with our students, we usher them through an evolving practice week by week, season by season, that sustains them.

Instilling self-efficacy

What is enlightenment if not being wholly, reverently present and engaged in one's life? Culturally, we're at a time when grounded presence, compassionate action and social advocacy, connection with nature (to which we belong as mammals), consent, and sexual reeducation feel like essential curricula if we are to evolve in a way that honors everyone and can resolve generations of wounding, abuse, neglect, injustice.

Yoga returns us to ourselves, helping us remove the conditioning of the mind and the imbalances within our body, and reconnects us to our joy and purpose. We remember our own wholeness, and as our practice unfolds, we discover a deeper understanding of self, and perhaps, begin to unravel the root causes of our own suffering. By regaining agency, we cultivate our ability to move more skillfully through daily life, enhancing our relationships and our purposeful work in the world with increased confidence. No one can "do yoga" for anyone else (Farhi 2018).

It is up to us as yoga therapists to discern which tools or practices will be most useful and relevant to the student in front of us, and to teach them with adequate information to practice well, yet titrate an appropriate dose of practice so as not to overwhelm them. What motivates them? How do we grow their interoceptive skill? Do they understand how and why the practices we've selected are relevant to their goals? How can we support them in identifying progress and staying the course? We want to set them up for the greatest possible success in their independent home practice, building their skill and confidence so they can feel deep, lasting benefits over time.

Recognizing each client as sovereign means we help them cultivate independence. They must feel able, ready, and willing to practice on their own for change to take place. In this way, yoga therapists serve as wellness coaches by using motivational interviewing, eliciting subjective feedback and discernment from the student, and clarifying and reassessing goals that propel the student forward with increasing self-efficacy.

My work with private clients has affirmed that through yoga therapy, students become willing to speak up and seek out the care they deserve, which can translate beautifully into comfortably and proactively receiving their pelvic exams and prenatal and postpartum care, openly discussing their symptoms and needs with their medical provider and partner, and pursuing mental healthcare without stigma.

Modeling and transmitting embodiment

The integrity and wisdom of a yoga therapist is sourced from within their own embodied practice, studies, and way of life. Our "beingness" is our calling card, the essence that draws students to working with us. I believe the same can, of course, be true for providers in other disciplines – we feel a tangible ease and trust when we're in the presence of someone who has walked the path ahead of us, comfortable in their own skin and glowing with vitality.

Asana practices can be chameleon-like, adapting to offer a variety of subtly different outcomes, depending on the baseline experience of the practitioner. Each asana can take on many different qualities based on our cues and how we apply them in terms of duration, repetitions, depth, sequencing, and more. We learn physical practice best through direct application, exploring trial and error on our mats. When it comes to knowing where to start or what a client needs, I always say, "Start somewhere useful." The most accessible training ground you have is your own body and life.

Over my years of teaching, I started to notice an unexpected trend of more and more teachers hiring me as their private yoga therapist and mentor. Looking back, it seems this way of being and my continual study created a certain magnetism for these relationships to flourish. I eventually moved into a faculty role, training teachers and yoga therapists, and here we are, coming together through the pages of this book. I've observed many instances in which highly trained body professionals, medical and otherwise, lack the embodiment of all the knowledge they hold. For example, when asked to describe the direction of the breath excursion, there's hesitation or confusion in their response, or we see the reverse of what we know to be anatomically true about the diaphragm.

What's movement efficiency? The ability to execute intentional and unconscious movements with minimal effort.

Our embodiment and physicality as teachers matter immensely as we attempt to transmit the teachings of yoga and movement efficiency with accuracy. That's not to say we can't have our own healing journey taking place concurrently with our teaching service – often pelvic-floor concerns may be exactly the reason we find ourselves here, compelled to serve others in this way. Knowing something cognitively is not enough. Yoga certainly provides intellectual and philosophical study, yet its richness lies in the felt experience and lived reality of these practices. Our capacity to eloquently convey this depth through verbal cues and skillful movement comes directly from personal inquiry. Yoga is meant to transform us.

I invite you, as you continue to read, to apply what you're learning to your own movement and life first and foremost, and secondarily to your professional work. As teachers of embodiment, we must cultivate our own sensate skill and sensitivity so we can teach others to speak the language of their body, too.

Every practice offered in this book has been tested in practice and in working with private clients and groups of students. It's one way I practice integrity, allowing myself to be a guinea pig, a student, always. Ultimately, yoga therapy and other movement-based contemplative practices (MBCP) call us to model the path forward for our students. Take this book as a resource for your own evolution and experiment with the content here in your personal practice before offering it to your students. You may be surprised by what you find, and you'll be nourished by your own devotion and care.

Let's take a closer look now at how yoga therapy differs from other pelvic-floor therapies, and the ways in which a yoga professional can team up with healthcare providers to deliver the best outcomes and care for a student.

What is pelvic-floor therapy?

Pelvic health remains a relatively emerging field, growing and maturing alongside the standardization of yoga therapy itself. Healthcare providers specializing in pelvic health can include physical therapists, occupational therapists, and physiotherapists, among others. While physicians, obstetricians, gynecologists, and midwives may know how to assess baseline health or screen for pelvic-floor dysfunction, they likely have varied levels of training and experience in the *treatment* of pelvic-floor concerns, making a referral to pelvic-floor therapy necessary.

Pelvic-floor therapy directly evaluates and treats PFM function. This may include internal vaginal and/or rectal palpation, as well as global assessment of movement and posture.

Internal pelvic-floor physical therapy, sometimes referred to as "hands-in" work as an offshoot of more conventional "hands-on" bodywork, may not always be indicated clinically. External, fully clothed assessment methods may give skilled therapists enough information to guide treatment, as can observing the recruitment of regional muscles and breath patterns during exercises, and eliciting subjective feedback from the recipient to attempt to complete the picture of their physical assessment. It can help put our yoga-therapy students at ease to understand internal touch may not be necessary, and that they always have the right to decline an internal assessment or treatment.

Observing global posture and movement patterns, including during weight-bearing activities, gives valuable information about how a woman moves her body, whereas internal pelvic-floor evaluations often take place supine, in a more passive position. From a clinician's perspective, it may be more convenient for observation and ergonomics to have a patient supine on a table in the exam room. As the patient progresses or depending on their concerns and goals, integrating more functional activities (internal assessment while squatting, for example) may provide more comprehensive results.

I appreciate when pelvic-floor specialists address the whole body, rather than becoming so engrossed in the pelvis that it can feel as though the rest of the body becomes neglected. Perhaps this is one unique way yoga therapy and other fitness or movement professionals can support a clinician's scope – by assisting in this integration process to restore confidence in activities of daily living and a return to exercise with peace of mind and improved function. This question can also help you vet other providers by understanding whether they take a localized or whole-body approach to pelvic care.

Credentialing of pelvic specialists

In the United States, the first women's health board-certification examination was administered in 2009 by the American Board of Physical Therapy

Specialties. As of June 2020, a total of 550 women's health specialists had been certified in the United States as a Women's Health Clinical Specialist (WCS) (APTA 2020). This designation lets consumers know these healthcare providers can ethically assess and treat pelvic conditions, which may include internal evaluation of pelvic-floor function, as well as external pelvic and overall postural assessments. In Canada, physiotherapists can become a designated women's health specialist through a similar certification process.

While it can be an important step toward developing professional competency, credentialing alone does not ascertain the biopsychosocial skill set required to meet the demands of pelvic-health clients. According to Carolyn Vandyken (2021), PT, Co-Founder of Reframe Rehab, and well-respected pelvic-health professional, many pelvic-floor specialist certifications are offered by private educational organizations (such as Herman and Wallace or physical-therapy governing bodies), rather than being fully integrated into academic or university settings.

Many skilled pelvic healthcare providers choose not to complete these certificates for a variety of reasons, and excel in their fields and patient care, while some who are certified may continue to practice in a more limited biomedical or biomechanical approach to pelvic health. Certification alone will not guarantee that clinicians have developed necessary competencies in an evidence-informed, biopsychosocial framework.

We need to diligently interview the providers we align with or to whom we choose to refer patients. Pelvic health warrants understanding the intersections of anatomy and movement science, pain science, trauma and the nervous system, mental health, hormonal health, and more. We may also need to shore up our studies and skills in these key areas to best support our students with pelvic-health concerns.

As a helpful adjunct to clinical pelvic therapy, students could receive therapeutic touch from other bodywork professionals to promote self-compassion, circulatory and lymph health, and general relaxation. The safe refuge of ethical, warm, skillful touch has helped me melt muscular holding patterns and unravel deep guarding, restoring glide and peace to the tendrils of nerves and vessels flowing through my pelvic bowl. Perhaps you'll also broaden your professional network to include skilled manual or massage therapists.

My personal, ethical standard is that I experience the service or touch of a provider first, when possible. If a professional and nourishing experience is received, I then feel comfortable referring my students. This requires vulnerability and an investment of time and resources that will likely benefit us immediately and our community of clients in the long run by properly vetting our referral network. When a student needs care we can't provide, we can rest easy knowing we have just the person in mind for their referral.

Other pelvic modalities

There's also a growing movement of nonclinical pelvic-health providers offering services like sexological bodywork, vulva mapping, vaginal steaming, and more, where a woman can learn to self-regulate, sense her pelvic space, and advocate for her own care with a witness they trust, often without the sterile, impersonal environment of a hospital or clinic. In any professional exchange, we hope and strive for reparative experiences. Somehow, when we enter the clinic or hospital doors, an unspoken authority may strip us of our voice, our capacity to say, "No, I'm not ready," or, "Can you please explain what's about to happen again, before it happens?" Remembering and actively reaffirming bodily autonomy is part of the inner referencing that takes place with yoga therapy. We can then bring that restored confidence with us into environments where we perhaps had surrendered some of our power in the past.

The act of negotiating consent, choosing to pause and wait, or potentially decline touch when the emotional charge indicates a somatic stopping point, can be a reparative experience for women. Each step of the way, they can relearn to register and honor their interoceptive clues, agreeing only to actions or treatments that allow a sense of safety to remain intact.

Skillful, loving touch may be one of the most effective ways to repattern or create change in our body through increased proprioception and interoception. If we can't feel or even connect consciously to the pelvic bowl, it may prove very difficult to effect real, lasting change. Touch may expedite this process of awakening through direct, tangible experience (Kent 2011, pp.29–82).

Internal and external genital touch are not within the scope of a yoga professional. Later in this book, we'll explore practical alternatives we can use to help our students gain access to the internal volume and curvaceous landscape of their own pelvic bowl through breath, imagery, and self-care practices.

When to refer to a pelvic specialist

Referring our clients to a trusted pelvic-floor specialist demonstrates care and discernment, and can give us valuable information that guides how we curate a student's practice. In short, I nearly always suggest students of mine consider seeing a pelvic-floor specialist for assessment and, if indicated, treatment. The natural limitations in our scope support considering a collaborative approach for folks with pelvic symptoms.

In Appendix A, you'll find sample forms to consider using with yoga-therapy clients. These screening tools give us relevant information about a client's symptoms and current pelvic awareness, further guiding our assessment process and practice, as well as indicating whether a referral may be warranted. You'll find more guidance around making referrals in Chapter 7.

Working together

When acquiring new client information, I ask who else they receive care from currently. I call it their "care team." This could include medical providers, such as the referring physician, urologist, or OBGYN (obstetrics and gynecology), the pelvic-floor specialist, and other complementary services, like massage therapy, acupuncture, fitness training, chiropractic care, and counseling. Understanding which results they've noticed from different modalities can give helpful insight as to what could be most supportive to their healing journey and how yoga can best dovetail with their existing care plan.

When we see an absence of diagnosis or other providers on an intake form, it may be prudent to help the student initiate contact with a specialist and encourage them to assemble their support team. Any time new symptoms pop up, symptoms worsen, or the student has acute or undiagnosed symptoms, it's best to work with a medical professional to rule out more serious conditions and get the information we need as yoga professionals to serve the student safely.

One morning, after a beginner yoga class in which I had mentioned the pelvic floor during our closing practices for the hips, a woman approached me. The room had mostly cleared out, and she seemed both hopeful and concerned. Her eyes were bright and open wide. She shared with me that she'd been experiencing fecal incontinence. I assured her that our conversation would be kept confidential, and thanked her for entrusting me with her feelings and experiences. We continued with dialogue around when it started, when she experienced the issue and what made it worse, and what she felt might be related to this somewhat new phenomenon. She'd given birth to her children vaginally years before (if my memory serves me, her children were both in elementary school by then) and she noticed the symptom only after having intercourse. Luckily, she felt supported by her husband and seemed to be left without added shame from his having witnessed the incontinence on multiple occasions. I explained the term fecal incontinence and how I felt it may be best for her to see a pelvic-floor specialist. I emailed her the contact information of two local colleagues I trusted, encouraging her to make an appointment. About two months later, she returned to class and thanked me, sharing that she had wanted to give time to the life and career transitions that had caused her great stress around the same time her symptoms began. They had since subsided completely. She added that she would contact someone if the symptoms returned.

As much as I wanted to support her personally with private yoga therapy, I again shared with conviction that getting an appropriate diagnosis was a pertinent first step. I gave her a couple of guidelines to be aware of as she continued to attend group classes. This exchange provided an invaluable experience for me in staying within my scope, respecting the role of medical providers, and practicing humility. She felt satisfied with our exchange, and I felt content knowing she was better equipped to seek care in the future. We can only help students when it feels ethically aligned and *when they express a readiness* to begin the unique work of cultivating a relationship with a yoga therapist.

Concurrent care

We can provide our services concurrently – where a client sees both a yoga therapist and a pelvic-floor specialist at the same time. It's important that we respect the client's privacy and share their information solely with explicit consent, and only with the relevant care provider. As yoga professionals are not yet bound by HIPPA, I've found it effective to simply request that my client cc an email between myself and the medical provider to give their consent that we exchange notes. Often, clinics and healthcare providers have a formal waiver that must be signed and documented.

Students often have questions about how to execute and when to regress or progress their exercises, as the time they get in a clinic is often limited by the clock. As yoga professionals, we can provide the quality of time and attentive cues needed to enhance interoceptive skill and improve overall movement performance. Although we need to take appropriate action (select *which* practices are most appropriate for a client), it's even more essential that we optimize *how* a practice is done. Receiving yoga therapy and pelvic care simultaneously can reinforce client education goals and treatment plans, as well as potentially fill any needs left unmet by another's scope or expertise.

Continuum of care

Another path is to work with people who have successfully completed or been discharged from their clinical therapy program. In physical therapy, the goal is often to return a patient to their prior level of functioning, addressing the diagnosis or targeted issue at hand. Yoga therapy provides a perfect segue to continue care with lifestyle awareness, maintaining one's home practice, and further observing and addressing the whole person's evolving needs.

Yoga often receives a cursory recommendation from physicians and physical therapists, valued for its capacity to create and maintain positive outcomes with very low risk of adverse effects. We can help facilitate these collaborative relationships by educating providers about the differences between yoga and yoga therapy. We can prime healthcare professionals to give more explicit referrals to trusted yoga therapists with more advanced training and specific skills in pelvic awareness.

What may not be immediately (or ever) indicated in a clinical setting, and thus not able to be treated and coded according to the current referral at hand, could show up as one of the more relevant pieces of the puzzle in a yoga-therapy setting. Sometimes, pelvic specialists only assess locally, whereas a full-body assessment may give clues that promote earlier results or more lasting healing. For example, we may see imbalances in the feet and legs that could contribute to, or stem from, a pelvic-floor imbalance. We can address this with a functional, well-rounded approach to asana and an active lifestyle.

We may learn that a student has recently lost their job, and that this was followed by a sense of insecurity, fear, and the onset or recurrence of urinary urgency and pelvic pain. Attempting to address only the physical symptoms would miss the key underlying drivers of stress and the lack of purpose they had found through their work. Restoring a sense of security through restorative sequences and breathing for autonomic regulation, self-compassion as a balm for one's grief, and eventually adding visualization for a renewed sense of purpose and direction may allow us to better address their needs and work beyond a purely musculoskeletal paradigm. We see and understand how the layers of one's being influence each other – never separate, and always in communication with each other. Of course, when physical symptoms persist, worsen, or reappear, resuming care with a clinically trained professional can help us discern if a new treatment approach may be indicated.

How to forge collaborative relationships

As we carry the torch of doing this work, it's imperative that we navigate and advocate through the medical maze, and forge collaborative partnerships. Seek out a board-certified WCS or other pelvic-floor specialists in your community to create a referral network to support your students. Also, build your team of allied professionals to deliver well-rounded care. You could provide educational resources or offer to teach an introductory workshop for their community on yoga's approach to pelvic health.

Although telehealth existed long before the COVID pandemic, many providers found themselves thrust into doing their work online when government-mandated closures took place. You could seek out telehealth pelvic care providers to include in your referral network and serve as a yoga therapist resource for their patients from all over the world. Of course, you'd first want to familiarize yourself with delivering services online to support patients remotely.

One way to expand your network is through social media. Cast a wide net by following pelvic-floor advocates and specialists. Spend time observing the quality of content they share and trust that you'll discern whom to reach out to directly. It also serves as ongoing, free continued education for us as yoga professionals to be updating our knowledge and further differentiating our scope of practice.

Providers can work together to support the same client on interdisciplinary teams. They collaborate on assessment, treatment, and goals using a shared biopsychosocial model, and conduct regular team meetings or correspondence to progress and review the case. My dream would be for women everywhere to have access to both the appropriate clinical diagnosis and treatment of their pelvic symptoms, *and* the holistic, compassionate presence of a pelvic yoga therapist to integrate their experiences and support lasting results.

Most importantly, allow professional relationships to bloom organically over time. Knowing yourself can support you in finding like-minded colleagues with whom you can build your dream team. I hope you'll use these suggestions to build your professional relationships, as it makes all the difference in the sustainability of our career and in the quality of care and support we can offer students.

Acknowledging shortcomings

Unfortunately, most physicians still receive very little training or knowledge about movement and exercise, and may even perceive pelvic-floor issues as an inevitable part of being a woman, childbearing, or growing older in a human body. Armed with the generalized advice of telling a patient to do Kegels, many patients walk away not getting appropriate care – and not even knowing where to look.

> Sheena had asked her doctor (years before meeting and working with me) about her nighttime urinary frequency. After a cursory pelvic exam and blood work, they confirmed everything was "normal" and suggested she simply try drinking less water or do Kegels. She thus continued to void her bladder every 15–30 minutes before falling asleep and multiple times overnight before trying yoga therapy. She struggled most of her life, frustrated with her "baby bladder," and suffered from decreased quality and quantity of sleep because of it. After only five yoga-therapy sessions across eight weeks, she could sleep through the entire night, stopped going to the bathroom "just in case" altogether, and reduced her night-time frequency before falling asleep. This was possible through simple yet highly targeted lifestyle changes, cultivating compassion for herself, and providing sound education about bladder habits and pelvic awareness. Through yoga therapy, she also discovered a direct correlation between her mental activity and stress level and the amount of urge and frequency she experienced. She no longer identifies with the phrase "baby bladder" and feels confident.

In terms of Sheena's concerns about bladder habits, the medical field had largely failed her. We can do better collectively, which includes educating providers about yoga therapy and how it can help women like her.

We must understand and articulate an evidence-based approach to garner respect as an emerging field and to help translate terminology for our students so they become proficient in communicating with their care team members. Let's also realize that we may even find ourselves educating healthcare providers about yoga therapy, exercise and lifestyle evidence, and pelvic care details. Trust that we have a powerful, unique offering to bring to the table.

Another woman messaged me online, having seen my posts about pelvic health. We had a brief conversation about options for care. Months later, she thanked me for explaining pelvic-floor therapy exists, and shared that she'd begun treatment with a local provider. She felt overjoyed to be learning about her body and finally getting the help she needed to improve her comfort, continence, and sexual health. Never underestimate the impact that our presence and expertise can make, even from afar and outside a formal teacher-student relationship.

An encouraging trend toward increasing public awareness and improving policies and recommendations for women's health seems to be taking root. For example, the American College of Obstetricians and Gynecologists released a report proclaiming that postpartum care needed to better address the multifaceted and intersecting needs of new mothers, and include an ongoing approach with multiple visits, rather than a one-and-done six-week visit (ACOG 2018). Although this book does not highlight postpartum care specifically, I recognize that many people in need of this information are women and may also be mothers. The inadequacies of care that new mothers experience is but a flashpoint for larger, systemic changes the healthcare industry needs to face before we can hope to meet the growing demand for pelvic healthcare. Pelvic-floor disorders affect millions of women around the globe, and one study estimated that demand for care for pelvic-floor disorders will increase by 35% between 2010 and 2030 in the United States alone (Kirby, Luber, Menefee 2013). This estimate is 72% higher than originally predicted in 2000 (Luber, Boero, Choe 2001), further illustrating the rapidly growing need for highly skilled pelvic care providers and the need to educate and train physicians to recognize pelvic-floor disorders and appropriately refer patients. It appears we have plenty of work to do before pelvic vitality becomes the new norm.

Thank you for sharing this important work to reshape how pelvic care is recognized and treated, and to help rewrite cultural norms. Share what you learn here openly with your friends and colleagues. The only way to normalize these conversations is to have them with candid honesty.

Ethics and preventing harm in yoga

Sometimes, trust gets broken. In guru-lineage, capitalist, patriarchal, and sexist environments, yoga has been used against people seeking healing, causing immense suffering. We've heard courageous recounting of victims' stories, and we've seen the dismantling of these power dynamics begin as the truth becomes more widely known (Dinsmore-Tuli 2020). To learn steps you can take to help eradicate these abuses in the yoga community, consider reading the second edition of *Yoni Shakti* by Uma Dinsmore-Tuli, Ph.D. You may also find *Practice and All Is Coming* by Matthew Remski and *Teaching Yoga* by Donna Farhi useful references.

The term "post-lineage" is used by yoga teachers who are consciously moving out of the hierarchical guru-lineage model and establishing more equitable and trauma-informed frameworks for their teaching. In taking up the role of teacher or yoga therapist, we step into a position of leadership and authority. Whether our students put us on a pedestal or we unknowingly find ourselves perched, we have a responsibility to respect the therapeutic alliance and return the power to our students through shared decision-making, self-assessment, and education. This paradigm shift needs to continue to take root in the conventional healthcare system and global yoga community so collaborative care and sovereignty can flourish and future abuse can be prevented. Our students and the tradition of yoga deserve this respect.

A full discussion around these allegations and the hierarchical methodologies that perpetuate harm is outside the scope of this book. Let's anchor this topic by defining consent as part of the solution moving forward.

Defining consent

My hope in describing the elements of consent is to help you create a respectful, nuanced framework for asking private questions, offering props, and working hands on respectfully with your students. This can be shared in writing within your intake form, as well as guiding your methods and interactions during yoga-therapy sessions. I define consent as an ongoing, fluid agreement between all parties involved in an exchange. More concisely, consent practices for touch or other interactions between a yoga professional and student must meet three key criteria: informed, voluntary and enthusiastic, and dynamic or ongoing.

The first, informed consent, means that you understand what's being proposed and feel sufficient details have been outlined to discern whether to give your consent or not. Asking a student "May I assist you in this pose?" doesn't elucidate what you want to do and why, or how you're proposing to work with or touch the student. Before we even approach a student, we need to discern our intent, and then it must be clearly communicated.

Second, permission cannot be coerced or persuaded; true consent must be voluntary. Beyond a flat, voluntary yes, we can look for enthusiasm as an indicator that the person truly gives their consent from within all aspects of their being. Rather than accepting a nod, muffled response, or a verbal "Yes," given without eye contact, we need to perceive the subtle, nonverbal communication going on while requesting consent – as well as throughout the duration of an exchange.

Last, consent is a fluid, ongoing communication process. During an interaction, our sensations fluctuate, our narrative may change, or we may simply change our mind about whether we wish to engage or perhaps be left alone to practice without intervention. At any time, a student must feel able to revoke their consent or ask a question to clarify the intent of action before continuing.

How we negotiate consent as adults may stem from childhood experiences or from past trauma. Learning to recognize our default patterns of response means that through this awareness we can change them. We'll talk about how this can play out behaviorally from a nervous system perspective in Chapter 3.

Baseline awareness: our first exercise

I imagine there may have been an activation building in your body while taking in the recounting of abuse that has existed in the yoga community. It may have also triggered memories or sensations related to personal experiences of such abuse. (Thank you for compassionately acknowledging if this feels true for you personally.) This highlights our very humanity, which is essential to doing good work as a yoga therapist – our desire to first "do no harm," according to the yogic principle of ahimsa.

Becoming aware without judgment or immediately "fixing" ourselves allows us to perceive accurately, wholly. From that baseline of clear perception, we can then respond skillfully, lovingly, articulately. It's a surprisingly deceptive skill for many folks, although it can be trained quickly with regular practice. Let's pause to explore this skill that you'll revisit throughout this book and which will be foundational to your ability to help students register their experience.

When you're ready, you'll take about one minute to become still and observe yourself objectively. I recommend putting the book down once you've read this description, and then standing up to begin. Do your best not to "think about" what you feel or don't feel, and instead allow yourself to perceive moment to moment the changing sensations, thoughts, and images arising internally. You might become aware of your posture, areas of tension or discomfort, as well as areas of your body that feel pleasant. You may observe the rate and quality of how your breath moves, where you feel your pulse, and when your mind becomes distracted, becomes attached to an observation, or returns to attentive witnessing internally. The goal here is not to "do" anything, but instead *practice being* and *observing.*

Notice if you closed your eyes or kept them open to do this exercise. Neither strategy is "correct" but know you'll likely perceive in subtly different ways depending on this choice. Perhaps explore it both ways and see for yourself, building skill with the opposite strategy of what you tend to prefer and the agility to change between them. You can use this baseline awareness exercise as a pre-test at the beginning of client sessions, as well as a post-test after an intervention.

Right relationship

Each encounter with a provider, whether clinical or nonclinical, can move a student toward healing and repair. Where there's been a rupture through past abuse or consent violations, right relationship can be like salve on one's wound, bringing relief with the simple yet profound recognition of our innate need to be respected and witnessed. Restoring safe connection can look like learning to say yes to what we want, as much as speaking a resounding no when we feel it pounding in our chest. As pelvic yoga professionals, we must do justice to the individuals and communities we serve by acknowledging the pervasive harm caused by sexual assault, rape culture, and all types of trauma.

We have a responsibility to recognize that impact, as determined by the observer or recipient of our words and actions, outweighs intent. By establishing practices of ongoing, fluid consent and dismantling the power dynamics that can exist between a teacher and student, we can greatly reduce the likelihood of such transgressions. And yet, sometimes people get hurt by what we say or don't say, or misunderstand our intent. Learning to acknowledge someone's pain when it has been perceived to be caused by your actions takes great humility. These are difficult conversations to have, yet we're seeing accountability come to the foreground in many industries. When we know better, we're called to do better. We further support right relationship by folding empathy, compassion, and social justice into professional conduct, policy, and organizational structures (Jain 2020).

The professional therapeutic relationship provides much solace and fertile ground for growth, and yet it falls short. We'll never reach everyone with pelvic-floor dysfunction by working in a one-to-one model of care according to the growing prevalence of these concerns and the relatively small number of certified specialists. We also need models for one to many, like group programs and circles in which peer support and nonclinical modalities live on the same pedestal next to clinical care. Let's create systems and offerings that honor a new paradigm – to value preventative, integrative care, honor rites of passage like menarche, pregnancy and postpartum, miscarriage and loss, and menopause, and develop inclusive care not yet readily accessible to all races, sexual orientations, classes, ages, and abilities. I'm hopeful we're seeing the rise of community care and interdisciplinary teams as a new norm.

The disparities that exist in healthcare (Hartigan and Smith 2018; Mandimika *et al.* 2015) impact us all, yet some of us benefit while others suffer from them. With privilege comes responsibility. We can ask, "What role can I play in creating more equitable and accessible pelvic care?"

As we personally practice reverence for embodiment, nature, expression, spiritual inquiry, and a sustainable pace of life through yoga, may it contribute to collective awakening, systemic change, and improved care for everyone.

CHAPTER 2

Philosophical Foundations of Yoga Therapy

Universal and timeless wisdom resonates with our essential humanity and recognizes the source power behind life and our capacity for change. We can come to know and befriend ourselves, relate better to each other, and generate healing when we embrace spiritual teachings. Nestled within the varied and vast tradition of yoga sits yoga therapy, the specific application of this philosophy and practice to alleviate suffering and cultivate wellbeing, meaning, and purpose.

In this chapter, we'll explore yogic philosophy that supports and differentiates our contemporary role as yoga therapists from the biomedical model of care, including a framework for why we suffer, how to support a client's wholeness, and the role relationships play as a crucible for self-reflection.

What is yoga?

Yoga provides a path to embodied living. The roots of yoga philosophy compel us to take up the weaving of our own lives, using threads from a trinity of practice, process, and end result. Yoga is action in the present, the process of which unfolds over time with repetition, and the state of yoga, or union and harmony, that we come to embody more reliably. We move to make the unconscious conscious, inhibiting habitual tendencies and conditioning to reveal new eyes with which to see ourselves and the world. In short, yoga prompts self-awareness and promotes integration.

Based in Samkhya philosophy, yoga appreciates the dynamic relationship between two features of our human experience: the oscillating, impermanent nature of our body, mind, and environment (prakriti) and the constancy of energy that enlivens it (purusha) (Pearson, Prosko, Sullivan 2019, p.70). Coming to the realization that we are both changing matter and unchanging spirit allows us to have hope, rather than misidentifying with a symptom or diagnosis, or viewing those as permanent or fixed. We can learn to take meaningful action toward fulfillment of our purpose, the expression of our unique aliveness that brings a sense of steadfast wellness and joy.

Yoga philosophy describes how the qualities of prakriti are shaped by our actions, as well as giving a methodology to more positively influence our perception, health, and wellbeing. Subtle, subliminal imprints may cause manifestations in our physical, material nature. What shows up in our body may be a result of cumulative history – a combination of past experiences, beliefs, personal, collective, and inter-generational traumas, and patterns of how we breathe and move that cause or continue to contribute to the current issue when left unchecked (Sullivan *et al.* 2018b). Becoming aware of habits through a practice of yoga therapy can support the creation of new ways to tend to and understand one's self. This can bolster our resolve to unravel the roots of our pelvic suffering.

Pelvic symptoms can also create changes in how one breathes and moves, postural guarding, emotional intensity or numbness, and the way one organizes one's daily life – our physical experience drives our choices, affect, and habits. Pelvic conditions (for most women) are rarely purely physical in nature and causation. Even when there's been a physical injury or objective tissue change, the subjective implications that result may permeate all other layers of the person's experience, which we will elucidate further in the upcoming discussion around the panchamaya model.

Yoga asana does provide physical benefits like exercise. There's also a need for future research to consider the intentionality of yoga as a movement-based contemplative practice – that *why* we practice postures and the intention we hold within this moving practice may be *how* change occurs (Solomonova 2015). Intention supports action. Studying how our goals and imagination enrich our lived experience may bring fresh insight to the questions behind how yoga therapy works.

As a complementary care modality, yoga therapy sees a student's agency and action as the drivers of change and resulting embodiment. We co-facilitate a student's experience, assisting them in refining how and what they practice both formally on the mat and integrated into their daily lives. I often tell my students, "You're in charge." This gives explicit reassurance to them that agency and self-efficacy lead the way during each session. When someone's experienced trauma, this continual reminder may help them take up the reins and remember their power.

How do we create change or healing? We must practice steadily, without interruption, and with sincerity and respect to see the fruits of our efforts. Sutra 1.14 includes the word asevita which translates as fully attended, completely served (Satchidananda 2008, pp.19–22). I love the image of attending to one's self fully, like how when caring for a newborn, the mother becomes absorbed into the present moment of meeting their needs with unconditional love – they remain enmeshed in those early days to establish a safe bond for life. Could we all learn to offer ourselves this totality of unconditional presence? We commit with faith that our practice will deliver a positive outcome – and the more reverent this devotion to ourselves and the process becomes, the more likely positive outcomes may occur.

Yoga therapy brings people home to themselves by creating a lifestyle that supports consciousness, compassion, and vitality. Embodied practice helps one listen and tend to the small signs of discomfort and dis-ease, as well as savor comfort and peace. This practice shifts our relationship to inevitable hardships and adversity, providing a container for integration to occur.

Lastly, these concepts permeate most lineages, schools, and modern methods of yoga practice and can create a shared language for yoga therapists, consumers, and collaborative care teams to work together more effectively. By understanding the embedded philosophy within its ancient texts, we further delineate yoga as a valued modality (Sullivan *et al.* 2018b).

Table 2.1: The eight-limbed path of yoga

Yamas	**Social behaviors or observances**
Ahimsa	Non-violence, do no harm, kindness
Satya	Truthfulness
Asteya	Non-stealing, sharing
Brahmacharya	Wise use of one's energy, including but not limited to sexuality
Aparigraha	Non-hoarding, non-grasping

Niyamas	**Personal behaviors or observances**
Saucha	Cleanliness, including physical environment, home, hygiene
Santosha	Contentment with what is
Tapas	Heat of cultivating one's focus, discipline, devotion
Svadhyaya	Self-study
Ishvara Pranidhana	Surrender
Asana	Physical postures, somatic inquiry, movement
Pranayama	Breathing awareness and specific breathing techniques
Pratyahara	Recalibration of one's senses, withdrawal of senses inward
Dharana	Focus, concentration
Dhyana	Absorption, state of meditation
Samadhi	State of oneness, flow, peace

We study, integrate, and apply the eight-limbed path of yoga, which has been outlined briefly in Table 2.1. This includes ethical foundations and habits developed by observing the ten yamas and niyamas, as well as physical postures, breath and energy techniques, clarification of one's senses, and various stages of concentration and meditation (Farhi 2000, pp.4–16). As entry-level yoga teacher trainings typically include discourse and in-depth study about these elements of practice, I'm not going to further define them here.

All these principles and practices hold immense value, none more important than another and all contributing toward wellbeing, or enlightenment. Through the therapeutic relationship between teacher and student, and after conducting a thorough assessment, we together determine which strategies or practices from this eight-limbed path to implement first to best address the student's goals.

Health is a continuum. A person's relative suffering or happiness, illness or vitality are inextricably linked to each other, tethered like two ends of the same rope. To teach with compassion and empathy, we must first acknowledge the validity of our student's experiences. The suffering they perceive is real, no matter our assessment or a lack of medical confirmation or diagnostic label. In recognizing their suffering and providing a framework within which they can self-assess and reflect, we help the student seek to understand "how they got here." Only then, with as clear a road map as we can get of their past and present circumstances, we watch and encourage them as, hand over hand, they pull themselves toward vitality.

This tradition paves a road to recovering our wholeness and worth, not in a vacuum free from suffering but by making us willing and skilled enough to embrace the adversity we inevitably will encounter with equal presence as the moments that leave us vibrating and weeping with joy. Our perceptions may determine, to a large degree, whether we suffer, cope well, or learn to thrive. Next, I'll take us through the five kleshas, or afflictions, to better understand, from a yogic perspective, why we suffer.

Why we suffer

Buddhism and Hinduism both speak about afflictions, or negative mind states, as obstacles to the path toward samadhi, or enlightenment. Some Buddhist traditions teach the three roots of suffering as spiritual ignorance, attachment, and avoidance (Tricycle 2021), while Patanjali's Yoga Sutras expand the causes of suffering to five possibilities (Satchidananda 2008, pp.83–93). Known as the kleshas, they're summarized in Table 2.2.

The word klesha translates as "affliction" or "poison." I appreciate another translation of the kleshas being like stains on our consciousness. Stains can be removed, albeit with diligent and repetitive awareness, to cleanse these habits of mind and inhibit the behaviors that stem from and perpetuate them.

Table 2.2: The five kleshas

Avidya	Ignorance, misperception, blind spots, illusion, separation from true self
Asmita	Misidentification of self – either inflated or deflated ego identity
Raga	Attachment, craving of pleasurable things
Dvesa	Avoidance, aversion, repulsion
Abhinivesa	Clinging to life; fear of death, transitions, or change

One can view either avidya or abhinivesa as the root of the other four afflictions. We'll start with avidya, referenced as the first of the kleshas in Sutra 2.4. When we do not know our true nature, we cannot move, act, and speak from that wisdom abiding within us.

Avidya, also defined as misperception or illusion, creates suffering by the fact we become unable to see reality clearly. Sometimes, this is explained as "what we don't know we don't know," or unconscious incompetence. For me, it's been helpful to also view avidya as the blinders we wear when operating from a feeling of utter and absolute conviction of something as right or true that is inaccurate. Not perceiving reality clearly (and never challenging those clouds to part to see the blue sky of clear perception) creates a sort of spiritual immaturity, whereas we can grow by considering contrasting opinions and referencing our ideas with close teachers and respected leaders in our field.

The other possible root affliction is abhinivesa, or fear. A more literal translation, fear of death, can show us the wisdom of the final closing practice we use, savasana (corpse pose). Each time we lie down and withdraw our senses, we can practice the ultimate surrender of our last breath. In revering rather than fearing death, we can learn to live out our values with more zeal and integrity.

We can also explore abhinivesa during any rite of passage or change in circumstance. If we resist or fear death, it's likely we also resist change. Any disruption to our identity and routine can feel like a death process – the loss of a job, a loved one, a relocation, even positive rites like marriage or entering motherhood – all require us to reintegrate who we know ourselves to be and establish new ways of living. Change is inevitable and constant. When we cling to life as we "know" it, even though the circumstances and context differs, we suffer. Yoga helps us learn to adapt and remain centered even within the great unknown mystery of life and death.

Misidentification, or perceiving one's self with either inflated or deflated self-concept, is called asmita. I attended a lecture with Amy Wheeler where this definition of asmita greatly clarified my understanding of this obstacle. Confidence and humility create two sides of the same coin. When either of these character traits goes to the extreme, we run into misidentification of our self, or ego. Confidence balloons into arrogance; humility collapses into self-deprecation and sabotage. We need enough faith in our sense of self to operate in the world, make decisions, and contribute in useful ways, as well as a healthy dose of humility that allows effective collaboration and seeing everyone's value in their different roles. As a newly defined field, yoga therapy is growing into its healthy asmita, and we're working to merge effectively within clinical care settings with a clear scope of what we can offer.

The remaining two kleshas represent a polarity of preferential conditioning. When we feel tethered by either strong attachment (raga) or repulsed by aversion (dvesa), we will continually suffer through intense craving and disgust or avoidance, the cage of duality that we've built for ourselves. Now, some attachment, like in parenting and familial bonds, serves us well as we develop and mature, just like a natural aversion to walking across a six-lane freeway during rush hour makes sense. These preferences can keep us safe and support thriving.

Our personalities though, when overrun with these opinions, can dictate a life that feels small and suffocating or endlessly hedonistic. Through our practice and awareness, we can take joy in the natural preferences that add quality to our lives, while weeding out the habits of mind created by the kleshas of avoidance and attachment. We can set ourselves free by neutralizing the emotional charge around preferences that prevent us from growing, exploring, and healing. After all, in order to heal pelvic dis-ease, we'll likely need to dissolve some habits while picking up others. When we merge the polarity of attachment and aversion, like the definition of yoga being union of opposites, we can reside in an openness to the present moment itself.

When we burn with passion for our mission to prevent and eliminate suffering caused by pelvic pain, incontinence, prolapse, and sexual dysfunction, it's easy to get on our soapbox and sing it from the rooftops. Public awareness campaigns and education have already changed the tide toward more access to pelvic healthcare and support being available, but let's be careful not to proclaim all pelvic symptoms are "not normal," as if to say the woman experiencing them is, herself, wrong or broken.

Not all women with pelvic-floor symptoms experience them as a source of suffering. When sharing the benefits of pelvic yoga therapy, we must be careful not to shame the use of pads or pessaries, demonize surgery, or claim that all symptoms warrant action or can be completely healed. Marketing to women's pain points can feel manipulative and degrading. Each woman decides for herself when to begin a practice or seek support. Let's cultivate trust and rapport by marketing instead to her innate wholeness and the possibility of healing, and hold her desires and questions with integrity.

Supporting the whole woman with the panchamaya model

Many models exist within the field of yoga therapy. One such framework is the panchamaya model, which describes the five layers, or sheaths, that make up who we are in this human form (Sovik and Bhavanani 2016, pp.20–22). Moving from gross to increasingly subtle in quality, these five distinct bodies permeate and continually influence each other; they are not separate. For the sake of understanding, we can study and assess each one, knowing they inevitably impact each other.

Physical body – annamaya kosha

The first and most tangible sheath is our physical body – what we can touch and see in material form. In terms of pelvic health, this sheath includes the anatomical bony structures and joints of the pelvis, the muscles and connective tissue of our pelvic bowl and core, the positional relationship of our pelvic organs, and the global organization of our posture and movement habits. We feed this body with food, water, and air, and thus, the outer world becomes assimilated as the building blocks for our inner cellular reality.

This body literally moves us through the world, and through physical postures on our yoga mat. Variety and efficiency of movement expression demonstrates health of this kosha – not just an absence of discomfort or dysfunction. Finally, this first kosha shows us how the care or neglect of the other sheaths impacts our physical wellbeing.

Physiological body – pranamaya kosha

Our vital life force, or prana, represents the animating, functional movement and processes inside our physical body. The digestive tube of the large intestine and its relationship to the pelvic floor anatomically can be viewed from the annamaya perspective, while the process and quality of our elimination displays the level of health in the digestive system within this second layer. This body also gives us clues from the quality and function of our breathing, our sleep, and our energy levels and is organized and influenced by the five vayus, or vital currents of energy.

When we experience pain, we're getting a "warning" signal by way of sensation that can show us what's happening within our many systems as it interprets the flow of variables and information coming in from all koshas. Lastly, the chakras or energetic centers also express this layer.

Psychological body – manomaya kosha

This third sheath represents our mind in the form of our thoughts and feelings. Pelvic symptoms can create rumination and fixation in this sheath

– overanalyzing our condition, checking visually with a mirror every day to judge tissue changes, or using the restroom hourly "just in case" and in the absence of signals from our bladder. Unfortunately, these mental-emotional stressors or hypervigilance will likely only perpetuate the cycle of physical or physiological dysfunction. Symptoms shape our thoughts over time, and those thought patterns further drive behaviors, breath, and motor control.

Psychological states also drive pelvic function and symptoms, particularly pain, so it's important to complete a thorough intake conversation to uncover patterns of mind that may be contributing to or causing related behaviors and pelvic symptoms. Changing circumstances or a new acute stressor in a woman's life can cause flare-ups of recurrent symptoms or can even correlate with new symptoms. Consider how identifying (or misidentifying) with a diagnostic label or believing a condition is permanent or unavoidable would then determine whether a woman ever seeks support at all, as well as the efficacy and results available to her from engaging with a care provider.

Think of this mental body like a stereo with many different radio stations and features, as well as a range of static and silence. This organ of perception, the mind, can transmit messages generated by the filter of ego, personality, and habits according to one's vijnanamaya kosha *and* receive "sensation messages" from the first two layers. The way my understanding of these interactions matured through conversations with a dear colleague, Leila Stuart, is an example of how we use our intellect to reach greater clarity. Yoga therapy helps us become compassionately aware of thought patterns, as well as consciously direct them, which we'll discuss next.

Witness body – vijnanamaya kosha

If the mind is the stereo, the vijnanamaya layer represents the person using it. Acting from present awareness and agency, we can reprogram the stereo. We can even compose new music as we design our lives in alignment with our values. When the stereo is playing static, or a station we don't enjoy, we don't throw the whole thing in the dumpster. We get out the manual, learn how to use the stereo, and make changes in how we engage in relationship with it – we choose the channel. Yoga gives us a guidebook for observing the mind, and this kosha is where we mature and develop our capacity to apply these practices and principles.

This kosha often gets labeled "intellect" or "wisdom" body, and when well developed, reflects our chosen, lived values. In this layer, we cultivate a capacity to observe ourselves without identifying as the messages being transmitted or received in the mind or the conditions or diagnosis playing out in our physical experience. Sovereignty and intuition are restored when we allow ourselves to act from the wise guidance of our higher self.

Living in accordance with one's values nourishes this sheath. Pain and pelvic-health concerns might push us to drop hobbies, sports, and artistic pursuits, or maybe we became so consumed by life, work, or caretaking others that we allowed our own needs to suffocate. This disconnection from what we value can leave us feeling like a ghost, barely present to the beauty of our own life. When we prioritize pleasure, creativity, and passion, we're more equipped to hold our own suffering, and may even experience less suffering because of the soulful nourishment we derive from self-expression.

Working this kosha can help women with pelvic concerns craft a compelling image of the life they want to lead, the life they believe is possible for them through healing their actual symptoms and suffering, and despite their suffering. In developing a rewarding vision and actionable goals to get there, we can motivate consistent practice, lifestyle adjustments, and a growing unconditional loving kindness.

As we cultivate integrity within self, relationships with others will be impacted. We may find during a pelvic healing journey that some friendships or intimate relationships wither, while others flourish. We may discover the limits of a current partner's compassion for our pain or shame, and thus grieve the changed relationship (or end it). A new community of like-minded friends may blossom as we start or resume a practice of yoga. Discernment always rests in the student's hands. As yoga therapists, we help our student anchor into the wisdom of her body, the truth of her Soul through exploratory, experiential practices. Through experiencing yoga therapy, she remembers she's in command of her happiness.

Spiritual body – anandamaya kosha

Ananda translates as bliss. Many teachers know this sheath as the emotional body, and it's often deemed the *causal* body – the one potentially influencing our liberation the most, as well as what manifests in the first two layers.

Our sense of connection to the ethereal, infinite realm of spirit may impact where we land on the spectrum of eudaimonic wellbeing (Lawrence 2020), the kind of peace and fulfillment that feels unshaken by circumstances or symptoms. Through this kosha, we connect to our Soul essence – we can catch a glimpse of our own purusha. Ritual, prayer, ceremony, and community expressions of spiritual practice can nourish this layer and support health in all other koshas. Some may add deep abiding joy and authentic gratitude to this kosha's list of gifts, too.

The five koshas allow us to observe and assess our student, accounting for the multitude of causal relationships and variables related to their pelvic-health experience. The integration that occurs in yoga therapy can reveal their true nature – the way they present themselves, the depth and vulnerability of stories they share with us, and a beautiful unfolding of their expression and thriving. If the sheaths represent veils that, when imbalanced, obscure or contain our inner self or soul, yoga therapy lifts each one to reveal new eyes, smoothing it away to provide a pure view and intimate connection to one's Soul. When all koshas function well, we are well.

Let's pause for a guided meditation in which you'll acknowledge and appreciate each of your five bodies through the panchamaya model.

Nourishing the koshas meditation

We'll be journeying from the most tangible to more subtle aspects of our being. All you need to do is allow yourself to notice what arises. Make a quiet space for yourself to lie down, rest, and receive this meditation.

First, notice how your body meets the surfaces under you. Feel your weight settling. Made of skin, fat, muscle, nerves, blood and bone, organs, and cells – this is your physical body, your home. Notice sensations that call your attention to different parts of your body. Where do you feel comfort? Discomfort? Neutrality or absence of sensation? Welcome all the messengers of sensation you feel. This body needs air, water, and food to live. The variety, color, texture, and taste of foods, how you lovingly prepare them, and how you consume them with intention – savor how they sustain you. What we take in makes up our material body. Thank your whole physical body now for being the vessel in which you live and express yourself.

Now bring awareness to your energy or life force, to the quality of your breathing. Is it smooth and even, choppy, shallow, loud or quiet, labored or soft? Can you feel your heartbeat? Where can you feel your pulse? Is your belly gurgling? The energy we drink in with each breath gets imbibed by every cell, fueling our many systems to reflect vitality in the way we breathe, circulate, sleep and wake, digest and eliminate, like the sun feeding plants so they grow and the moon calling the tide back again – our energy body is fed by nature and rhythm. This is the movement of life within you.

Next, we'll watch the fluctuations of our mind. Simply notice what thoughts, narratives, or emotional signatures are present. Do these thoughts and feelings persist? How do they evolve as you become still and quiet? Can you feel the activity of your mind become slower, like a waterfall that plunged down into a pool, spreading out over the surface of the water like a smooth mirror? There will always be thoughts – no need to try to stop them. We can also attune to the spaces between thought and feeling. Getting still can help us find that space. Boredom can birth curiosity and creativity. Novelty challenges our mind, repetition reinforces learning. Our minds can grow and change like our body. Offer sincere thanks for your mind and all it does for you.

We learn to witness the mind stuff, our cyclical nature, our physicality and know that we are that and we're not that. The yearning for something more, or a deeper truth and purpose, beckons us. We acknowledge now the wisdom kosha – our intellect, discernment, intuition – the part of us that learns to choose and respond with integrity, agency, and vision. What does your deepest Knowing hold to be true right now? We hone this kosha through self-reflection, conversation, reading, making art, and by the devotion to remain a student of life until our final breath. Offer your unique quirks, personality and identity, and inner wisdom deep thanks, and be willing to hold it all lightly as you craft yourself anew with each practice. Let your life come alive guided by what you value most. Be thankful that you can come to know yourself intimately and express yourself completely.

The fifth and most subtle kosha, closest to purusha or our unchanging spirit, our meaning-making, fulfillment-seeking, spiritual self, receives nourishment from connection and belonging, love, truth, justice, purpose, and intimacy with the very source of our one precious life. When we derive satisfaction and joy from this ephemeral, infinite part of us, it is unwavering – we are well no matter what happens to us in this life.

This kosha nourishes, colors, and permeates all other aspects of our human experience. Can you connect to the part of you that has always belonged? Can you feel the warmth of unconditional loving kindness? Rest a few more moments, lingering in the presence of your own being. Worthy because you exist, you are love itself.

Distinct yet one, these five koshas represent the many aspects of who we are born and live to be in human form. Like five perfectly cut facets on one precious gemstone, we polish them through the practice, process, and state of being that is yoga. Feel these five layers of you merge now, take in the totality of you in this moment. Feel your body resting, supported. Take a few moments now to wiggle, yawn, hug your knees into your belly, and roll to your side. This practice is now complete. Write down any insights, sensations, thoughts, or images you want to remember from this meditation. May they serve you well.

Yoga therapy nourishes each layer of the individual as an inherently comprehensive, BPSS model of care. We apply this inclusive lens to honor the biomechanical, psychological, hormonal, social, spiritual, sexual, and relational aspects that co-create a woman's current pelvic experience. In Chapter 9, I'll share some key questions you may wish to include in your assessment process from a koshic perspective.

Relationships – a crucible for self-reflection

With pelvic-health concerns like fecal incontinence, painful sex, or the confronting visual changes to one's vulva that can occur after childbirth, for example, women may stay silent, not realizing support is available. Cultural conditioning tells us to keep private matters hidden, that bodily functions are shameful, disgusting, embarrassing. Many women suffer in isolation, when in fact their symptoms may be very common – and often treatable. As yoga therapists, we can hold space for people to share their experiences and thus realize they are not alone, they are not broken, and they are worthy of being witnessed with compassion.

A few months before my second daughter was born, a girlfriend had chosen homebirth for her first. Her mother provided live-in care for weeks prior to and after her delivery. When relaying to my own mother how beautiful and special it felt to be welcomed into this dear friend's postpartum cocoon, complete with observing her vulva as her mother lovingly checked her sutures, my mother drew in a breath and remarked that she felt this act of care was, in fact, "undignified."

In that moment, my compassion grew for the level of avoidance or disgust my mother had been taught or learned, whether explicit or implicit, familial, societal, or ancestral. The source mattered less than the reality that suddenly pressed its weight on my heart. This saddened me, yet I then understood and accepted that I may never experience the kind of care I witnessed between my friend and her mother during such a crucial rite of passage as becoming a mother.

Some of the cultural awakening we're now experiencing is generational; the groundwork has been laid for women's sexuality, consent and accountability, pelvic health, and a return to undisturbed, non-medicalized birth and postpartum practices. Yoga therapy is well poised to serve in a nonclinical role to support dignity and wholeness through the various life stages a woman may experience. I hope to do my best to hold my daughters' intimate questions and to perhaps be invited one day into their most pivotal moments.

We can do some of our healing work alone, privately. We may heal more deeply or completely when being held, heard, and witnessed. Many distinct types of relationships work together to support personal wellbeing, including family, friendships, community, a beloved partner, a formal teacher or mentor, and nature itself. Here, I offer a few ideas of how we might support students with this inquiry.

Right relationship with a teacher accelerates the embodied learning experience of yoga therapy. Deepening relationship with a primary teacher and exploring contrasting viewpoints with multiple teachers enriches our path. The professional teacher-student container provides a safe, accountable space to nurture growth.

The role of a partner may not include sexual intimacy yet most certainly honors a depth of emotional intimacy – a place where you allow your self to be seen and secrets to be known. What I refer to as The Beloved, this relationship fulfills the intimate role of bearing direct witness to one's daily lived experiences.

The social-spiritual nature of observing the yamas and niyamas (Table 2.1) and studying the kleshas (Table 2.2) can support students in self-reflection around cultivating more explicit, expressed gratitude for the relationships they do feel supported by, as well as identifying areas for more conscious expansion and closeness. Conflict tempts us to negate, blame, avoid, or lash out at others, only causing more suffering for everyone involved. It requires honesty and vulnerability to admit where we've faltered in relationships or where and how we've found ourselves feeling disconnected or lonely. Applying these foundational inquiries allows us to take responsibility for our role in each relationship or organization we belong to, giving us ways to understand our habits and get creative about new ways of relating.

Lastly, if or when adverse childhood experiences or traumas become unveiled through reflecting on relationships, or while working directly with pelvic imagery and movement, we respect our scope of practice and remind our student to further unearth and integrate those experiences with a qualified mental-health professional or trauma therapist.

Using these inquiries as a tool for self-study can help clients develop the skill of resourcing – bringing consciousness to the places, people, and support they can currently access. This way, when swimming in less familiar or turbulent waters of conditioning, habits, memories, and sensory patterns, they have the buoyancy of friends, professional support, and a resourced environment to keep afloat.

CHAPTER 3

Body Wisdom

Long before I knew yoga therapy existed, movement captivated my personal and professional attention. Dance, improvisation, rock climbing, and trail running presented opportunities for creative expression and adventure, and illuminated my limits – real and perceived. As meditation in motion, my body has allowed me to perform on stage, run 52 miles in a single day, grieve losses, navigate conflict and effective collaboration, and treasure moments of ecstatic joy – what a wise, capable vessel we've been given. Welcome the diversity of your experiences and trust they fuel your distinct contribution to women's wellbeing and pelvic health.

Support for MBCP continues to grow. An estimated 300 million people worldwide enjoy the benefits of practicing yoga (Yogi Times 2021). We're all seeking peace and wellbeing. The body knows and shows us our needs better than we can often conceptualize or articulate. Women sometimes share that their pelvic symptoms seem to function like a canary in the coal mine, showing up at the first signs of depletion, conflict, or stress. We can learn to listen to the body's clues and patterns, and understand the physiological and psychological patterns found in practice and mapped by science.

Asana supplies forms within which to study ourselves. I invite you to expand the definition of asana to include somatic inquiry, strength training and exercise, restorative postures, and the power of walking in nature. Asana could simply mean "a practice of moving your body in attentive service to wellness." In this way, we also come together from a variety of lineages and perspectives, using a shared language of movement. This may require us to rewrite our methodologies from the inside out, letting go of ideologies that profess there's one right way or such a thing as "correct" and "incorrect" alignment, in exchange for a more open-ended process of mutual discovery. We reconsider imposing aesthetics or a lineage's opinion about how a posture is to be performed, and learn instead to activate the student's unique impulse to generate the practice from within.

It's important we see our role as yoga therapists in this broader therapeutic context. We bridge philosophical foundations (that can feel at times esoteric and ephemeral) and emerging scientific research to better understand the mechanisms of how yoga works – this is a somatic practice held in social context by therapeutic relationship. This chapter attempts to illustrate the kinesthetic and relational intelligence available to us by understanding the autonomic nervous system (ANS) through polyvagal theory (PVT).

What does it mean to feel safe?

None of the body's systems function in isolation. Yet our fundamental safety and security, understood also through the subtle energy of the muladhara "root" chakra at the base of the pelvis, may boil down to the perception of safety or unsafety that we register internally, often subconsciously. Think of your nervous system as a kind of operating system or programming. No matter how effective we are in delivering a pelvic-floor practice, it's likely our student's progress would only be fleeting if the governing message from their body is one of danger, risk, or threat. This visceral, physiological, and often subconscious scanning of our environment and circumstances has been labeled neuroception (Porges 2004). A kind of registering of the totality of our experience, neuroception is our real-time radar of whether we are safe.

Self-regulation asks us to tend to our own perception of safety, while co-regulation allows us to learn through the transmission of another's reliable presence (Porges 2017, pp.9, 25). In the therapeutic relationship, we act as a kind of tuning fork, assisting our students in finding a sustainable frequency through connection. Self-regulation can be a viable path toward healing. A starting point and vital principle to return to, we can only control our own actions and choices. Yet it's no longer enough to tout self-care as the answer. Feeling safe becomes then both an internal referencing and a communal responsibility.

As educators, healthcare providers, and yoga therapists, we must consider systemic injustice and the very real possibility of trauma having been experienced by our students. We consider these facts when designing our physical spaces, communicating our offerings clearly, making our work accessible, and formulating procedures and policies for client care and mutual safety. Building our referral network also acknowledges the depth and breadth of approaches sometimes required to improve or resolve pelvic concerns. Feeling supported and meeting our needs together in community amplifies co-regulation.

Being together, whether physically or virtually, requires that we set the tone together for a platform of mutual respect and safety – we share the responsibility of co-regulation.

Although the stress or discomfort associated with a pelvic-health concern may cause someone to seek support and spark change, in general, stress can inhibit our ability to learn, connect, breathe and move well, and rest and recuperate. Imagine what it might be like to deal with incontinence or persistent pelvic pain on top of economic hardship, racism, or gender discrimination. We need to listen to students and see the big picture of stressors they face, allowing them to make connections and directing them toward resources aimed at improving access and inclusion.

What a student can experience during a yoga-therapy session may be very different than what plays out in their body (and thus pelvic floor) when they're presenting during an important sales meeting, dealing with personal finances, or navigating familial conflict. In this way, consider how limited our effect may be in providing care if we only take an isolated and localized, solely physical approach to pelvic health. The pelvis can act as a protective space. The psychosocial and spiritual elements of learning how to feel safe can support students in maintaining results after they leave our presence and reenter life at large.

Nervous-system education is one way to offer this wisdom. It's also a brilliant model for body-based self-reflection to see beyond pelvic state and symptoms to the underlying messages communicated within one's body. Let's step back and review the basics of the ANS.

Inner governance – a conventional view

In conventional understanding, the ANS has two choices – gas or brakes (Sapolsky 2004, p.48). The gas pedal metaphor represents our "GO" system, what's known as the sympathetic branch of our ANS, or fight and flight responses. Sympathetic activation allows us to wake up in the morning, focus intently, exert ourselves physically – it's our ability to mobilize or hold a certain level of "charge." When we feel threatened, circulation shunts away from digestion in favor of flooding peripheral skeletal muscles, while our pulse, blood pressure, and breath rate increase to prepare us to fight or run to safety. You're likely already aware of the negative health impacts of chronic stress or persistent sympathetic arousal (Ross and Michalsen 2016, pp.471–483). Optimally, when a threat subsides, our physiology returns to a state of calm.

The relaxation response often gets touted as the magic elixir that yoga serves on a silver platter. This is the parasympathetic branch of the ANS that functions as the brakes of the body-car, allowing us to slow down, rest, and digest. Activation of the parasympathetic ANS lets us fall asleep at night, serves our digestion and elimination, decreases inflammation, and facilitates quiet solitude and connection.

It was believed that the sympathetic and parasympathetic branches of the ANS tended to have an inhibitory effect on each other – if we have our foot on the gas, it cannot also press the brakes or vice versa (Sapolsky 2004). This either-or perspective may provide a compelling, clear path to better manage one's lifestyle. Many people perpetually swing between these extremes, whereas yoga therapy can help us modulate energy and live more sustainably.

In summary, both sympathetic and parasympathetic functioning are necessary and healthy. This outdated duality, however, doesn't show how we function with far more nuance. We need to have access to and shift easily between *many* states to respond with context-appropriate coping. We function along a continuum, which PVT illustrates more clearly.

The polyvagal theory (PVT)

Dr. Stephen Porges' polyvagal theory merges evolutionary biology, neuroscience, and psychology (Porges 1995). Some have scrutinized his theory as an oversimplification, as human behavior requires multiple complex and overlapping mechanisms. Primarily adopted into the mental-health and trauma-therapy domains, PVT has more recently made its way into the field of yoga therapy (Sullivan *et al.* 2018a).

Porges' approach offered long-awaited validation of our body's wisdom, evidenced by the fact that the vagus nerve contains around 80% afferent fibers, which allows the body to send important insights to the brain. More research is yet needed to clarify the exact mechanisms behind how our body registers safety and the complex drivers of our emotions and behavior, yet this theory seems to back somatic or "bottom-up" approaches to therapy that view physicality as elemental to lasting healing. ("Top-down" approaches might include talk therapy and meditation, working with the mind as the driver for change. Yoga can be used to address both.)

PVT states that the ANS has three primary channels: ventral-social engagement, sympathetic-mobilization, and dorsal-immobilization. The vagus nerve offers distinctly different response patterns depending on whether we access the ventral branch in the face, middle ear, voice, and heart, or the dorsal branch's role within our viscera and limbic system (Porges 2017). Both branches of the vagus activate parasympathetic dominance, while we also still have access to sympathetic activation. All three states can function defensively under threat and while we feel safe. The scope of this topic goes well beyond what can be offered in a single chapter; what I've included intends to give a sound framework for supporting therapeutic relationship. View the three primary ANS states according to PVT in Figure 3.1.

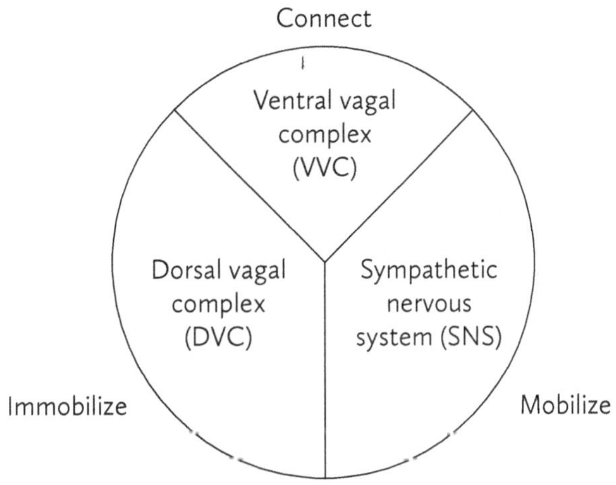

Figure 3.1: The three primary ANS states according to PVT

These three modes of ANS function typically get placed in a hierarchical ladder metaphor (Dana 2020, pp.7–18). With ventral vagus at the top as the most evolved response to stress, PVT demonstrates how we use connection, facial expressions, and communication to mitigate the negative impacts of the stressor and return to a calm state. When we're faced with imminent danger, we go to the next rung on the ladder and mobilize our defenses with a sympathetic response. If the threat grows too great, or we're trapped, we collapse into the last, most primitive state activated by the dorsal vagus. I choose to use a circle to show the cyclical nature of how we can access all states when warranted, removing the potential judgment and shame that could come from the hierarchy imposed by the ladder.

The myelinated ventral vagus branch remains unique to mammals who raise live offspring. Think of the attachment behaviors we naturally participate in with a newborn baby, like cooing, smiling, and exploring exaggerated facial expressions, or how we observe a mother cat bathing her kittens with touch. When we have access to sufficient safety and care as young children, our ability to accurately register social cues develops (Dana 2020, pp.8–10).

When we feel threatened or unsafe, practices like singing and speaking, being spoken to, meeting someone's eyes, or feeling the warmth of someone taking our hand can help us return to a sense of connection through social engagement. Ventral vagus activation represents this movement "toward" or "being with," highlighting Porges' contribution of the social engagement platform to our understanding.

Sympathetic activation shows how resources mobilize to help us meet a stressor, preparing us to fight or flee (also known as the flight response). The physiological changes that play out here largely remain true according to what we discussed in the conventional model. Here, we see movement "against" or "away from" the other.

The more primitive, unmyelinated dorsal branch came first phylogenetically speaking, and is common to all animals, including fish. When faced with a life-threatening stress (real or perceived) this dorsal branch can cause us to collapse, freeze, shut down, or "feign death." This shows how our system can be overwhelmed, shifting from an "I can" mentality of meeting a stressor with sympathetic mobilization to flipping a switch to "I can't." A complete movement "inward" on one's self or "escaping" through dissociation shows the immobilization response of the dorsal vagus complex.

Two additional "blended" ANS states

In addition to the primary channels of response (ventral-social engagement, sympathetic-mobilization, and dorsal-immobilization), humans can access two other states, play and intimacy. They show us how fine-tuned our mammalian biology has become and offer additional ways to cope with stress and express ourselves in relationship. We can modulate sympathetic and dorsal vagal responses by maintaining a sense of connection through ventral vagal activation.

Watching my husband play with our daughters, complete with wrestling, loud growling, and teeth snarling, I came to understand this blended state of play in a new context. Without the smiles and laughter, this physicality could easily be perceived as aggression. These same behaviors from a stranger would likely register as danger. The power of relationship makes it play (Porges 2015).

The second blended state, intimacy, involves a merging of ventral vagal social connection, with the deeply restful immobilization of a dorsal vagal response. Intimacy here does not necessarily imply sexual activity, although this calm contentedness may create a certain receptivity to sexual response. By attending to intimacy, we can melt into the arms of a beloved or thoroughly rest in our own loving companionship, be moved by art, and commune with nature (Dana 2020, pp.91–103; Porges 1998).

In Figure 3.2 you'll see all five states according to PVT, as well as arrows that show the increasing activation on either side of the spectrum, integrating our earlier conventional understanding. Our aim is to understand and build skill, tracking somatically which states are dominant or current in our ANS function.

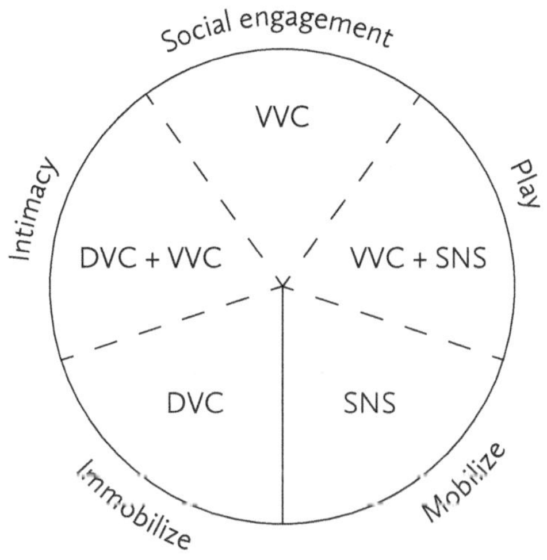

Figure 3.2: The five states of the ANS according to the PVT

Shifting states through therapeutic relationship

Over the course of a yoga-therapy session, our client likely experiences several, if not all, of these ANS states. Consider how a student may arrive wide eyed, short of breath, and consumed with life up until the minute your session begins (excess sympathetic charge). Then, we guide them to flow through active breath-based movements, harnessing their attention (dissipating the excess sympathetic charge).

Upon conclusion of their closing meditation or rest period, they may even seem reluctant to speak or move, eyes soft and body melted into a pure state of contentment (healthy dorsal vagus immobilization). Finally, they rise to seated and we make eye contact, have them verbally recount how they feel, and review their home practice to help them safely reenter the world, alert enough to drive home (ventral vagal activation through social engagement into healthy sympathetic mobilization). Through keen observation, we discern how to employ varied cueing methods and practices, different types of touch, and intelligent sequencing to support our students' expanding capacity, gradually exploring contrast and novelty.

Regulation includes "dysregulation"

While relaxation may be a foundational, necessary state for learning and healing, it's not the only nervous system state we want students to practice. Recognizing one's "dysregulation" may be the first step. When we're perturbed, off balance, or sense a threat, how easily and perhaps quickly we can return to a sense of safety, ease, and belonging demonstrates the health of our nervous system. (Just like how biomechanical stability must be defined as a dynamic, adaptive response to a stimulus and the agility needed to return to a stable state, rather than a fixed point or state without response. More on that in Chapter 4.) True resilience is an ongoing, dynamic inquiry.

One possible application with pelvic-health clients might be to have them list a few of the triggers they currently experience. By bringing attention to reactions they feel are default coping methods, we can help them anticipate the trigger, armed with body awareness, compassion, and strategies that may, over time, help generate a new response (Dana 2020, p.38).

For example, one client had no trouble relaxing into restorative postures with the supportive environment and my presence in a yoga-therapy session, but felt like her household was a volatile, anxiety-driving force exacerbating her pelvic symptoms. She'd struggled with pelvic pain and stress incontinence for many years after the birth of her daughter.

We established relaxation in the safe context of our therapeutic relationship first, then began to introduce new contexts through her imagination. I'd guide her into imagining she could be at home feeling this safe and content, observing the sounds and presence of others in her home while simultaneously watching her breath. At first, even this proved difficult, but over time, she not only established a home practice – she also felt able to regulate herself internally through this compassionate awareness during everyday moments. Identifying the spaces, sensations, and thoughts associated with her perceived dysregulation and anxiety gave her the power to then choose a new response.

Prone savasana helped her find that frequency initially, and the true testament to her results from yoga therapy were that she could tap into her somatic state and change it without needing to spend 20 minutes face down over a bolster. She restored resilience. Soon after our first few sessions, this client reported that she no longer experienced any pelvic pain or stress urinary incontinence (SUI). We hadn't done any pelvic-floor "exercise," and instead focused on guided imagery to connect to and trust her pelvic bowl. Being a yoga teacher, she did well at integrating the practices and concepts we explored into her other practices, teaching, and lifestyle. Around a year later, she had resumed riding horseback comfortably, and even started to write again after a years-long creative dry spell.

The window of tolerance

The ANS functional range we have access to is known as the window of tolerance; either excess or deficient arousal (sympathetic or dorsal vagal in nature, respectively) takes us outside this window. A wider tolerance indicates increased resilience or capacity to cope.

Persistent pain and trauma, especially the impact of early childhood adversity, can narrow a person's window of tolerance. Pelvic concerns also shrink one's world. Favorite activities get dropped for fear of having an accident in public, intimacy may suffer from shame and embarrassment, and pain limits what we perceive to be possible for our quality of life, fitness, and sense of normalcy. An attempt to spare ourselves suffering, we create cycles of avoidance, hypervigilance, and anxiety that can perpetuate our pain, tension, disconnect, or pelvic dysfunction.

A narrowed window of tolerance could be observed as increased mental-emotional reactivity, physical tension, fear and avoidance, inactivity or decreased adherence to their home practice, frequent flare-ups of symptoms, or delayed healing or progress. A multitude of reasons could contribute to this smaller "window." Also, be mindful that lifestyle, financial or familial circumstances, existing comorbidities, and other factors could be driving these behaviors or outcomes due to temporary circumstances. It's essential to address the whole person with a BPSS approach to identify next best steps to increase their capacity.

Effective yoga therapy can widen one's autonomic resilience (Brown and Gerbarg 2009; Sullivan *et al.* 2018a; Tyagi and Cohen 2016; van der Kolk 2014, pp.265–278). We may see our student become braver in their movement vocabulary and/or intensity, emotionally more available, and more creative, hopeful, and resilient in their life off the mat. We present challenges they can meet successfully, thus restoring a greater capacity or increased threshold for coping. This can include both physically active or stimulating breath practices that challenge mobilization thresholds, as well as calming practices like meditation, breathing, or restorative postures that increase capacity for rest and stillness.

Patterns serve a purpose

Working with the physical body provides a tangible, material ground from which to observe habits and their outcomes, and the framework of PVT provides a certain objectivity, trusting the body is doing its best to keep us safe. The word maladaptive gets used to describe residual responses that are no longer context appropriate in the present. Our brain and body, however, don't care whether a stressor is real, imagined, or remembered; when triggered, a very tangible psychophysiological response plays out in the present.

Trauma may make it difficult to focus, perceive sensation accurately, or complete a home practice regularly and can lead to significant physical and mental-health issues (Dana 2020, pp.9–10). This may show up when working with trauma or sexual assault survivors. Bringing this to light can support us in offering compassionate, ongoing guidance and reassurance during practice and giving concrete instructions to encourage successful home practice. These students may feel stuck, wanting to make change yet failing to act. They may present with concurrent diagnoses like depression, anxiety, gastrointestinal issues, insomnia, or post-traumatic stress disorder (PTSD); collaborate with their primary care and mental-health providers. To be held in loving kindness through our therapeutic relationship and by executing appropriate postures or sequences, a student can learn to regulate and mobilize safely. They contact their ability to harness the attention, breath, sensation, communication, and sovereignty needed to move forward.

We may also observe overactivity, insomnia, or anxiety in our students. Whether due to a trauma being kept at bay, or simply as a product of our cultural conditioning that we must stay productive, rest can feel challenging. Stillness holds gems of insight and regeneration but often can feel very difficult to surrender into with great depth. A necessary, counter-cultural skill, yoga therapy can gradually instill in students more capacity for attentiveness, rest, and how to create space between a stimulus and response.

Resilience means cultivating physiological agility, receptivity, and choice, becoming more able to both mobilize and rest, activate and discharge. Although we still have much to learn about the mechanisms behind sexual response (Meston n.d.), we may be beginning to understand how sexuality illustrates this physiological range and adaptability beautifully (Stanton *et al.* 2015).

When we work closely with our students, they can learn to identify their physiological state, and establish familiarity and a felt sense of safety through practice. Encourage connection and nonjudgmental awareness first, and then investigate capacity gradually. Pelvic yoga therapy, and the introspection and prana it generates, churns our inner world, inviting us to till the fertile soil of our life.

Trauma-informed methods

For the many reasons explored throughout Part 1, I invite all pelvic-health professionals to seek additional training in trauma-informed care and consider the needs of sexual violence survivors (Yamasaki 2021). Here are some ideas to help you begin to make your practice and language more trauma-informed.

- Outline and employ informed consent practices; include them on intake forms.
- Learn to guide your students in developing a Resourcing List (professional and personal relationships, places, objects, habits, and practices that help them maintain or restore a sense of safety during challenging times).
- Create your own Resourcing List to help you with challenging cases, expand your own capacity, and address vicarious trauma.
- Use invitational language and inquiry-based methods; normalize modifications and props.
- Seek explicit consent before sharing testimonials or stories – even when they're positive!

As yoga professionals, part of our ongoing certification may include operating within a formal code of conduct (IAYT 2020). Individual schools and lineages may have similar documents in place. If you function as a school director, training program faculty, or studio owner or manager, please consider developing your own ethics culture and explicit consent practices to support survivors and prevent additional harm.

A few words about shame

The pelvis is one place in the body ripe for personal and collective unlearning. Women have long been objectified sexually, and yet there's still intense debate (and outright censorship) over our sexuality, reproductive rights, birth, pelvic health, and nudity. Many women may still feel that talking about pelvic symptoms is shocking, dirty, or disgusting, leaving them feeling isolated and broken, without the hope of getting professional help. Others may have been taught explicitly or learned culturally that desiring sexual pleasure and celebrating sexual expression would be immodest, worse yet, immoral. The female pelvis has historically been shrouded and misunderstood.

Defined as a distressing, humiliating feeling, Brené Brown describes shame as a belief that something's deeply *wrong with us*, not our behavior (Brown 2010). For many women, this extends to their anatomy. Pudendum is one name for the external female genitals. The etymology of pudendum, and thus the pudendal nerve within the pelvis, comes from the Latin verb *pudere* which means "to be ashamed" (Draper 2021).

We know shame's making an appearance when we'd rather disappear into thin air than have someone see our red flushed cheeks and fresh tears stinging our eyes as our skin crawls with awkward embarrassment. It's not a matter of *if* shame will ever come up during a yoga-therapy session, but *when*, and we can learn to hold it with compassion, even reverence, as a messenger of where healing may be possible.

Secrecy allows shame to persist. Community and conversation may be possible antidotes as we invite clients into a portal of curiosity and gentle self-interrogation.

Three essential threads of self-inquiry

The questions here intend to help you and your students reflect on patterns of behavior and create ground-level safety and "resourcedness" that can support the at-times uncomfortable, tender work of yoga therapy.

SHAME
What elements of pelvic health, sexuality, menstruation, hygiene, or nudity bring up shame for you? What names for the genitals cause you to react? What's one small step you could take toward releasing this shame to invite more loving compassion or celebration into your body?

SAFETY
How do you behave when you feel completely safe? Take a moment to feel this in your body, and then write down several examples – do you laugh wholeheartedly, get silly, share personal stories easily? How can you weave more of this joyous participation into your life?

SUPPORT
What kind of support do you long for? How would having this kind of support impact your pelvic health? How would it impact your creativity and sexuality?

As these questions may have caused sensations, narratives, images, beliefs, and emotions to surface, let's close with a simple body-based practice.

Orienting

The following practice stems from work I've experienced in the realm of nervous system reeducation and polyvagal inquiries (Johnson 2021; Lyon 2019). Really, it's about using our senses and physicality to cultivate presence. Yoga practitioners, and sometimes others who practice mindfulness, meditation, or somatic modalities, tend to "go inward" when asked to become present to what they feel, which often includes closing their eyes. While that can be useful to register subtle clues from interoception, it may prevent them from bringing full presence into movement, daily tasks, and interactions with others. This inward-only focus excludes awareness of the environment, while embodiment and resilience are also *relational.*

We need skill to simultaneously track inner and outer environments, as it may increase our functional capacity for daily activities. From a therapeutic lens, this exercise can support folks coming from either hyper or hypo-arousal to find better regulation. Let's try it.

Stand up when you're ready.

Take a moment first to observe your current sensations and state without changing anything.

Begin to feel your feet against the floor. Spread your toes and shift your weight from side to side and through different parts of your feet. Eyes open, please. Notice where your gaze lands, what do you see? What are your eyes drawn to? – color, texture, light, and shadow... What do you hear? Spend a moment seeing the objects around you while adding a small, rhythmic bounce with your legs.

Now let your eyes scan to the right, eventually looking over your shoulder behind you. Let your eyes lead and feel your body follow, creating a spiral through your torso and hips. Bring your eyes back to gazing straight ahead, let your body settle here where you began. Then, when you feel ready, scan your eyes to the left, allowing your body once again to follow into rotation as you look behind you. Register that you're fully aware to the objects, people, and shape of the space you're in right now. As you feel your exhalation, bring your eyes, and then your body, back to a centered position. Let your gaze be soft and open to the periphery. Let yourself take in the truth of this moment – "I am safe here. I am safe within myself." Can you awaken a kind of three-dimensional awareness, feeling the space around you through your skin? You're fully calm and in command. You know where you are, and you've taken up your rightful place through cultivating this presence. You've oriented to your own power.

Invite this skill of tracking sensation also as a method of identifying your ANS state. With that baseline awareness, you can better discern which practices or tools to implement.

Whenever conflict or anger tries to consume us or shame tells us to hide, we can open our eyes and mobilize our physicality to reorient to the environment and present moment. We can learn to return to a more regulated state with practice. With the philosophical, ethical, and physiological foundations of yoga therapy now embedded in our consciousness, let's dive in to Part 2.

PART 2

WHERE ARE WE? WHAT DOES A PELVIS REQUIRE?

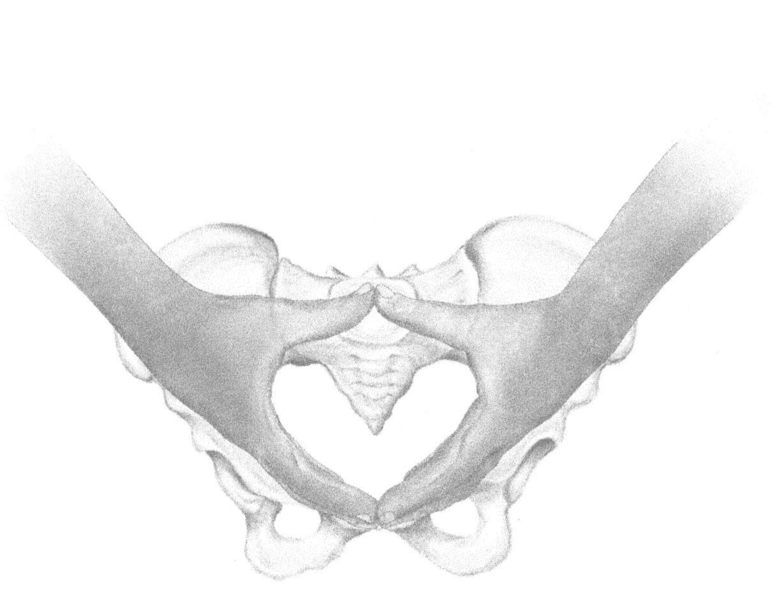

CHAPTER 4

Local Anatomy

The pelvis is a busy place. Compressive forces from the upper body and spine need to stream down through the sacrum into our legs efficiently. During weight-bearing movements like walking, the reverse is also true. The ground reaction forces and leverage from each stride need to translate from a sagittal plane orientation up into the beautiful swish of spinal rotation and counter rotation with our arms swinging freely. The efficient function of our pelvic bones help make this movement possible – what we often perceive as a centered, graceful quality.

A great paradox exists here, as the pelvis must simultaneously manage containment and opening. Relaxation allows us to use the toilet, have sex, and birth babies (not necessarily in that order!). Active coordination and strength of these muscles maintain continence and support organs, and yes, even while exercising, sneezing, and living our later years as wise women. A common metaphor for the pelvis is a bowl or bucket, except ours literally has holes in it. The pelvic muscles need enough finesse to contend with gravity and manage intraabdominal pressure (IAP) *and* release what needs to come out or in when we choose.

Not to mention this is home to our reproductive organs, digestive and excretory functions, and an energetic, sexual, and spiritual center. Our pelvis provides a foundational level of core stability, and even acts as a sump pump to help circulate blood and lymph.

Through this great portal, all human life begins.

We'll tour the pelvis by covering skeletal and soft tissue anatomy and briefly overview the corresponding organ systems. To enhance your learning, please participate in the experiential inquiries, and then adapt and apply them as you see fit for your students. Touch awakens proprioception and interoception in ways the mind alone cannot. It's also helpful to familiarize the bony landmarks and the muscles of the abdomen, hips, and pelvic floor. This can be offered as a verbally guided self-touch experience or given as an open-ended invitation for a student's private home practice after learning pelvic anatomy with pictures or models. If offered in a yoga-therapy visit, I typically participate by touching my own body to normalize the activity, provide visual demonstration, and clarify questions as they arise. You could consider integrating soft balls and other props to provide a medium to touch through if using their hands feels too vulnerable. Let's begin.

The bones

When teaching group workshops on the pelvis, I ask early on, "What are the bones of the pelvis?" Most of the time, participants name the ilium, ischium, and pubis. Indeed, these terms name distinct areas within the pelvis, and they can help us begin to know our way around the landscape we're traversing. What I find curiously absent, and rarely understood or named, is the distinct relationships of the pelvic bones and joints that create a functional picture of how the pelvis moves. Let's take a closer look.

The ilium, ischium, and pubis identify three "geographic regions" within the "continent" of the *same bone*. In young adult life, when we've finished growing structurally, these regions fuse together to form the two pelvic innominates, or the pelvic halves. Understanding the pelvis has two distinct sides can help illustrate functional concepts.

I'll never forget feeling how this clicked again for me, gazing at my then 18-month-old daughter as she played. It dawned on me with newfound clarity – her little toddler pelvis needed to become a much larger, wider grown-woman's pelvis. Of course, these pelvic bones were still growing and needed to not solidify until adulthood. The three "zones" of the pelvic innominate bone come together inside the acetabula or hip sockets, fusing in several gradual stages (Howard 2017, p.35; Wobser, Adkins, Wobser 2020).

If you happen to work with young women or children, know that how we move and the daily demands we put on our structure – which is especially important to consider when working with committed young athletes – can influence the still-developing bones and joint articulations of the pelvis and hip for the rest of our life. Adult women, those with a bony pelvic structure mostly predetermined in shape and form, still have some capacity for plasticity in terms of functional relationships, especially in the soft tissues.

A few words now to ensure we're on the same page. Prominences or bony landmarks include rough, bulgy, or "end-point" places where soft tissues attach – unique names for different areas of a bone based on their purpose. Knowing key terms of pelvic anatomy will make applying the imagery and exercises in this chapter easier. You can look up images or terms to clarify, and palpate them on your own body or a skeletal model. Consider having your favorite anatomy reference near you as you read on, and start to appreciate the contours of the pelvis as shown in Figure 4.1. Keep in mind anatomy illustrations can differ.

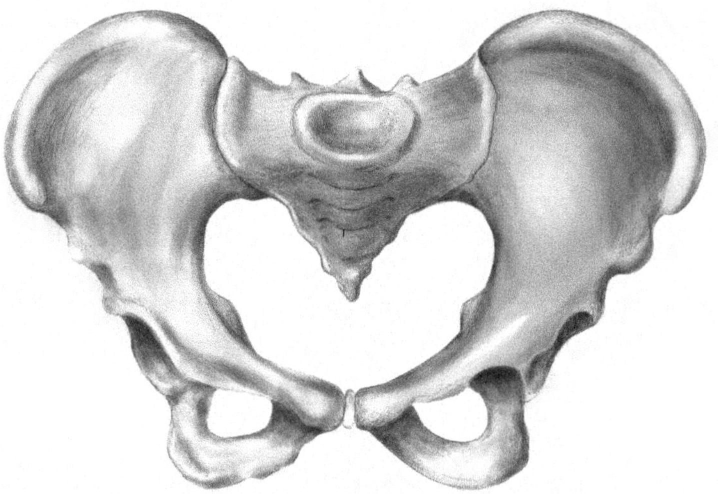

Figure 4.1: The basin of pelvic bones

Let's define now the bones that make up the pelvis. We have four in total: the two pelvic halves or innominate bones, the sacrum, and the coccyx. For some reason, anatomists chose "innominate," which literally means "no-name" bone. How boring for such a beautiful, central part of our body! It could certainly have received a more creative moniker for its spiraled shape and complex contours.

If you have access to a full-size skeletal model, I highly recommend getting your hands all over that beautiful plastic pelvis. Standing behind the skeleton, cup your hands around the top of the pelvic bowl to hold the "wings" of the ilia on either side of the sacrum. This broad, bony structure in the posterior makes a sturdy place to land when we lie down on our back or our side. How your hands scoop around to embrace the iliac crests can give a nice feeling of your organs being held and supported. The anterior support at this same level comes from the integrity of our abdominal wall muscles and fascia and the anterior bony rim of the pelvic inlet. This broad, upper space in the pelvis funnels into the pelvic inlet where a baby's head engages to move through the birth canal (Calais-Germain 2003, pp.12–33).

Now bring your hands up from underneath the pelvis, placing your fingertips on the pubic symphysis. Cupping along the inferior pubic rami, rest the heels of your hands on the outside of the sit bones or ischial tuberosities. Feel how the pelvic outlet at the bottom is closed in the front and opens to the space behind you. See if you can envision and feel the V-shape your hands are tracing within your body. This inferior space is supported by the layers of pelvic floor, sometimes called the "back wall" of the pelvis, as we can imagine muscular support fanning outward from the relatively upright sacrum to connect to the inner surfaces of the pelvic bowl.

Draw a diamond shape with your mind's eye, like in Figure 4.2. Begin at your tailbone, the posterior-most point of this space. Then trace the diagonal pathways forward to feel both sit bones. Lastly, acknowledge your pubic bone at the front. We'll come back to this metaphor later to add detail.

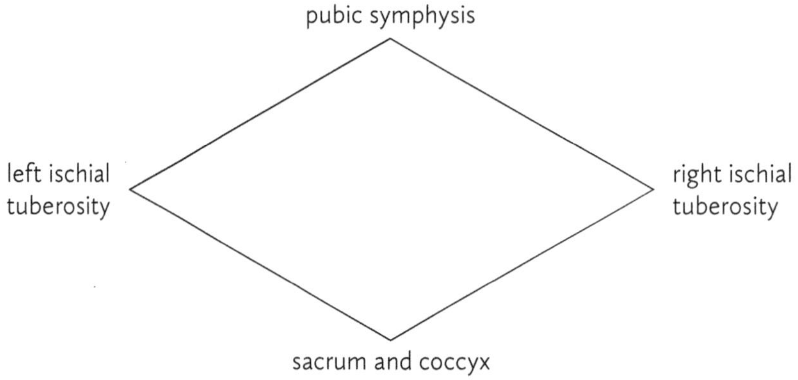

Figure 4.2: The pelvic diamond

Let's complete the tour of bones by palpating the sacrum and coccyx. First, come to standing.

Take one hand around to your back and slide the heel of your hand down until you feel the top, broad surface of your sacrum. Take in the fact that its name translates to "sacred or holy." Your palm and fingertips conveniently cup around the natural curve of your sacrum, tapering into a narrower shape at the bottom. Comprised of three to five fused vertebral bones, the sacrum has a curved keystone shape that is concave to the interior of your pelvis. Some women feel bumps down the back of their sacrum, like tiny spinous processes – keep this in mind for helping students find comfort when lying supine. A little softness from a blanket or squishy, slightly inflated ball can do wonders for breath excursion, relaxation, and peace of mind. Let your legs bend and notice if you can feel your breath descend into and influence the sacrum. Change hands any time and spend several breaths here.

Step your feet out a bit wider now, keeping your legs active and supple, and let your fingertips trace the right and left sides of your sacrum. Many times, one side feels more accessible than the other, or we discover some tenderness in the surrounding tissues. If you find tissues that feel tense, sinewy, or denser, gently rub them with a circular motion, encouraging them to soften. While you do this, you can move your leg by rotating your femur in and out in the socket or making circles with your leg draping down from that same pelvic half. Be gentle and curious.

Walk your fingers lower until you find your coccyx, palpating lightly to either side. To finish, brush down your sacrum or shake your hands out, and then rest in standing. Take a little walk to feel how your brain map of the pelvic bones has improved – you might find you're more aware, you're moving more fluidly, or there's a greater sense of volume and support from your center. Celebrate whatever you're discovering.

The coccyx is comprised of three to five tiny segments, most commonly four (Woon *et al.* 2013). Even though it can become fused independent of age and gender, the joint between sacrum and tailbone can play a role in muscular balance and dynamic imagery. Movement here is very subtle, if present. We can discern whether to cue students to visualize the movement of the sacrum, and by default feel the tailbone at the distal end or imagine the tailbone itself. For folks with tailbone pain, we may simply invite them to cup this area gently and envision the soothing warmth of their hand helping the posterior pelvic floor relax.

In review, we have four pelvic bones: the right and left pelvic halves (the two innominates), the sacrum and the coccyx. Now let's dive into the functional joints!

The joints of the pelvis

At the front of your pelvis lives the pubic symphysis. The right and left halves of the pelvis join here, with a cartilage disc and synovial capsules on either side. What this means functionally is that the two sides of our pelvis can move independently, albeit a very small distance or glide. This micro-movement at the center can allow for greater ease in walking and a slight springy rebound when squatting or landing from a jump.

For clients with symphysis pubis dysfunction (SPD), it's often most helpful to start with yoga asana that includes simplified, bilateral lower-extremity weight bearing to maximize comfort and efficiency rather than emphasizing more complex asymmetrical or unilateral postures. We may also address imbalances in adjacent muscles, like the iliopsoas, hamstrings, adductors and others, to promote integrity and balance the loads affecting this joint. We can then gradually reintroduce movement variety necessary for daily life (single leg stances, asymmetry) with the goal of desensitizing a possibly over-sensitive pain system as they restore trust and become more skilled in their physical practice. Lastly, consider again the complexity of pain, taking a whole-person approach and not solely biomechanical.

Around the back, we come to the gloriously stable sacroiliac (SI) joints, where the sacrum meets each pelvic half at the ilia. Constructed from varied concave and convex surfaces, they fit together snugly like a puzzle and are surrounded by robust ligaments and muscular support. The pair of dynamic joints allows forces from the spine to transfer through the curves of the pelvis into the legs and vice versa. Minute motions of rotation and translation, or sliding, occur at the articular surfaces of the SI joints. We'll practice them experientially as an act of embodied education and befriending one's pelvis.

Manual assessments of SI movement may hardly be detectable, let alone clinically reliable (Goode *et al.* 2008). They may provoke pain but don't necessarily tell us *why*. Also, pain does not imply movement dysfunction as causation, regardless of the pervasive language around instability. This limited approach has persisted despite years of research suggesting a change in course (Palsson *et al.* 2019).

We may hear students proclaim, "My SI went out," or, "I have SI instability." Perhaps more likely than joint subluxation or instability, motor control and imbalances of surrounding tissues may be culprits of SI pain. Also, remember any time pain persists, we'll need to investigate the role of the nervous system, sensitization, and psychosocial emotional components (O'Sullivan 2015). As yoga therapists, we can positively affect pain responses through adequate rest and relaxation, provide psychosocial coping strategies, and refine recruitment patterns to increase efficiency. Muscle activity influences the integrity of the joints and their movement, and can be organized more efficiently through intention and dynamic imagery (Franklin 2012, pp.31–74).

The SI joint has been labeled (even marketed) as unstable and in need of protection, and intensive, virtuosic asana or deep, static stretching held the blame and responsibility for injury, long-term laxity, and even hip-joint replacements.

In some cases, this may be plausible or even true. As yoga therapists, we do our best to educate and empower students, which means language is paramount.

Fear-mongering and nocebo cues create tension and stress (Palsson *et al.* 2019), which further override clear thinking, receptivity to subtle sensations, and good motor coordination. We may only rarely see such extreme performances from our students – unless they happen to be athletes, dancers, gymnasts, or yogis.

Nocebo and placebo defined: Nocebo: Cues that reinforce a perceived negativity bias and can promote or maintain negative outcomes; example: using language like, "Do this to protect your SI joint from degenerating or eroding." Placebo: Cues that reinforce a positivity bias and can support the greater likelihood of positive outcomes, often using skill-based language; example: "Press into both feet and feel how your legs and hips activate – they know how to support your pelvis!"

Students may also self-select these physical activities if they inherently have more joint range or hypermobility – and then perpetuate that trend by practicing forms that glorify flexibility beyond normal functional ranges. We may be able to help prevent suffering for hypermobile practitioners by increasing movement integrity with two principles. First, ask that they avoid practicing at end range, which may pose a larger inquiry around expectations and identity. Second, require the student to engage actively within the posture to switch on the necessary neuromuscular support and prevent loads from negatively impacting ligaments and joint capsule tissues.

When we encounter these students, it can be useful to diversify their practice by introducing active engagement or external resistance as complementary training, along with helping identify what causes increased symptoms or brings relief. Yoga therapy can also address adequate sleep, active recovery, movement efficiency, and mindset. This is often a slow process of trial and error to build greater trust with subtle somatic perception, cultivate strength and resilience, and examine their allegiances to their form, sport, or lineage. Many asana shapes hold very little functional equivalence – they don't directly reflect the range of motion or skills we need to live comfortably in our physical body. Like the old saying goes, just because you can doesn't mean you should.

Although I agree that aggressive, forceful, repetitive actions beyond current training thresholds or tissue capacity, or with inadequate rest and recovery, can negatively impact the joints, let's paint a more encouraging picture that pelvic joints are inherently quite stable. Words matter, and we want to help students build a trusting relationship with their body as capable and safe. We facilitate this by employing skills-based cues and education.

Redefining stability

Stability can be defined as a robustness that allows someone to return to homeostasis or "center" after being perturbed or taken off balance. It isn't a static phenomenon in which we force ourselves to remain perfectly still. To the contrary, true stability comes from being able to perceive and respond accurately, adapting in the moment to restore a sense of equilibrium no matter what gravity or life throws at us.

The joint movements we study here, while small, allow us to navigate the fact that we are living, changing beings. They allow us to transfer and disperse forces instead of accumulating or concentrating forces into localized places, which can lead to inefficient movement or tissue damage. It may serve us well to move beyond the polarity of deciding between whether to "mobilize or stabilize," and instead see that focusing on movement efficiency is capable of training both.

Efficiency means we can orchestrate movement with the appropriate amount of effort to accomplish the task. Too little effort and our movement can become disorganized, and we may rely on joint structures and connective tissue for support they're not so equipped to give. Too much effort, and the excess tension can alter joint mechanics and load certain aspects of the joint surface more than others, and overuse some neuromuscular patterns while neglecting other nerve and muscle fibers waiting in the wings for their chance to help. Efficiency allows even complex movements or high-load activities to appear effortless and smooth, and may promote longevity as we learn to skillfully use our body.

A multidisciplinary approach to movement (not solely practicing asana) can help make sure we don't fall prey to a limited, dogmatic approach. Understanding movement science principles helps us design a home practice that can instill the rich benefits made possible by the dynamic partnership of stability and mobility.

Next, we'll begin to investigate how the pelvic bones move.

The bone rhythms

A bone rhythm shows us the dance that happens under the skin's surface within each joint. This X-ray vision freshly illuminated my embodiment through studying with Eric Franklin, and coincidentally, one of his teachers has also been mine – Bonnie Bainbridge Cohen, founder of Body-Mind Centering. Anatomists have long understood joint mechanics theoretically. Somatic modalities choose to teach this science experientially to enhance awareness and movement function (Calais-Germain 2003, pp.28–33; Franklin 2012, pp.149–178).

We try to break down movement into linear, mechanical, "correct and safe," or "incorrect and unsafe" dualities. It makes learning and teaching more straightforward; it *feels* simpler. In reality, the body is built for variety and variability – alignment is dynamic. Our bones dance when we move, and what appears to be linear or taught as two-dimensional is often multiplanar by design. The more ways we move and load the body, the better.

You could also refer to this as a study of arthrokinematics, or how our joints move. We study these movements as an act of anatomical *satya*, or honesty, to uncover the truth that exists under the surface. One of the yamas, honesty can be applied as we assess a student's baseline function or imbalances. We simply want to get clear about what's happening (or not happening) in the present and move toward functional awareness through the objectivity of bones. The complexity of these bone rhythms can require intellectual *tapas*, or disciplined focus. When the mental load becomes greater than your somatic felt sense, pause and regroup. Then simplify your imagery back to a singular plane or image. Let these bone rhythms integrate with repetition.

We're bringing attention to actual joint movement, like shining a spotlight with our consciousness, not making or forcing something to happen with voluntary movement. Our pelvic floor thrives on this subtle, necessary shape-shifting. When the image is hard to form mentally, or difficult to sense kinesthetically, it usually implies you may need more embodiment with that function – practice there more. It can be useful to introduce images to students one plane at a time, otherwise this knowledge acts as an internal operating system in my mind as I adapt cues for relevance to a specific action or asana. Anecdotally, I've also seen it rewire more balanced functioning where asymmetry had existed.

Next, we'll try experiential exercises to attempt to feel the three planes of action for pelvic bone rhythms. If you don't "feel anything," it could be that you're learning to form imagery and sense subtle sensations – this might be a new way of practicing for you. It could also mean that the exercise simply isn't what you need right now (it could be functioning fine already!). We'll use a weight-bearing stance, but take note that these anatomical actions happen whenever we explore the movements of our hip joints. We'll do more asana-based applications together in Chapter 11.

Frontal plane

Stand with a comfortably wide stance, allowing your feet and legs to take a natural amount of slight external rotation. Reach behind to touch your sit bones, or ischial tuberosities, and massage around them to increase interoceptive awareness. Land your fingertips gently yet firmly back on your sit bones. Now, begin to move down into a slow wide squat or grand plié.

What do you feel happening under your hands? Do your sit bones move or do they not move?

Become curious about your sit bones in the frontal plane. See if you can tap into the inherent widening and narrowing excursion they take to allow you to squat and stand back up. As the sit bones move out, the ilia do what's called "in flare" – remember, this is the pelvic innominate bones in action, so what happens down at the sit bones is mirrored with a counter movement above at the ilia. If you're not convinced, you could try keeping your sit bones where they are in a standing position (don't let them widen) and attempt to squat. I don't recommend practicing repeatedly this way, as you're voluntarily overriding the pelvic bone rhythms, which could create tension, confusion, and dysfunction over time. This inquiry is simply a teaching tool to help you sense and discern through contrast.

If you tried the static imagery of your sit bones not moving, be sure to complete a few repetitions of your wide squat with freedom for your sit bones to slide apart and return toward each other each time. You could imagine them as smoothly sliding French doors or like they're roller skating away from each other for you to sit back and then rolling or even actively pulling themselves back together to stand up. When you finish, shake out your arms and legs, rest in standing, or take a walk to observe any changes you feel.

Please note, this is one key bone rhythm I often see lacking in students who have habituated to a posterior pelvic tilt or a learned voluntary cue of "tucking their tail." It's often the easiest plane for students to feel the bone rhythm, too, so that's helpful. When teaching this inquiry, especially if you have a student take a more parallel, narrow stance, at times they'll attempt to "make the bone rhythm happen" by way of abducting the thighs on the way down. Beware of this and continue to track the knees and feet in a similar spatial intent, while highlighting the pelvic bone rhythm through imagery awareness or palpating one's own bum.

Lastly, for folks with prolapse or symptoms of heaviness or pressure during squats, suggest they explore this bone rhythm with a parallel stance, perhaps placing a block between their thighs to help engage more pelvic support. Another option to further reduce demand on the pelvic floor could be to explore this supine or with legs up the wall, allowing the feet to slide against the floor or wall through a closed-chain movement. Every exercise can be adapted to meet the current needs of the student and then progressed gradually as symptoms are managed.

Transverse plane

Remember the shape of the pelvic half or innominate bones from superior to inferior – the bone itself is twisted. Each pelvic half takes a spiraling journey top to bottom, which is important for the pelvic micro-movements that help absorb and transfer force.

Trace this dance with your hands now free from the skeletal model. Hold up your palms to model the broad ilia top of the pelvis, then let your hands descend inferiorly while bringing your fingertips together to reflect the pelvic outlet. Do this a few times to anchor the image in your mind and attempt to feel these contours in your pelvis consciously.

Now hold the right side of your pelvis between both hands and imagine the femur head in the acetabulum, or socket. Do a small plié or squat, focusing your attention on the right side. When the pelvic half spirals in or medially from the anterior superior iliac spine, remember the sit bone swings out laterally. As a subtle, relative counter rotation, the femur head spirals outward or externally when moving into flexion. To stand back up, feel the opposite happen as the femur spirals in on its axis, and the pelvic half rotates externally or laterally (the socket swirls back over the femur head to return us upright). Counter rotations give our body time to absorb and transfer forces over a greater surface area, creating perhaps better efficiency and longevity. This exercise in the transverse plane allows you to better embody the coupled motion of hip flexion with slight femoral external rotation – potentially giving the pelvic floor a better chance to move through its full range. (Admittedly, this subtle dance of transverse plane pelvic motion can sometimes feel elusive.)

Sagittal plane

Finally, we move on to the sagittal plane. I find it most useful to bring attention to the tip of the tailbone for this inquiry. Use your fingertips if touch feels helpful, and begin to take the same small squatting motion up and down. Can you feel your tail move at all? Where does it go as you descend into your plié or chair pose (utkatasana)? Where does it venture to when you press the floor away and come back up to standing?

When we bend or initiate moving down into a squat, the sacrum nutates. Nutation means the top, broadest part of the sacrum nods forward into the body, while the tip of the tail swings back in space, creating more eccentric loading of the PFM – they lengthen. When we stand back up, the sacrum counter nutates or returns to its starting position, and by default, so does the tail. I make note for students that this return of the tailbone swinging back underneath us is not an active tucking action that creates a posterior tilt or gripping and clenching in the buttocks or pelvic floor. Simply observe how this active use of dynamic imagery creates more power, sometimes even more depth of range in your squat.

Lastly, if the anatomical imagery makes smoke come out your ears, imagine instead a metaphorical tail of your own design. How might a thick, heavy dinosaur tail feel compared with a feathery, fluffy tail that bushes out even more when you descend into a squat and gently comes back to midline, smoothing those silky hairs down as you stand up? From the diamond metaphor, you could visualize and feel the distance between the tailbone and pubic bone elongating as you bend and descend, and then that distance shortening on the way up to standing.

Remember, the joint actions are still happening in the other two planes. If you're game, see if you can imagine them all swirling and moving simultaneously to allow you to bend and straighten your legs. From embodying these micro-movements, we may begin to feel a beautiful, responsive elasticity within the PFM.

These bone rhythms may help us more reliably recruit the pelvic muscles the way they're designed to be used – in a dynamic, ever-changing context. In short, if the bones move, the muscles attached to those bones will be moved, too.

What about the hip joints?

It feels warranted to add that the hip joint, albeit essential to embody for pelvic health, is different than the joints we discussed above. Often in workshops, this is named first, as if the pelvis itself is understood to be one static object and the only joints are below (at the hip) or above (the spine). It is not one solid piece, nor would I encourage you to embody your pelvis as one plastic bucket or one stable brick of your body to be stacked with other bricks into "correct alignment." We live in dynamic, changing bodies that respond to our environment and gravity in each moment – at least the hope is that we can ebb and flow easily, right?

Take a moment to feel your femurs rising into their sockets, carrying you and your pelvis through the world with ease. Hip joint function and hip muscle balance does impact pelvic-floor health and vice versa. Just be clear in your own embodied understanding how the hip is the connecting joint between the pelvis and legs – not a joint within the pelvis itself. In Chapter 6, I address how to find and feel support from the femurs.

The soft stuff

We went into skeletal anatomy first, as it gives a tangible map of the terrain to begin. Now, we'll come back up to the surface and address the tissues layer by layer – skin and genitals, fascia and muscles. As we affect the plentiful ligamentous structures less directly with yoga therapy, we won't study them in this text. Please browse illustrations of the connective tissues at the SI, pubic, and hip joints, including the sturdy sacral interchange of the thoracolumbar fascia. Seeing these fibers of support may instill appreciation and faith in their role.

This section is called "The soft stuff," because historically, we've obsessed over muscles. Looking at many anatomical books or illustrations, you'll often see drawings of cleaned-up, stripped-down deep fascia (maybe) and the muscles. Bright red, they beckon to our desire to study the concrete and tangible, the lesser taboo of these tissues. Maybe muscles also represent that which we feel we can control, bending them to our will through voluntary training, sculpting, and manual therapy. Even though this *is* a book about pelvic-floor health, I want to consciously take down the hierarchy that this reductionist approach might represent. We must remember the pelvic muscles are invested in the health of their surrounding neighbors, and vice versa, and they belong to a woman with very real feelings and opinions about this part of her body.

I noticed how curiously absent the genitals can be, even from books on pelvic health, which is why I've included them here. If this feels triggering to you or your client, know you can take time to normalize and welcome new terms into your experience with a titrated approach. Omit or alter your vocabulary as a process of co-creation with your student.

Sensing the skin can help distinguish external parts – the vulva, mons pubis, pubic hair (or lack thereof if that's your preference) – and internal parts – like the vagina and cervix. What touches our clothing is considered the whole vulva, the internal canal is the vagina, and the space where they meet, or transition, is the vestibule. I say outer and inner labia instead of labia majora and minora because some women have larger inner labia (minora) that protrude beyond the outer labia. Labeling these aspects of genitalia based on location and relationship rather than presumed size can help destigmatize the natural variations that exist between bodies. Every vulva is unique and beautiful.

The skin also covers a highly proprioceptive layer of our body called the superficial fascia, which includes connective tissue, capillaries, fat, and nerve endings. Our fascial matrix communicates six times more proprioceptive information than muscles (Schleip 2015). This can be important to note when using foam rollers, myofascial release balls, or pelvic wands; these methods should not create a pain response. Less is more. When we employ the sense of touch, we're accessing the brain and nervous system, too (Miller 2019). Compassionate, skillful self-massage may provide a better sense of safety and relaxation than stretching alone, which may lead to more positive, lasting tissue changes (Capobianco, Mazzo, Enoka 2019).

We study by differentiating tissues by name and type. Functionally, please remember that the fascia surrounds or envelops all other tissues, anchoring them to the bones. My favorite way to see this is through fruit! Peel an orange and notice how the outer peel and inner white pith or fuzz are continuous with the membranous lining of each juicy segment and even every tiny pod of nectar. We're bound together by the interwoven, comprehensive fabric of our fascia.

Self-touch can play a role in both desensitizing pain or resensitizing a woman to her body in potentially therapeutic ways. Soft, fleshy contours cushion bones, pad around nerves, and transmit pressure, stretch, and vibration messages back to the brain. Practicing imagery (imagining doing a specific movement, for example) can improve the body maps in the brain, differentiating each part from the next to grow one's capacity to focus, feel, and move well (Blakeslee and Blakeslee 2007, pp.60, 65).

Of course, the process of awakening what has been "lost" and soothing "on-alert" areas from chronic or acute pain mechanisms can also be facilitated by relationship with a clinician specialized in pelvic-floor manual assessment and treatment. As yoga therapists, we can help students feel equipped to negotiate consent and communicate with their specialist before and while internal touch occurs. This can help restore autonomy where it had been taken away or threatened, strengthening a woman's ability to speak up in times of conflict and intimacy. Internal manual therapy may restore glide and suppleness to scar tissue, release trigger points, and give a woman great insight about her holding patterns and current function. Receiving touch from a pelvic specialist also allows the patient to practice full body relaxation, finding a level of surrender that may be challenging to cultivate if they're attempting to reach down and release their own internal trigger points, for example.

As yoga therapists, we might support this through imagery, as awareness can touch every part of one's body. The ease with which we speak about the pelvis could become as normal as scratching an elbow or feeling a hamstring sensation. Culturally, we're becoming more adept at these conversations. The clitoris has basked in the spotlight of media attention far more often since its full internal anatomy and beauty became more widely known through MRI studies (Gross 2020; O'Connell and DeLancey 2005).

The clitoris and its erectile tissues embrace the urethra and vagina, nestle within the layers of PFM, and can engorge with blood when aroused, like the penis. I'd feel remiss if I left out the powerful role of sexuality in pelvic health and embodiment. If someone is numb or averse to arousal and sexual exploration, it may make sense that having a happy, healthy pelvic floor may then also feel elusive. The opposite effect may also be possible through mindfulness. As individuals begin to embody the pelvis, womb, and genitals through platonic practices of self-study, they may find new inroads to pleasure.

If a student becomes surprised or triggered by newfound sensations that could equate to arousal in their perception, especially if they've experienced sexual trauma or childhood sexual abuse, we must be ready to respond with compassion and clarity. Be impeccably clear with yourself and your student that while these sensations are valid and normal, even welcome, it may serve their continued healing to find a professional, qualified party to help them sort through past experiences, reignited traumas, and arising desires. Meaning making is the student's terrain, not ours. We may offer yoga philosophy frameworks for self-reflection, leaving the interpretation ultimately in the student's hands.

As yoga therapists, we hold the present moment with equanimity, embodied practice, and compassionate witnessing.

This, I hope, brings credit to the importance of having a sex therapist, sex-positive psychologist, or mental-health professional skilled in trauma resolution on your referral team. At the very least, allow students to express their goals, concerns, and needs inclusive of their sexuality within your confidential therapeutic relationship. We can be a witness to her wholeness in this way, and help her get appropriate support.

Capacity for expression and communication can be supported by the tangible, physical strength and resilience we cultivate through embodied practice. The physical kosha both supports and reflects the subtle layers of self.

Now, on to the muscles!

Some sources say the pelvic floor consists of two layers and others claim three; many of its fibers interdigitate. It helps to know that anatomical references can vary widely – as can our human forms. Leave room for variability in each student's experience and physical reality, and cross reference multiple anatomical illustrations.

What's most important is that we understand relationships and function. We can often leave minutiae and direct treatment of specific muscles to qualified clinicians – and tailor the dose of how much anatomy detail we teach our students so it remains relevant and accessible. Whatever we teach intellectually, we also experience and practice somatically.

Moving beneath the skin and contours of the fascial, fatty matrix, we come first to the superficial layer of the pelvic floor, often referred to as the urogenital triangle. Shown in Figure 4.3, this layer often lists the bulbocavernosus, ischiocavernosus, superficial transverse perineal muscles. I include the external anal sphincter, representing the posterior aspect of the figure-eight image in the anal triangle. You can also see the horizontal fibers of the deep transverse muscles on the drawing's right side.

Next, we come to a membranous middle layer. This thin pouch bolsters the anterior portion of the pelvic outlet and contains the erectile bulbs of the clitoris. It contains urethrovaginal sphincter muscles and the deep transverse perineal muscle within its glistening fascial sheath, with the perineal body at the center. The perineal body is a fibromuscular structure between the vagina and anus, and can be correlated to the central tendon of the thoracic diaphragm. If you've never palpated your perineal body, please do so now or when you're next in a private, comfortable space.

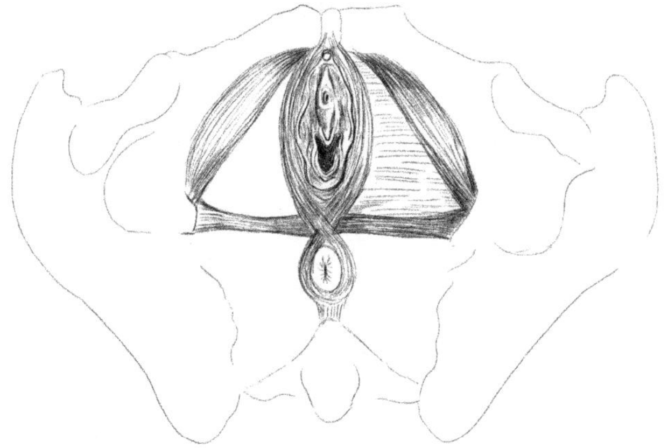

Figure 4.3: Superficial muscle layer, inferior view

As an imagery exercise, I find it useful (and quite fun!) to track a vertical axis inside my body, aligning the perineal body, respiratory diaphragm, the soft palate in my mouth, and the crown of my head like a slithering inflated tube like we see drawing attention to car-wash stations and the like. Consider this like a myofascial comparison to the energetic central channel, or sushumna. Undulating, whipping, and writhing freely – what if we could all access this level of adaptive posture instead of the static strategies (stacking body parts like blocks, for example) that have been slow to fade from popular language? Pelvic embodiment lends a levity to everyday movement, exercise, and one's mindset. A dynamic central axis will guide you through life with fluid receptivity.

You can get a felt sense of this anterior, more superficial portion of the pelvic floor by vulva cupping, a term I first heard from Kimberly Johnson. Simply place the heel of your hand at the pubis, and allow your palm and fingers to drape back around your vulva. Let your touch be broad and soft with no agenda. If the geometry of your body allows, you may feel the tip of your middle finger resting ever so lightly on the central perineal body. Rest your attention here and notice if you can feel your breath ebb and flow under your hand.

As these more superficial layers assist with closure, continence, and excretion, the deepest layer of the pelvic floor provides strong support to the entire inner pelvic space. Called the deep pelvic diaphragm, this dome-like structure (Hjartardottir *et al.* 1997) consists of the powerhouse team of the levator ani muscles. This includes the puborectalis, pubococcygeus, and iliococcygeus. It can be useful to sense the few inches of vaginal (or rectal) canal, and visualize how the depth of that space is surrounded and supported by the layers of levator ani muscles. Seen in Figure 4.4, this deep team of pelvic tissues buoys our organs upward.

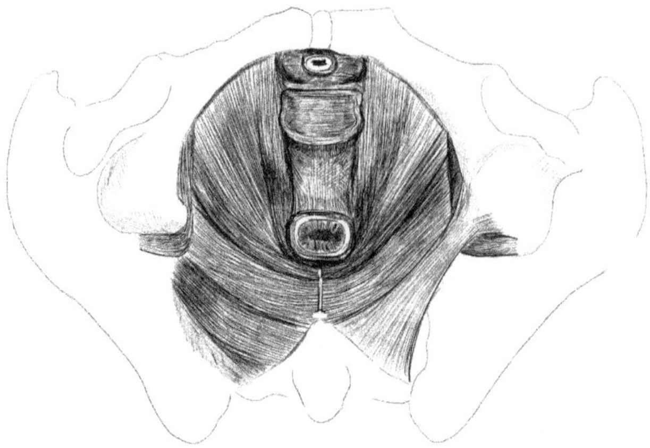

Figure 4.4: Deep muscles of pelvic diaphragm, inferior view

When the PFM contract well together, they create a closing (the squeeze) and an upward support for the organs (the lift). We'll look closely at pelvic-floor engagement and creative cueing in more detail in Chapter 8. Also, the anterior skeletal bridge (formed by the superior pubic rami) of the pelvic inlet may help reduce the load on our connective tissues and PFM – provided we allow dynamic spinal curves and efficient movement.

In yoga, students often get taught a "neutral-pelvis" position. These well-intended cues can become an obsession, interpreted as the "right way" to stand or move, leading students to adopt a posterior pelvic tilt, muscular bracing, and breath holding. This over-correction can increase downward pressure into the pelvic floor and thwart efficiency. Acknowledging and allowing a small anterior tilt and the accompanying lumbar lordosis provides a bony "shelf" of support to the organs, while breathing naturally helps manage pressure.

The obturator internus (which is connected directly to the deep pelvic-floor layer through the arcuate tendon levator ani, or ATLA) and other deep hip rotators, piriformis, iliopsoas, and the gluteus group give us a literal lift when moving about our daily lives. One study with a simple hip-rotation exercise program, performed in five minutes twice daily, generated similarly effective outcomes as PFM training (Tanner 2015). Creating regional hip muscle strength and balance can work wonders in reducing excess effort in the pelvic floor and indirectly trains the pelvic tissues, improving global movement efficiency.

Pelvic imagery

To help you locate and feel the pelvic space, I'm going to share a variety of imagery strategies. By no means is this an exhaustive list, and for imagery to be effective it must be personally relevant, accessible, and pleasant for the participant. Substitute new metaphors as you come to your own conclusions or when helping students find language for their own felt sense of their PFM.

Remember the diamond? The superficial, urogenital triangle supports the front half of this space. The entire diamond shape is then filled and supported by the deeper levator ani muscles fanning out from the posterior. The perineal body lands approximately at the center of the diamond, with this whole network riding up and down with each breath.

It may serve women as a self-assessment tool to evaluate their experience in each of the four quadrants of the diamond – dividing front and back, left and right sides. You'll see in Figure 4.5 a vertical line from pubis to coccyx and a horizontal line between your sit bones. Many women have asymmetrical patterns of function in their pelvic bowl, myself included, historically speaking. Simply doing Kegels or bilateral movements for the sake of "balance" won't always target this imbalance. We may end up perpetuating our habits instead of changing them. Change requires novel inputs.

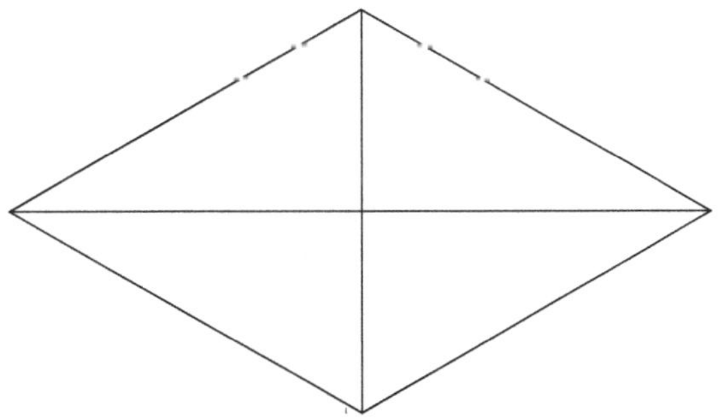

Figure 4.5: The four pelvic quadrants

With the quadrants in our awareness, however, we can focus our intent and efforts, and start to regain command over blind spots. Focus on restoring embodiment where there seems to be decreased capacity to feel, sense, or move. Seeing a pelvic-floor specialist for internal touch can also help instill new habits.

You could also explore the metaphor of a strong, supple trampoline instead of the more common image of a hammock or sling. One study confirms the pelvic floor may function more like a buoyant dome (Hjartardottir *et al.* 1997).

Even though the most visible dome shape was found during supine ultrasound assessment, this may be useful imagery for weight bearing, especially for women who'd like to regain a sense of lightness on their feet and improve organ support.

Organs and systems

The pelvic organs live under the peritoneal sac containing the abdominal viscera, what's called subperitoneal, yet they clearly interrelate with organs elsewhere. Take, for example, the kidney-ureter-bladder relationship. This organic team follows the muscular river of the psoas major, connecting upper and lower body, back body to front body. Similarly, the intestines and their health can impact not only the rectum and posterior pelvic floor, but also the neurobiochemical environment in which all these organs live, like in the cases where pelvic symptoms coexist with digestive conditions. The complex interplay between symptoms and diagnoses is outside the scope of this book and may create subspecialties within the pelvic-health field. Always consider symptoms could be related to a systemic health issue or infection. When in doubt, refer your student appropriately.

Let's look at the pelvic organ systems now.

Bladder and excretory system

An adult bladder can hold about 2 cups or 16 ounces when completely full, and usually has a small residual volume – similar to how we don't completely empty our lungs on each exhalation but keep a bit of breath to maintain the inner space of the organ rather than having its walls collapse in on themselves. Filling a balloon with this volume of water can give a lovely visual and tactile sense of this organ's capacity.

As our bladder fills, its muscles stretch and the brain registers these sensations to create the feeling of needing to urinate. When voiding, the detrusor muscle of the bladder contracts to bring the bladder down in size, while, simultaneously, the urethral sphincters and PFM at large must relax to allow free passage of urine out of the body. This coordination can get scrambled if women are constantly Kegeling – especially if they've been taught to practice Kegels to "stop the flow of urine." Hovering over toilets in a squat and frequently peeing "just in case" can also disrupt this relationship between brain, bladder, and the PFM.

We may not be able to control our bladder muscles voluntarily, but we can learn to consciously encourage our pelvic floor to relax and create an easeful stream. Urgency and frequency can often be caused or worsened by up-regulation or chronic sympathetic activation, lending strength to the results possible with yoga therapy to down-regulate and calm. Key takeaway: Toileting is a relaxation practice.

The bladder snuggles behind the pubic symphysis at the front of the ring called the pelvic inlet. Palpate the broad, anterior surface of your pubic symphysis, then move your fingertips up to the superior surface, approaching the mons pubis. Be gentle here. Cup your hand and hold this circular interior space in your attention. Breathe deeply. Visualize your bladder balloon as calm and relaxed, floating happily in the pelvic bowl.

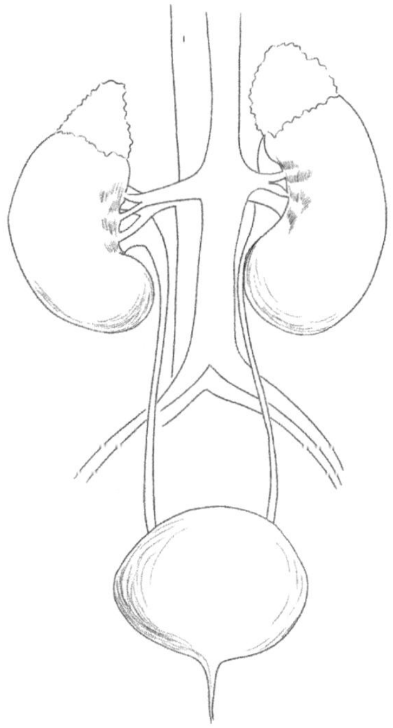

Figure 4.6: The excretory system

Here's a bonus embodiment for the excretory system: While bladder cupping, bring your other hand around your back ribs, seeking the warmth of your kidney on that side. Imagine your kidney, lower back, and iliopsoas muscle on that side melting and flowing easily into the central bladder, while the ureter tube creates a lightness and buoyancy for the bladder, tethering it upwards. Enhance your experience with the visual aid of Figure 4.6. After a few breaths, brush your hands down and pause to notice how that side of your body feels. Then repeat the process on the other side.

The uterus and creative force

From a physical perspective, the uterus has bilateral ligamentous connections to our sacrum, ischial spines, and pubic symphysis, and sits saddled between the bladder and rectum. Our womb moves back when our bladder has filled, and forward if the rectum becomes full. If both neighbors need space, the uterus generally moves upward. Increases in IAP propel the uterus downward – good reason to learn breathing and movement strategies that help us manage inevitable pressure changes in this dynamic human body. If you've ever experienced pregnancy, you know first-hand just how magnificent this organ is – she can expand from being pear sized before conception to a proud watermelon stretching from pubic bone to the lower ribs at full term.

This ever-adapting organ also reflects nature's wisdom of cyclical living. Just like seasons and the moon phases, our womb moves through periods of fallow and full harvest, incubation and emergence. The hormonal shifts women experience with each menstrual cycle, and again at menopause, can support them with a reliable way to respect equally work, play, and rest, and alter her activities and the pace of her life to respect how these hormonal changes impact pelvic-floor performance and overall energy. Pregnancy impacts the pelvic floor not only through the changes in one's center of gravity and IAP, but also with hormonal shifts impacting elimination and constipation, blood volume, and overall pelvic-floor contractility. Culturally, we don't like to slow down or stop – an embodied way of living invites us to reconsider, and I am on this road with you, dear reader. Our life's pace can either prevent this kind of awareness from ever surfacing, or serve us well by making space to pay attention.

A woman's uterus likely holds, at the very least, stories and beliefs based on what they were taught (or not taught) related to menstruation, sex and pleasure, and the choice or ability to become a mother or not. In addition to personal narratives, we've been riding a collective growth curve as we unlearn conditioning around womanhood and motherhood. Our womb space sits at our center, and as we start to reflect on our relationship to her, we can unveil great potential for integration and healing.

I always felt a deep knowing that I would become a mother in this lifetime. It wasn't embellished with the kind of little-girl pretend games and feminine yearning and longing that I've seen expressed by others – I just knew. What I didn't foreshadow was the depth of grief I had inherited and held in my womb that excavated itself during and after the birth of my oldest daughter. Birth and motherhood remade me – once by miscarriage and next by unexpected cesarean. My next pregnancy and birth journey revived me, affirming our need for full-spectrum expression, the power of pleasure, and connection, and restored safety and autonomy. Experiencing a swift, transcendent labor culminating in homebirth left me intact and lucid, steeping in rich evidence that we can reclaim our resilience. For women choosing not to have children or those unable to, and women now post-hysterectomy, this space still carries our creative spark and speaks to our capacity to be in flow with our emotions, contributions, and sensuality.

Exploring themes like receptivity and release, holding our creations and mothering them to fruition, and then fully expressing those gifts may be useful lines of dialogue for a svadhyaya practice supported by yoga therapy. The womb space may offer an invitation into relationship with our vijnanamaya and anandamaya koshas. What do we most value? How do we express our unique purpose? Can we live in a way that is more connected to our source and spirit? Again, we provide a prompt – the student reflects and determines the meaning and possible course of action to express and integrate these parts of her identity. I bow to Tami Lynn Kent's work, *Wild Feminine*, as a beautiful resource for revealing the spiritual and energetic fruits of exploring the womb realm.

Let the imagery of Figure 4.7 wash over you. Then, place your hands over your lower belly and take three deep breaths into this womb space now. Be with what arises, whether as emotion, imagery, words, or sensations. Give your body thanks for the receptive and generative forces that live here.

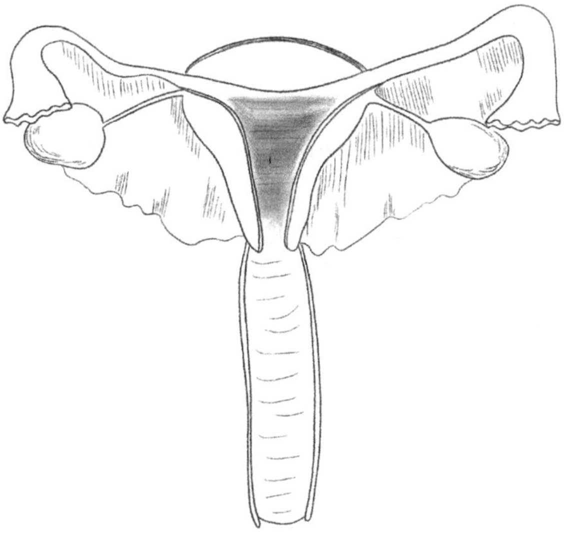

Figure 4.7: The reproductive system

Bowel and digestive system

The journey of our digestive system begins in the mouth. This tube-like pathway from mouth to anus represents another connection to the outside world, like an inner skin. We take in and assimilate that which is "not us" – thus the outer world becomes part of us as we feed our very cells. We'll explore accessing postural support from this system with the developmental pattern of mouthing in Chapter 10.

It seems we still hold more collective shame around feces and the anus than other aspects of pelvic health (believing this part to be dirty, disgusting, or untouchable), although that may not be true for everyone. Like bladder voiding, bowel movements are a normal, recurring event that we can relax into, welcoming a chance to pause the pace of life. For posterior pelvic-floor health, we can investigate themes like asking for and receiving support and how we can be more aligned with our gut wisdom, integrity, and intuitive knowing.

One of the most common causes of pelvic-floor strain over the long haul is how we poop. Or, in fact, whether we actually can poop in the first place. Constipation may be a culprit that leads to the development of pelvic-floor issues and is something to eliminate (pun intended) altogether for women with pelvic-floor concerns. Luckily, a mindful or yogic lifestyle can work wonders on one's regularity. Make sure you check out Appendix C for more insight about constipation relief.

Anatomically, let's sense this relationship together now. Place the palm of your hand over your sacrum, with your fingertips draped very low toward the coccyx. (This may be easier or more comfortable if you can lie on one side and relax your legs and hip muscles.) Palpate to either side of your tailbone very gently, and notice if one side feels different or more sensitive than the other. We're not massaging with any agenda, other than becoming gently acquainted with this part of our pelvis. Cupping your sacrum, take some deep breaths and visualize how your rectum follows the curvilinear pathway of your sacrum and coccyx, surrounded by the depth of support from the levator ani group. If your body agrees, move your hand lower to cup the tip of your coccyx and anus, allowing your middle fingertip to lightly contact the central perineal body. Perhaps you can even feel the wave-like swell of each inhalation under your hand.

Shift position as needed, placing your hands on the front and back of your pelvic bowl. Visualize the anterior to posterior volume of these organs in order – urethra, vagina, anus – and then move your attention internally to sense the bladder, uterus or cervix, and rectum. Each of the organs has a place, shown from a cross-sectional side view in Figure 4.8. Nestled and even gliding over each other as we move, they accomplish their interdependent functions.

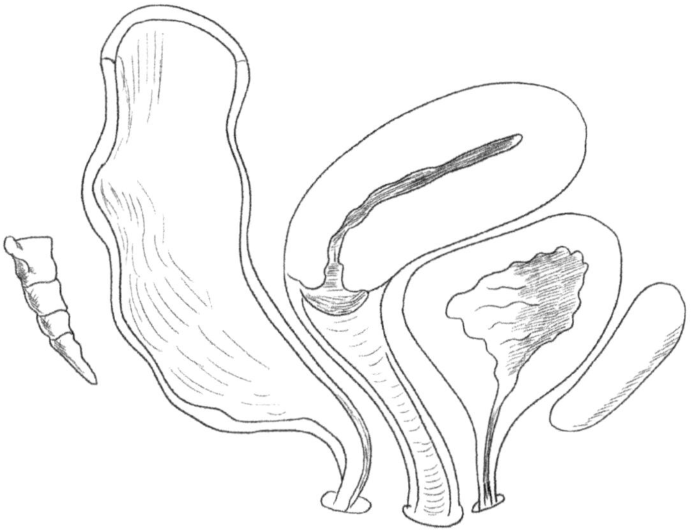

Figure 4.8: Nesting pelvic organs, side view

Fluid system

One essential function of the pelvic floor is to circulate blood and lymph, often referred to as a "sump pump." Gravity encourages pooling of fluids into the pelvis and lower extremities – and you may have noticed an indented sock line around your ankles toward the day's end. The more sedentary we stay, the more this pooling becomes reality. I grew up in Wisconsin, so dampness and flooding in basements when the spring thaw and rains came feels familiar. The mechanical pump draws stagnant water out of low pit-like places to keep them clean and dry. We want our pelvic tissues to remain juicy and supple instead of congested, clogged, or dry, and so we must learn how to enhance circulation.

One survey states approximately 68% of people with diagnosed pelvic-floor dysfunction experience a worsening of their symptoms with prolonged sitting (Cozean 2018). This is a shared trait of individuals with varying diagnoses, so we can guess intelligently that a sedentary lifestyle may increase symptoms and delay healing for many different types of pelvic-floor conditions. Prolonged sitting may also exacerbate pelvic symptoms due to other causes like placing pressure on bursa and nerve tissues, and postural or breathing habits, in addition to the congestion or stagnation due to inactivity.

Receptivity in our pelvic bowl, and the mobilization of pelvic tissues through both breathing well and physical movement, allows any stagnation or cellular waste to be moved from the pelvic bowl space back through the trunk for cleansing via lymph and blood. Walking encourages circulation by mobilizing the pelvic girdle, hips, legs, and spine in a beautiful dance, as can yoga asana practices, dancing, *and* relaxation.

Think of a sponge. If we clench that sponge in our fist, and dip it into water, it will only absorb a small fraction of what it's capable of drinking in, compared with if we allow the whole sponge to submerge. Tension prevents movement and fluidity – relaxation precedes and invites flow and efficiency. How would we make soap bubbles in our sponge? Squish, twist, and move the sponge within our hands. Movement lubricates, hydrates, and heals.

Pausing for integration

We have the power of consciousness at our service through meditation practices. One's awareness can venture into known and not-yet-known territory, bringing the gift of insight.

To complete our study of local anatomy, I invite you to rest. Make yourself comfortable, and allow your mind to meander through the newly highlighted contours of your pelvis, and the volume of space within it. Trust what you're learning will integrate and serve you and your students well. Take several slow, low breaths into your pelvic bowl now.

Once you've completed a restful pause, you may notice that your pulse and breathing have slowed down or become quieter, your face has relaxed, or your muscles have softened. You may even feel revived energy from having taken a rest. Now, you're ready to explore the power of diaphragmatic breathing, sound, and pranayama.

CHAPTER 5

Breathing, Sound, and Pranayama

Breathing brings life, expanding and condensing our lungs around 20,000 times each day. Most of this takes place without conscious control, thankfully sparing our attention for other tasks. Practicing yoga, however, means living with greater consciousness. We can use breath and sound to voluntarily enhance this otherwise innate, unconscious function and provide crucial benefits to pelvic health.

Healing has happened when what used to cause strife or suffering no longer has a hold on us. Breath practices act as a bridge between our physical body and more subtle aspects of energy, personality, communication, and affect. As yoga therapists, we can help people with pelvic issues slowly step back into the fullness of life that is their birthright.

The definition of pranayama asks us to cultivate attentive, disciplined use of our life force energy. Preceded by the yamas and niyamas that guide our lifestyle and relationships, and after a certain level of mastery of physical postures called asana, pranayama takes us deeper into the eight limbs of yoga practice by regulating and understanding our physiologic and energetic self.

Patanjali understood the mind and breath reflect each other (Satchidananda 2008, pp.51–52, 57–58), and how lengthening our exhalations allows us to tap into the restorative power of parasympathetic function in our ANS.

I often see yoga therapy perceived or marketed as The Great Down-Regulator. Yoga practice can skillfully help us regulate and relax, and how we use our breath is key. Down-training may be the first essential step for working with many different pelvic conditions, especially those with a non-relaxing pelvic floor. These students are often in a state of what's called "up-regulation." Stress and excess sympathetic activation can perpetuate inflammation, muscle tension, and pain, and limit the movement of breath.

If only it were as simple as giving down-regulating practices to all pelvic-health clients. We also need movement to proactively restore safety and agency, increasing our threshold for sensation from gross to subtle. Sometimes, pacifying or down-regulating ends up being a strategy of enduring what we don't like or want – always responding to the symptoms. Parasympathetic activation often gets touted as if it's the medicine for all modern-life malaise, when in fact some students may first benefit from measured doses of up-regulation.

We need regulation *and range*. Learning to hold more "charge" allows us to invite in more prana and pleasure, and may also help address root-cause material by teaching us to stay present to discomfort or intensity. Greater capacity means we're more able to switch channels in our nervous system and that we can experience more activation or stress and still cope effectively, learning to embrace all states of being.

Conscious breathing, for many, can jumpstart this process of attentive self-regulation. Yet sometimes, our best attempts at "calming down" or "trying to relax" fail. In the pages ahead, we'll lay the foundation for what functional breathing looks and feels like anatomically, and then move through a series of practices intended to help shift common compensations that may prevent a student from breathing well.

Included in this chapter are sounding explorations, which create a base for more complex mantra practices. We'll inquire about how the shape and sound produced can influence the activity and relaxation in our pelvic basin.

Lastly, we'll look at a few pranayama techniques. This provides a framework to assist you in discerning and selecting from the myriad other pranayama technologies we have at our fingertips, according to your needs or the needs and goals of students.

Breathing anatomy

In the previous chapter, we took an in-depth look at the bones and tissues of the pelvic bowl directly. Now, we'll familiarize ourselves, perhaps again if this feels like a review for you, with the structure and function of breathing.

The diaphragm muscle connects inside the circumference of your ribcage, descending with a concentric contraction on each inhalation. This creates the pressure change that draws air into our nostrils and fills our lungs. As the diaphragm relaxes, it returns upward into its dome-like shape inside the ribs.

This passive recoil is reflected in the elasticity of the lungs themselves – when we're at rest it takes little effort to exhale.

The central tendon of the diaphragm flattens and gets pulled down, and the entire parachute or dome moves downward as the muscle fibers slide together in concentric action. The whole diaphragm gets tethered into the front of the spine by the crus, or tendinous tails. This connection blends – interdigitates – with the beginnings of the psoas major and the anterior longitudinal ligament of the spine. This area around the thoracolumbar junction is busy, home to major blood vessels of the abdominal aorta and inferior vena cava. The adrenals and kidneys also anchor to either side of the spine there, resting into the psoas major behind them (Bordoni and Zanier 2013). Practice wise, we can mobilize, undulate, and free this area and upwards through the whole thoracic spine to create suppleness that serves our pelvic health and daily movement. During restorative postures and especially supine core exercises, this place begs to be broadened, released, and grounded. As you view Figure 5.1, rest your attention behind your abdominal viscera into the inner back wall of your body. Sense how your torso's entire cylinder is connected and moved by breathing.

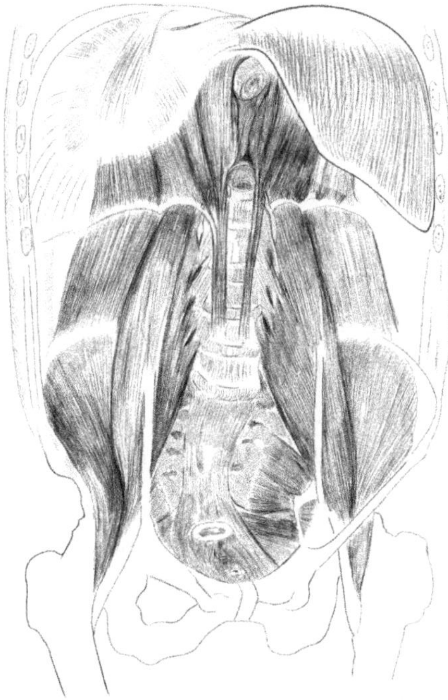

Figure 5.1: Intricate, dynamic support: respiratory diaphragm, the iliopsoas team, and the pelvic bowl

Touch your ribs, tracing along the rib angle in the front – from sternum and xyphoid process in the center, following the diagonal border downward. Be gentle. Palm these front and side ribs as you move into side bending both directions. Can you feel a natural elasticity or rebound in the ribs? These slender, curved bones are meant to move freely from their cartilaginous connections into the sternum.

Now follow the lower ribs around into your lower back. The last two floating ribs will take you back to the spine. Find your spinous processes with your fingertips, and move your awareness up about 1 inch from where you traced the lowest ribs. You'll land approximately at the level of the spinous process of your 12th thoracic vertebra. Now, drop attention into your touch here and guide your awareness forward, sensing deeper inside your body by about two to three inches. Welcome to the front of your spine, where the crus of the diaphragm anchor. Take a few breaths and imagine your lungs and diaphragm descending toward this area with a calming wave on each inhalation.

The diaphragm works in concert with the body wall muscles that allow for expansion of inhalation and can assist exhalation. This dance may be overridden by accessory or secondary muscles of breathing like the sternocleidomastoid (SCM) and scalenes if a compensatory breathing pattern (or simply, stress) has taken hold. (Do you have students with unrelenting jaw, neck, or shoulder tension? While this is common, locally massaging or stretching these areas often only brings short-term relief. It may be better resolved by addressing breathing habits, stress, and ANS states.)

Lastly, the breathing cycle has stillness built into its rhythm. Bringing attention to the small, subtle pause after each exhalation might help entrain patience, curiosity, and a more regulated experience than breathing with control or seamless continuity between exhale and inhale. Notice now how you become quiet and pause at the end of an exhalation, and allow your body to spontaneously inhale when it becomes necessary. Let your body lead.

Paradoxical breathing shows a departure from this natural coordinated rhythm, which can be remedied with education and experiential guidance (Calais-Germain 2006, pp.133–157). We'll soon explore key practices to help unlearn these compensations and restore diaphragmatic breathing. Let's look more closely at how breathing involves the pelvic floor.

The breath excursion

The action of the thoracic diaphragm compresses and shape-shifts our abdominal viscera, and echoes this pressure down into the pelvic floor, which is referred to as the breath excursion. This "excursioning" goes missing when one breathes with a shallow or restricted quality. Although we know air only enters our lungs, we may explore imagery to access the breath's subtle influence elsewhere.

During inhalation, both the thoracic and pelvic domes descend. On exhalations, they rise. What's fundamentally different, however, is the fact that on inhalation, the thoracic diaphragm contracts concentrically, while this downward nudge on the organs creates a release or eccentric allowance in the pelvic-floor tissues. Then, during the exhalation, the pelvic floor takes on the more active, potentially concentric role, supporting and buoying the organs upwards as the thoracic diaphragm relaxes (Anderson 2015; Talasz *et al.* 2011).

The effort of breathing cycles between many key muscles, rather than all of them relaxing or working at the same moment. While our skeleton does receive support from postural muscles that resist the pull of gravity, the health and volume of our breath also supports us from the inside out, oscillating effort from one place to another. Innately intelligent, our body collaborates to distribute the workload. The message of sustainability is with us by design.

During quiet, natural breaths, this rhythm is quite subtle. We may sense it more clearly when taking deep conscious breaths and in certain positions more than others. For example, when we increase the demand for stability and support on our core system, like in a plank pose (variation of chaturangadandasana), we may be less aware of these oscillations, even though they're still providing underlying support for the isometric nature of the activity. Even more subtle in contrast could be comparing a standing or sitting breath awareness to supine, or lying down on your back, which affords more ease and a tangible experience of breath movement. If we lie prone, giving the soft underbelly the firm boundary of the floor, we can amplify the breath excursion into the pelvic bowl and back ribs.

Inversions, such as downward dog (adho mukha svanasana) or wide leg forward bend (prasaritta padottanasana), can strengthen respiration and may amplify the calming effects of the exhalation. When we take the pelvis higher than the heart or head, gravity works against our thoracic diaphragm, requiring a more robust inhale. The abdominal and pelvic organs then get drawn out of the pelvic bowl by the assistance of gravity during the exhalation, potentially creating an even more down-regulating and decompressing effect by lessening the load on pelvic tissues. Remember, too, the circulatory role of breathing – moving blood and lymph to prevent stagnation of womb and pelvic energy. Every breath cycle helps bring nourishment and remove waste on a cellular level. We can select positions to enhance how gravity assists this process.

Writing this book through the onset of the COVID pandemic, I longed to travel. At least my organs and diaphragm got to keep traveling with each breath! In all seriousness, stress isn't going anywhere. We can always find a reason to worry. Well into the future, we'll likely see students who experience breath holding, decreased breath excursion, and pelvic-floor tension. Good thing we can shift our perception, utilizing practices of yoga therapy and our relationships to buffer the effects of stress. Restoring this internal dance between the thoracic and pelvic diaphragms could be the source medicine that reduces pelvic symptoms and other perceived stressors to greatly improve a person's quality of life (Prosko 2016).

Sensing pelvic coordination

For students feeling perplexed by breathing in general, let alone attempting to feel their breath subtly rippling into the pelvic bowl, it can be useful to remember the principle of progression. You may consider starting with simpler and less demanding postures in terms of postural support to help them find a relationship to their breath excursion. Then, incrementally increase the demand of gravity with more active positions to see how well they can maintain full, three-dimensional breaths with pelvic awareness.

For those who seem to require vigor and intensity before welcoming stillness, we could also argue the opposite: that an active or stronger practice (even a brisk walk instead of asana) may lead them naturally into this breath awareness once they rest. Placing enough demand on the respiratory system can make it easier to sense and sometimes give it the workout it needs to give in and relax afterwards. This may be their entry point, and we can work to gradually invite them into more awareness or rest over time.

The following three practices can offer a baseline experience of breathing, as well as increasing interoception of one's pelvic floor directly. You can also layer the self-touch inquiries into many other asana practices to support a student's ability to sense the pelvic breath.

Sit bone or vulva cupping

Using a sturdy chair with a blanket or bath towel for padding underneath you, have a seat. Feel your sit bones and the quality of awareness in your pelvic diamond. Warm your palms by rubbing them together, and then sit on your hands. Let your palms cup around and support each sit bone. The pinky edge of your hands, just medial to your sit bones, may begin to contact the pelvic floor. Breathe here, imagining your sit bones dripping into your hands and down into the earth, allowing all the muscles between your hands to melt and soften. Let yourself take little micro-movements of a seated cat-cow (marjarasana) action or with small shifts of weight side to side. You may even take a few audible exhales, letting your jaw relax and mouth hang open with a bit of slack. After about one minute, take your hands away and compare your seated awareness to your prior baseline. Acknowledge changes you feel with gratitude. (You could, of course, explore this self-touch strategy lying down, as well.)

If sit-bone palming feels like you're moving in the right direction, but a little too subtle, you can make contact more directly to the perineal body. Fold a small washcloth into a diamond shape to sit on, or roll it and place it between your sit bones lengthwise, with the volume or height of your roll right at the center. This should not create discomfort or pain; you can scrunch your washcloth roll to gather it in toward the center, so as not to create too much pressure directly on the pubic bone, clitoris, or sit bones. Remember how the posterior of the pelvic floor has more soft tissue? You might prefer to focus contact there, and guide attention inward and upward anteriorly.

Once you're situated, take several deep breaths, sending the inhales downward into the rolled cloth, and then allow the full recoil of your exhalations. Continue with your deep breaths as you take a small, slow circling action of your pelvic bowl, a few times in either direction. Spend no more than about a minute exploring the washcloth contact. Return to center, let your breathing become quiet again, and rest. Remove the washcloth, and again, acknowledge what you feel that might be different than before.

You could instead sit on a large, inflated physioball, as it will not only allow the downward excursion of the pelvic floor during inhalation, but also press back against the perineum for extra feedback. In this way, a ball might provide more dynamic, variable feedback than an inanimate washcloth.

Vulva cupping

Touch facilitates focused attention and can increase our felt sense of the parts of us making contact. The warmth of our own hands, and the immediacy of control we retain by owning this as a self-touch inquiry, can strengthen resolve, agency, and confidence. Some women I've worked with have never held their body in this way; encompassing one's perineum front to back can surface strong emotions. Always offer techniques as an informed invitation, which might first be explored privately in a student's home practice and then witnessed or further integrated within the safety of a yoga-therapy session.

Holding the volume of space that is our pelvic bowl can be useful to encourage the breath excursion to descend deeper. You can try this practice first in a relaxed position like sidelying or lounging in bed and then bring it into a seated inquiry once you've found some clarity and comfort.

Place one hand on your lower belly, with your fingertips on your pubic bone, and have the other hand cupping around your sacrum with the tip of your middle finger approximating the tip of your tailbone. You might choose to remain here for several breaths and omit the next step.

If your arms are long enough to allow comfortably, cradle your vulva in both hands from front to back. Your middle fingers might connect around the central tendon, or perineal body, just in front of the anal opening. (You could alternatively suggest a student laces the fingers together, and place both hands with the palms over the mons pubis and fingers gently draped under and around the vulva.) Breathe normally and notice what you feel without judgment. When it feels like enough time has passed with this inquiry, release your hands and rest.

As this practice closes, remember the cupping sensations and imagine they create a kind of soft harness of support that carries your pelvis as you walk and move about your day.

Supported forward bend (salamba paschimottanasana)

We're going to practice allowing our anterior abdominal wall to fully release. It can feel so counter-intuitive to let it all hang if we've been taught to "support" or "engage" constantly. Voluntary core engagement tends to create over-recruitment, which can impede our natural breath and force absorption; it can also increase pressure on the pelvic floor. Doing this exercise should not cause any low back discomfort or any concerning pressure or bulging sensation into the perineum. Keep in mind, this is a practice of undoing and allowing, not actively pushing your belly out forcefully.

The function of our lower extremities influences our pelvic floor, and to take a triple-flexed position (ankle dorsiflexion, knee flexion, and hip flexion as required by basic movements like walking, squatting, and more) from active to passive can be a boon for our nervous system, breath excursion, and pelvic-floor relaxation. For this practice, you'll need a chair, a sturdy table or wall, and something to hug like a pillow, bolster, or firmly rolled bath towel.

Scoot toward the front of your cushioned seat like you see in Figure 5.2.

Place your rolled towel or pillow on the table in front of you. If you have a bolster, it can be placed in your lap and provide support all along the front of your torso as you lean into the table. Sit tall, and then exhale and fold forward from your hip creases, letting your sit bones pivot behind you and widen a bit as you bring your chest toward the table. Wrap your arms around your prop, and rest your upper body weight into the sturdy support of the table. You can rest your forehead into your hands, or turn and rest your cheek against the prop. Spend several breaths here, allowing the forward fold to draw your attention inward and downward, emphasizing the downward current of energy called apana vayu.

If you have active diarrhea, you may skip this supported forward bend. When it has resolved, trial this pose for a few breaths as a test run to determine comfort.

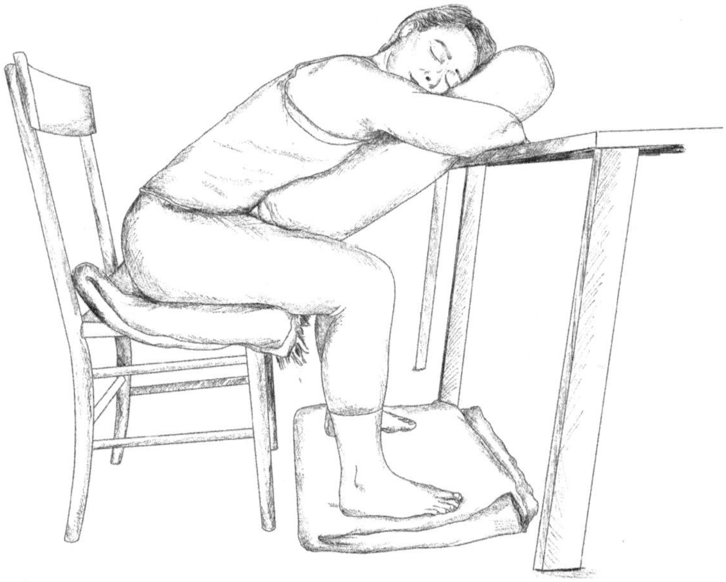

Figure 5.2: Supported forward bend

Now, over the next several breaths, feel your belly hang slack toward the ground or spread into the bolster. Let your belly rest and notice if you can feel your back floating ribs being moved by your breath. You may be able to feel this letting go in your pelvic muscles, too, as your tail seems to swing with each breath. Notice or imagine how your tail can sweep back subtly on each inhalation, coming back to rest as you exhale. Explore these suggestions while maintaining a relatively neutral spine (versus moving into deeper spinal extension or flexion).

Throughout this practice, feel the soles of your feet grounded. You can explore whether your legs stay parallel, perhaps lending a bit of pressure to your lower abdomen during this practice, or instead abduct your legs apart to increase the awareness on the widening of your inner thigh muscles and their attachment into the front of the pelvic bowl. Turn your head the other way for a balanced amount of time, resting and yielding your body's weight into gravity.

When you're ready to come out, press your arms and feet down and begin to lengthen up into the crown of your head, elongating your spine. Move through some dynamic cat-cow, side bending, and circling. As you move, notice how your core reflexively knows how and when to support more or less – rather than you having to cue it cognitively. Your body knows what to do.

Return to a vertical seat and feel the effects of those few precious minutes of quiet awareness. If, after completing the above inquiries, you assess that more change may be necessary to create optimal conditions to free the breath, and therefore sense its excursion, you can select from the corrective practices in the next section.

Corrective strategies to help restore breath excursion

Well-intentioned cues sometimes get in the way of natural, three-dimensional breath excursion. For example, instructions like "engage the core," "lift up," or "pull your navel toward your spine" can create gripping or holding in the abdominal wall, which can result in increased downward pelvic-floor pressure, decreased breath volume and excursion, or both.

Culturally, these cues have worn grooves in many women's minds, perceived as the fix for back pain, leaking, and belly pooch, and to look slimmer. These holding patterns might be one of the very causes of these concerns. Starting from a relaxed state and allowing the abdomen and pelvic floor to coordinate their efforts may improve continence, posture, and more (Smith, Coppieters, Hodges 2007).

Other widespread postural habits can contribute to dysfunctional diaphragms and pelvic-floor confusion. Consider how often we see forward head posture, hyperkyphosis, and anterior rounding of the shoulder girdle, which can create a sense of collapse into the abdominal cavity, increase pressure on the pelvic floor, and impede both diaphragm excursion down and the filling of the upper lobes of the lungs.

Excessive or prolonged lumbar flexion and posterior tilt of one's hips presents frequently, too, from commuting and desk-bound work. This puts the PFM into a shortened or contracted position and increases weight-bearing load into the sacrum and tailbone, rather than allowing the sit bones to provide their namesake support.

If you're serving pregnant or newly postpartum women, consider the effects of carrying a growing baby (and birthing said baby into the world) and cultivate the opposite. This can include pressure-management awareness, restoring the reflexive nature of the pelvic floor after delivery, maintaining an active lifestyle, and countering the effects of breastfeeding postures and the deep fatigue from sleep deprivation. Considering the life stage a woman is in, or has recently experienced, provides essential information for designing their yoga-therapy practice.

No one position or movement is "bad," but when it becomes our default norm, or worse, our body's only known or presumed safe option, we need to restore variety and variability. Our body will come to display how we've used it over our lifespan. We conform to what we most often do so it feels wise to weave movement and variety into daily life, as well as select a customized practice for our pelvic health.

Why restore diaphragmatic function before teaching pranayama manipulations?

It may be prudent to work toward restoring diaphragmatic function and the breath excursion before giving specific pranayama techniques to students. This way, we can affect the quality of other more complex breath practices to come. Breathing impacts the quality of our movement, too. One study showed even "healthy" participants may exhibit disordered breath patterns, which correlated to lower functional movement scores (Bradley and Esformes 2014; Chaitow 2016). We can help students enhance breath awareness first in relatively low-load, static positions like constructive rest position (CRP) (outlined in Chapter 6), and then progress into higher-demand, dynamic practices like breath-based vinyasa work, activities of daily living, and higher-load tasks like lifting and jumping. A staged training approach to breath coordination has shown promising results for incontinence (Hung *et al.* 2010).

Crawl, walk, and then run. (Pun intended for women wanting to jog who may benefit from revisiting these breath basics.) Explore the following exercises to feel what you may encounter with students and critically reason which might be most useful in their home practice.

Rib circumference feedback

Get a strap for this next inquiry, or even better – grab an elastic band instead of the more static woven-cloth yoga belt. If you don't have a strap or band, and don't mind the warmth, you could also use a firm yoga blanket snugged around your back and held up securely under your armpits. The prop's contact will emphasize lateral and posterior rib awareness.

Consider doing this activity in standing when possible. After observing your baseline posture and breath quality in stillness, add the prop.

Bring the strap around the back of your ribcage, right around the inferior angle of your scapula, and cross the ends of the strap in front of your body to make an "X." Hold the ends of the straps just taut enough, and take a small bend in your legs to begin. Focus on expanding the strap's circumference with your inhalation, especially through the sides and back of your body, as many of us are familiar already with how mobile the breath can feel in the anterior structures and core layers. Gently cinch the strap smaller as you exhale, allowing it to support your ribs on their return trip inward. As you begin to inhale again, remember to let the strap loosen just enough to follow the natural increase in volume. An elastic band will give you variable resistance – strengthening your inhalation and assisting your exhalation!

Only a short practice is necessary, so after four to eight breaths, release the strap and see how your embodiment compares now to your baseline.

Prone breathing

One of the practices I missed the most while pregnant was lying face down, flat on the earth. Many yogis or exercisers have been taught belly breathing, and while that may be useful, it can also create a false sense of expansion through misguided efforts to push the abdomen out rather than allowing the breath to work in a more three-dimensional capacity. Lying prone gives the abdomen a firm boundary that can redirect the influence of the breath into the sides, back, and "basement" of the core cylinder – the pelvic floor.

Depending on where you are in your menstrual cycle, or if you experience digestive disturbances, this practice might not be accessible to or comfortable for you on certain days. Be honest and kind with yourself; proceed only if the result is one of pleasant relaxation.

Find a firm but comfortable surface to lie face down on, like a carpeted floor, or place a few layers of folded bath towel under your whole torso.

Yield your body weight into the floor. Quietly observe your breathing with no agenda. Then, begin to direct your attention and the flow of breath into your side ribs and then your back ribs. Feel how your sacrum and pelvis start to rock back and forth on the wave of each breath. You may also notice your PFM releasing and widening with the wave of each inhalation downward.

This can carry on as a luscious afternoon siesta of practice. Trust that you'll know when to finish, letting an exhalation have all the time it needs to come to completion. Curl onto your side for a few minutes of rest before getting up off the floor, or roll onto your back for a savasana. We'll explore a more detailed prone savasana inquiry later in Chapter 10.

Supported bridge (salamba setu bhanda)

Lying supine in a supported bridge with the pelvis slightly elevated can offer a fast track to restoring diaphragmatic breath excursion and for centering the femur heads down into their sockets, reducing gripping or holding in the hips, thighs, pelvic floor, and belly. Here, we don't have to contend with gravity to hold ourselves up. Instead, gravity assists us on each exhalation, letting the weight of our abdominal and pelvic organs slide toward the ribcage as the lungs empty. A higher support for the pelvis makes this decompression even more amplified, which may be useful for those experiencing prolapse. Customize the height to your student, taking into consideration their menstrual cycle and any other contraindications to being inverted.

You'll need either a bolster or a thick blanket for this practice. If using a blanket, fold it into a rectangular shape to support the full width of your pelvis. If students feel any eye strain or pressure into their throat or face, you can decrease the height of the prop, or simply use these cues in supine position. See Figure 5.3 for visual reference.

Find CRP first, placing a soft support under your head and neck if you wish. Spend a moment scanning your body for your baseline sensations. Start to press into your feet, and feel your pelvis leave the ground. Rise high enough that you can easily slide your prop squarely under your pelvis, centered at the sacrum. Support the full width of your buttocks, and feel or see that your pelvis is level.

Imagine melting your thigh muscles. Feel them stream down through your hip creases and pool into your hip sockets. Let the femurs rest in gravity. Soften the muscles around your tailbone and sit bones, and allow the thigh streams flowing downward to create a deep pool at your sacrum, deepening your imprint into the blanket or bolster. You may imagine what it might be like to roll your metaphorical tail out like a red carpet between your feet.

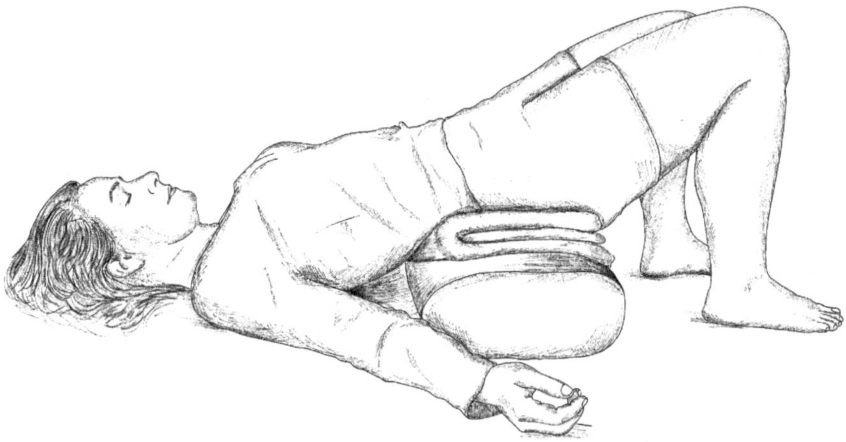

Figure 5.3: Supported bridge

Spend a few minutes here tracking your breathing. If it feels welcome, you can draw your inhalation deeper, lungs filling downward to move your viscera toward your pelvic bowl, and then allow a fully passive recoil to occur on your exhalation. Let yourself sink, spread, and release as your body exhales, and feel how your pelvic bowl becomes hollow, lighter again, as your organs have ascended.

After several rounds of conscious deep breaths, let your breathing become quiet and natural again. Take in your whole self and how your body meets the floor. Feel your feet. When you're ready, press down into the floor to lift your hips just high enough to remove your props and return to the floor. You might linger in a supported savasana or roll to your side and continue reading.

Diaphragm shimmy and bouncing

Stand up, and let your legs yield into a small bend. Spread through your feet and relax your jaw and mouth. Take a breath in, and on the exhale, let yourself sing, "Ahhhhh," with an open mouth. We do this once to hear our own sound and to practice releasing tension throughout our whole body, and importantly, through the abdomen and pelvic floor. Notice the calm continuity of your voice here in stillness.

The next time you exhale audibly, begin to shimmy or shake the juicy volume of your organs, continuing now to produce sound as you rebound. Feel your inner contents being stirred, swirled, organs sliding and slithering on each other, noticing how your sound becomes percussive, punctuated from this inner movement. Take your next inhale whenever it feels necessary, and play with adding planes of movement to your shaking – shimmy through a small cat-cow, wiggle with a side bend, celebrate with circles of your wagging tail.

Using your feet, create a rhythmic, pulsing bounce, or even take tiny jumps if you feel ready for it, continuing to sound as you rebound. Have fun cutting loose, and when you've had enough, rest in standing. Notice how you feel, including the quality of your breath or amount of prana circulating in your system. It only takes about 30 seconds of effective diaphragm dancing to get the benefit.

This technique requires and can teach yielding or embodied ease; if one remains tense, it becomes a sort of hammerhead shark, robotic dance with the voice sounding strained. Drop down into the soft depths of your viscera and support of the earth to let it go. This can provide great feedback for the pelvic floor's reflexive support – a prerequisite for increased impact, like when bouncing, hopping, and jogging.

Understanding intraabdominal pressure (IAP)

First, a few key ideas about IAP: we need some, we need to train it wisely with gradually increased demand, it varies task to task and woman to woman, and breathing manages it (Wiebe 2018).

While decreasing IAP may be a natural first response to heaviness, prolapse, or incontinence, we must remember that some pressure is needed and healthy. Generating enough IAP or core pressure supports our spine from the inside out and allows us to safely do things like pick up our kid and go for a jog. Our body needs enough stiffness or stability, and not too much. Learning to manage or regulate pressure well may allow students to progress further and perhaps faster than simply teaching them to decrease pressure demand altogether.

One of the most common questions we'll hear from students is, "What exercises are safe for my pelvic floor?" The answer is that it truly depends, yet the response women usually get at a postpartum or post-surgical check-up consists of general statements to not lift anything more than ten pounds or to avoid certain movements altogether. What a disservice to tell people what not to do, creating fear and avoidance that can further perpetuate dysfunction, without giving them any wisdom as to how to regain function and safely return to daily life activities and exercises they enjoy.

It's essential to understand how relative IAP can be, as it varies person to person even during the same exercise (O'Dell *et al.* 2007). How we execute a movement matters for IAP and pelvic symptom management (Prosko 2017). Assessment and progressive exercise principles are so important, and yoga therapy can shine here. We need to recognize women's desire for certain activities and help them both with developing patience and acceptance for the current stage of training or healing they find themselves in and creating a systematic approach toward their goal.

Every task or movement can be modified, both through regression strategies to meet the student's current capacity and through progressive loading to gradually foster greater confidence and fitness. Training and educating about pressure management will help women discern whether to include, modify, or exclude an activity. We can give our students the context they need to practice skillfully.

Getting a full excursion, three-dimensional inhalation allows the core system to expand with increasing IAP, elongating or sliding apart the muscle fibers of the pelvic floor and abdominal wall, which readies them for a more effective concentric contraction. Committed exhalations allow us to "blow off" excess pressure, especially during exertion, deepening the contractibility of the core system.

Coughing and jumping often produce the highest maximal IAP (Cobb *et al.* 2005). Consider this progression: clearing your throat, blowing your nose, sneezing, coughing, jumping. This list moves from lesser demand to more force, as well as from deliberate acts like throat clearing to more sudden blasts of IAP. Just before any of these, a full three-dimensional inhalation can prepare one's core cylinder system. The exhalation ideally provides containment from the foundation (pelvic floor) and walls (abdominals), making sure the action has an up-and-out pathway – expelling air or mucus from the nose or mouth instead of squeezing urine, gas, or feces out the bottom.

When I was about four days postpartum after my VBAC (vaginal birth after cesarean) delivery, I stood in the shower and realized I could gently blow my nose without feeling my pelvic organs want to drop out of my body! The few days before that, I naturally tried to prevent myself from blowing my nose or coughing and instead practiced mindfully breathing in, getting my lungs and diaphragm to descend as much as possible, and then used the exhalation to clear my throat a little at a time. This heightened example of the immediate post-delivery window hopefully illustrates how simple day-to-day events can be infused with conscious, embodied awareness and become a training opportunity for pelvic health.

Give yourself one minute to explore reflexive core support. Sit or stand tall, and place your hands around your perineum front to back as you did in the vulva cupping practice. Allow your inhalation to expand and descend, start your exhalation, and then clear your throat two to three times while completing your exhale. Do you notice a natural response or feel a rebounding, increased tone under your hands? This is the innate wisdom of your core system at work, pelvic floor included. If a student feels instead a bearing-down sensation during throat clearing, they can learn to consciously coordinate the pelvic-floor engagement and relaxation with their breath. Start here before progressing to breath or movement activities with a higher demand for IAP management.

Pressure outcomes vary widely from student to student. This critical reasoning process can help prevent us from making dogmatic, generalized recommendations and instead practice observing the student's performance in real time. Using sound provides ways to further explore pressure management and the state of one's pelvic floor.

How sound builds resiliency and confidence

If breathing represents a powerful agent of change, sounding is its supercharged counterpart. Using our voice can activate the parasympathetic branch of the ANS. It requires us to modulate and elongate our exhalations, creates resonance in the face and throat through sound vibrations, and focuses our attention.

If we chant with music or sing with friends, we also engage our listening, and perhaps our eyes to make contact, which further supports ventral vagus activation, or part of our social engagement system, like we discussed in Chapter 3. Moving from simple to complex sounds, alone to partnering, private to public with these practices can coax us out of our shell, cultivate confidence, and widen our window of tolerance, all while offering an enjoyable, gentle way to influence pelvic-floor tone (Rudavsky 2020; Wiebe and Clinton 2018). Enjoy the visual similarities seen in Figure 5.4 as we compare the larynx and vocal cords to the pelvic floor.

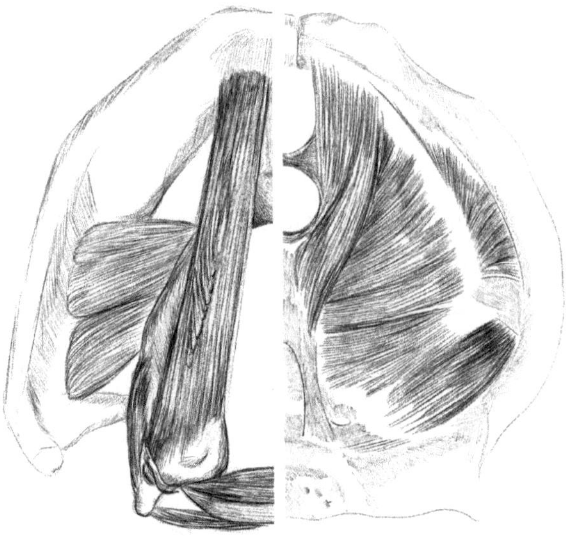

Figure 5.4: similarities between vocal cords (at left, superior view) and deep pelvic muscles (at right, superior view)

A few words now about ujjayi pranayama: Be curious about students with pelvic concerns who also practice yoga asana regularly, especially when their chosen practice focuses on a pronounced, loud performance of ujjayi. While ujjayi can certainly hold benefit by helping folks measure or modulate their breath during vinyasa, it can also easily be overdone, creating tension in the neck and throat, constricting the voice, up-regulating the ANS, and possibly limiting breath excursion. To gain command without as much tension, I've found the sounding techniques below more useful for some students.

Sounding strategies

For closure and containment

When a student needs to relearn connection to, and restore strength in, their core system – especially when meeting a new load or demand with a movement task – encourage them to use an audible exhalation. For this purpose, implement a hissing "SSS" sound or "Shhh," or a low humming vibration with the lips contacting each other for an "MMM" sound. Notice how the shape of your mouth and lips creates tension to produce the sound, mirroring the closure or drawing together that happens deep in the pelvic bowl.

Personally, I feel a hissing "SSS" sound most in the front of my core system, from clitoris and urogenital diaphragm up into my transversus abdominus. The

"Shhh" sound resonates more in the center, drawing my perineal body upward as the exhalation concludes. Lastly, a low humming "MMM" vibration seems to connect my pelvic, thoracic, and soft palate diaphragms, helping me sit tall from my rooted foundation and clear my mind with the buzzing sound. Most importantly, try it and feel for yourself – and let your students come to their own conclusions about which strategy they feel serves the intent or action chosen.

For relaxation and release

Horse lips simply sounds funny and often lightens the mood in the room during group workshops or classes. To do it, draw your breath in through your nose and then exhale out through your mouth with closed but fluttering and relaxed lips and cheeks. Sometimes, when a student has perpetually clenched their jaw or ground their teeth, it can take some practice to allow this kind of flapping in the wind to take place. It's worthwhile practice. If you want to really get after it, stand up and let your legs bend some. While you exhale into horse lips, wiggle your bum side to side and see if you can also let your buttocks be free. Giggling welcome!

My other favorite breath and sound strategy for pelvic relaxation is to let your jaw drop slightly open, producing a relaxed "Ahhh" sound for the duration of your exhale. This "slack in the drawbridge" of your mouth and jaw will mirror a slight drop and release down into your pelvic bowl. A breathy sigh (like how you would fog a mirror) doesn't quite get the same effect, so chant or sing the "Ahhh" tone instead. Let go of producing the sound and rest just before it creates any strain toward the conclusion of the exhalation.

For exploring IAP management

A simple way to explore modulating IAP comes from singing. I thank my friend and colleague Emily Greenleaf for her brilliant invitation to explore crescendo and decrescendo to feel what's happening in the core cylinder. To try it, simply start your sound quietly, amplify to a peak of your loudest volume, and then modulate back down to a very soft sound. Feel what happens muscularly while you investigate through volume.

Finally, natural human behaviors give clues about nervous system state. After a long day at work, we may find ourselves yawning, tearing up, drooling, or sighing (Dana 2020, pp.131, 257–261). Animals and babies never stifle yawns like we may as adults. You may explore snarling, baring your teeth with an audible exhalation or roar, and then rest – safe like the predator relaxing under a large shade tree.

These exercises create physical, physiological changes, and we should place equal trust in the psychosocial and emotional changes that can occur when a student discovers or reclaims their creative range, confidence, and agency, and capacity to play. The pelvic floor reflects this virtuosic, adaptive capacity by responding in nuanced task-appropriate ways, supporting a varied approach to breathing and sound (Aljuraifani *et al.* 2019).

What to do if making noise feels weird (and how to support clients feeling the same)

As yoga therapists, we get the benefit of embodying the practices that we may eventually give to our students. If dancing, wiggling, and making sounds generally feels weird to you, congratulations. You've allowed yourself to begin exploring, and thus you can embrace and shift your shame, awkwardness, or inhibitions. If any of the techniques here (or in this entire book for that matter) create hesitation or embarrassment, practice alone at home consistently. Watch yourself in the mirror. Video yourself, and then play it back and see if you can watch and listen without contracting physically, looking away, or judging what you witness. Just observe. (Then, if you wish, delete said video.) Rinse and repeat until the water runs clear – there's no longer a charge or residue of self-judgment muddying your view of self.

Once you've become comfortable sounding, shimmying, and more within the safety of privacy, you might coax yourself into new arenas, like offering these techniques at the end of your usual classes with familiar students, practicing at a public park, or sharing on your website or social media, as relevant to your audience. Your embodied ease will facilitate a direct transmission to students *and* they can personally explore the benefits of these strategies.

We first explored single-syllable chanting, because I believe in simplicity. This may support your student's compliance through concrete, easy instructions. The simplicity of a practice also leaves mental bandwidth free to notice how different sounds or apertures relate to the core cylinder, allowing observation of the different levels of engagement created. See Chapter 13 for a melodic, full mantra practice I adore and teach often, and use it as a progression from what we've done here.

Pranayama practices

Who breath – pacifying

I learned this practice first from my teacher Donna Farhi, when assisting her in Austin, TX. Pacifying and calming, this practice naturally elongates the exhalation by using a gently pursed lip position to create the "who" sound. Remember to use minimal tension in the mouth and jaw to create the shape, finding ease within the specificity. Alternatively, you could simply place a straw in your mouth. Breathe in through the nose as described, and allow yourself to slowly exhale through the tube of the straw.

To practice, sit tall and focus your attention on your natural breath rhythm to observe its baseline qualities. Let yourself exhale completely to mark the beginning of the who breath practice, and then allow a full expansive inhale to enter your body through both nostrils. At the top of the inhalation, make your pursed lips shape, and exhale through your mouth like you're blowing gently toward a candle flame without extinguishing it or making it waver. Your exhale takes as long as it needs to come to completion, and then relax and close your mouth to begin the next in breath. Stay with the who breath, using the candle-flame imagery to focus your mind's eye and modulate the force with which you exhale.

After about a dozen breaths, let yourself rest and notice any effects. Observe the quality of your mind or mood and any changes in the quality or rate of your respiration, as well as the resting tone through your core muscles, specifically the lower belly and pelvic floor. Although this pranayama can have a very calming effect on your nervous system, it's likely that by prolonging the exhalation, you may find an aliveness arising in your deep core support.

"Blow before you go" – embracing exertion

Exhaling with more intent and vigor may improve IAP management during a movement task. Just prior to initiating and throughout exertion, like standing up from a chair or lifting a heavy bag of groceries, blow out through pursed lips (Wiebe 2015). Called "blow before you go," this strategy has helped many students, and me, learn how to activate (or reactivate post-injury or postpartum) support from the bottom up during exertion. This is a short-term strategy – once core activation feels sound, move on to breathing normally throughout activity.

Alternate nostril breathing (nadi shodhana pranayama) – balancing

Subtle energetic differences exist between the left and right sides of our pelvic bowl. Our right side manifests active and heating solar qualities, while the left represents cooling, lunar aspects (Kent 2011). This corresponds well with the pingala and ida nadis, or channels, respectively, that the yogic tradition teaches. Interesting to note, too, that these body representations and nadis link up to the opposite hemisphere of the brain – pingala is associated with the left hemisphere and ida with the right (Werntz *et al.* 1983). Of course, when activating and balancing these contrasting channels of energy, we also feel bolstered through our central channel, or sushumna, creating a relaxed yet attentive quality of mind.

This practice can remind us of our innate ability to regulate and create resilience quickly and easily. Let's start with a simplified version of the classical alternate nostril technique, and then we'll dive down into the pelvic bowl for a creative, fun adaptation.

You'll be using your right hand, with only the index finger extended. Sit tall and notice your breathing and sensations before we begin. Allow yourself to exhale completely through "both barrels" as I call it, or out through both nostrils. Then, gently close your right nostril to inhale on your left side. At the peak of your inhalation, shift your finger to close the left side, and then exhale out the right nostril. Pause briefly, stay on the right side with an inhalation, following with your exhalation over to the left nostril. This makes a bit of an upward arcing image in my mind, like following a rainbow up and over, and then beginning at the same side of the rainbow to breathe in, sliding down the other side with the exhale. That marks one complete cycle. How long you practice here can depend on familiarity and comfort with the technique, attention level, and conveniently weaving this practice into your day.

Complete this practice by exhaling through your left nostril, and then rest your hands in your lap. Let your breathing do what it wants and zoom out with your attention, noticing the outcomes you perceive.

If you've just completed your asana practice and feel rather fancy-free, especially throughout your tongue and jaw, back body, and posterior PFM, you might investigate this pranayama practice as a tail-initiated one (without the mudra). Start your exploration in a supported supine position so you can release and explore allowing your tail to swish side to side, and then later attempt to engage with this imagery and sensate reality from a seated position. Rather than using the mudra or fingertip pressure to close and change nostrils, imagine swinging your tail to the closed side and breathe through the opposite. To complete the practice, let your tail float back to your midline. Notice how you feel afterwards, and perhaps even take a short walk to observe this newfound awareness in action.

I've had such fun exploring this, and clients have found it to be challenging as well as enlightening that they can learn to perceive their pelvic bowl on such a subtle level. Try it and report back to me, will you?

Applications

Remember to include an initial breathing assessment for individuals you support. Observing the baseline of their breathing function, both at rest and with static and dynamic postural assessments, will give you clues about how well their diaphragm and pelvic floor coordinate through the full excursion, how well they manage pressure in a variety of contexts, and the overall state of their nervous system.

Also, during the intake process and ongoing conversations at each session, watch how their digestion, sleep, energy levels, and mood patterns may provide further insights as to how to refine and guide their home practice according to the needs of their pranamaya kosha, or physiological body. Each person represents a complex and beautiful puzzle, and deserves a unique combination of practices and self-study prompts to support their wellbeing.

Breathing holds so much power. We can't survive without it, and we can't truly thrive when it's compromised. The thoracic diaphragm draws our heart down on each breath in, as the pericardial sac is attached to its central tendon, and buoys it upward as the lungs empty. The heart does not function as a solo artist. The whole body dances with breathing, which helps pump and channel blood through the circulatory system, supporting our heart muscle in its role.

Pranayama, sounding, and mantra provide great opportunities to enhance these subtle skills. I like to think of specific strategies like temporary scaffolding – they can provide us with a form to follow, a structure to create a specific result. The outcome I believe we most desire, however, is to free the expansive cyclical wisdom of our breathing and being; to no longer require formal practices to feel present, alive, or peaceful. Rather than relying on pranayama as a crutch, we use it to liberate each breath and embody its power – our power. As imbalances fade into the past, we can then choose practices to amplify fitness, capacity, or pleasure.

In the next chapter, we'll give this life force energy clear pathways to animate our wholeness by examining global relationships in movement and their impact on pelvic health.

CHAPTER 6

Global Functional Relationships

The human body has long been divided into pieces and parts, differentiated by labels and examined with scrutiny and scalpels. The process of discriminating through contrast provides a useful road map to understand structures and speak a common language. Yet we impose separation where there's none. Fascia represents a prime example of how reductionist and mechanistic our models of understanding were for decades, and now we're beginning to understand how our soft, outer contours communicate about and respond to this lived experience between body, mind, environment. Every part of our body can affect others through the kinetic chain, the two-way communication of the ANS, and the intelligence of our body's many interrelated systems.

Although we're going to focus on improving awareness, coordination, and relationships within the musculoskeletal system, we influence and inevitably move our organs, nerves, vasculature, and fluids as a result. These practices, and all asana, can be adapted to more directly influence nerve gliding or "flossing," circulation, and digestion, for example.

In this chapter, we'll seek to restore or enhance function throughout the body in service to pelvic health and liberating our physicality. Movement doesn't happen in isolation, rather in patterns that flow through our body sequentially. Like a collaborative team with many members, when everyone knows and fulfills their role, everyone wins. Our body community can thrive when we tend each part, knowing them intimately, distinctly.

Some might view these activities as corrective exercises, addressing common imbalances or "embodiment blind spots" caused by any combination of our modern way of life, inactivity, illness, injury, or having been neglected over the lifespan. Unfortunately, we're still not really taught these body-care skills in primary school or even in higher education, unless we specifically seek out studies like exercise physiology, dance, or physical therapy. We can help people make fitness and movement an integrated part of their lifestyle.

Consider the material in this chapter "pre-yoga" (Anderson 2010) (or what's called "pre-hab," an abbreviation for pre-rehabilitation) as a preventative approach. Some of the practices were influenced by self-myofascial release and somatics and informed by my study of the Franklin Method. Instead of doing "stretches," enjoy how dynamic movement can recalibrate effort and ease (Association for Hanna Somatic Education Inc 2021). The practices can act like a "tune up," perhaps making asana more accessible and effective.

This is by no means an exhaustive list – I've selected key practices that have served clients well. And this isn't a cookie-cutter plan – there's no magic protocol for any one pelvic symptom or diagnosis. Our observations guide us in determining which body areas or exercises to prioritize. Optimizing global function can help decrease the student's obstacles to efficient breathing, pelvic function, and force absorption, thus supporting the pelvis in fulfilling its many roles. Let these practices open further exploration, as there are many ways to embody movement function in each area.

Protocol for practice

With each exercise, it will be useful for you to pause long enough to feel your baseline pelvic sensations, posture, and breathing before doing the intervention. Afterwards, come back to a neutral posture and observe yourself in dynamic stillness. In this way, you engage systematically in a process of change (Hackney 2002, pp.19–26). Take note of changes you feel, and write down which two to four exercises seem to make the biggest impact on your sense of pelvic awareness and overall strength or ease. Once you've identified what feels most useful, make a pact to weave those few practices into your week ahead for continued benefit and more lasting embodiment of those changes.

This whole sequence takes approximately 30–40 minutes, allowing more time as needed to become familiar with the techniques and if you'd like a longer rest in the final posture. I've assumed a baseline of anatomical knowledge here, and simply named the landmarks or muscles referenced. Have your favorite anatomy book or application open to help you form the mental image of what part of your body is being touched or moved.

Find your head

It can prove difficult to organize the breath and core cylinder's function when we hold our body with excess tension or in a forward head posture. These positions are not inherently wrong or injurious when visited as a temporary, dynamic state. What may be problematic is when compensations get "sticky" through chronic inactivity, habitual repetition, or prolonged working positions. The following two suggestions may help melt neck tension and realign the weight of the skull with the central axis. To make these inquiries more functional, please stand.

Releasing neck tension: mastoid massage and sliding the sternocleidomastoid (SCM)

Find the mastoid processes, which are the two large bumps of your skull sitting directly behind your ears. Once you're touching the mastoids, slowly massage them in a circular motion with your fingertips. Make micro-movements with your head, nodding and turning. Find a centered resting place and imagine a line, like an axis, between your fingertips. Move this imaginary line forward and back in space, allowing your nose to reach forward, and then draw your jaw back in space, like trying to make a double chin. A few repetitions are sufficient.

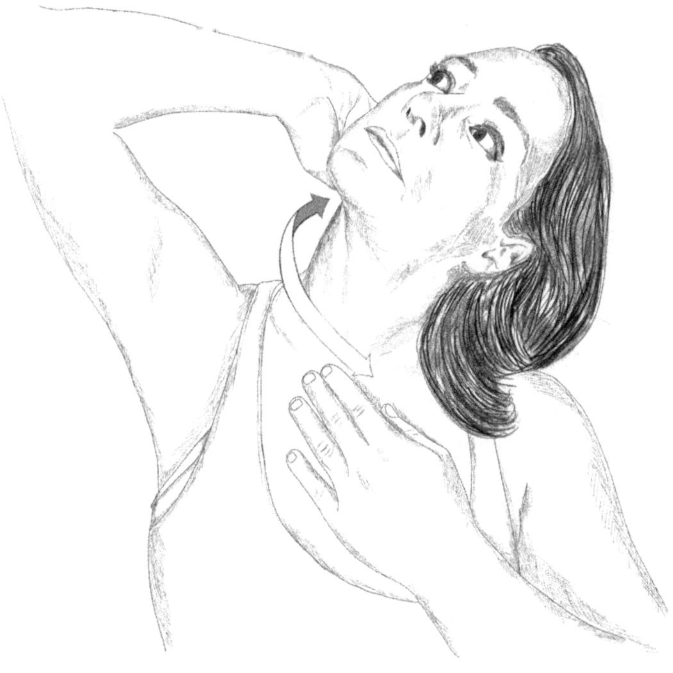

Figure 6.1: SCM sliding

Using Figure 6.1 as your guide, now trace from one mastoid process down in a spiral-shaped path around your neck to land at your medial collarbone and sternum. Visualize and attempt to feel this pathway slippery and melted, allowing the SCM muscle to soften. You can also gently move your head and neck while you "paint" your SCM. After a few breaths exploring, do the other side. Finish this practice by gently nudging the flesh at your sternum down while extending your neck, and then lift your mastoids up with gentle pressure from the heels of your hands while letting your jaw hang slack with a tiny nod "yes." Drop your arms and rest for a beat before continuing.

Chin tuck

As you pause, take a little walk or explore a standing posture. Notice how your muscular recruitment of the midline or deep core changes if you allow yourself to momentarily slip into more of a forward head posture or if you better relate your skull back to the central axis dynamically. For many, a gentle chin tuck can help find this relationship. A small activation of the anterior neck flexors can switch on a connectedness from throat to abdominals down to the pubic bone.

The amount of effort needed (mental and/or physical) or actual movement of the head and neck will vary from person to person and with movement context. Some people exhibit beautiful posture when they're standing still, yet may lose this postural relationship when in motion, especially when attempting to control speed or impact forces. Be careful not to overdo any cue, and let this be a living inquiry that suits the needs of the individual.

Unwind inside

Jaw tension and teeth grinding present commonly in contemporary society, and there's a high correlation between jaw and mouth tension and pelvic guardedness (Franklin 2002, pp.98–102; Koch and Johnson 2019). Ask any birth professional about this connection, and they'll affirm that relaxing the jaw, tongue, and throat can greatly support pelvic relaxation. One potential solution involves embodying the mouth directly and, perhaps more specifically, the soft palate (Anderson 2010, pp.44–45). Let's explore this together.

Melting jaw tension: the mouth cavern

Many techniques focus on the solid matter of our form – this one explores space. Take a moment now to become aware of the inside of your mouth, where and how your tongue lands. Allow your tongue to begin moving, slowly touching and gliding over each inner surface of your mouth, teeth, and the insides of your cheeks. If you wish, you can gently massage your jaw with your hands from the outside simultaneously. Let this be a luxuriously slow process, and if you start to salivate more, know that's your parasympathetic system saying thank you.

Drop your arms back down to your sides for this next part. Move your tongue as far to one side as you can, reaching into your cheek pocket. Pause and breathe there, relaxing your eyes and jaw as much as possible. Return through center for a moment, and then reach your tongue across to the other side, feeling it elongate to press the tongue tip into your inner cheek. Move your tongue to each side once more, and while you stay there for a breath or two, allow your eyes to look in the opposite direction. If it causes any discomfort or eye strain, cut your effort in half and find more ease. Once you've done the tongue-eye counter movement in each direction, please rest. Notice how the inside of your mouth or face has changed.

To finish this inquiry, feel the roof of your mouth toward the back, which is the soft palate. This place could be viewed like a spreading sub-floor to the brain. Let your soft palate broaden like a beautiful umbrella blooming inside your mouth. Rest your brain down into this buoyant, expansive support. If you'd like, see if you can also feel your pelvic bowl responding similarly to this suggestion from above.

Tongue to tail improvisation

This next practice can be done either seated or standing. If standing, allow your legs to have a slight bend in them. If you sit in a chair, you might add a layer of blanket for softness and sit toward the front of your chair. Before you move, sense the quality of your pelvic floor.

Sense internally the soft volume of space that connects the root of your tongue and throat down into your tail. You can add a metaphorical tail that suits your fancy, or gently touch the tailbone for a moment to locate your awareness. Begin with slow motion flexion and extension of your spine, letting the swish of your tail back bring you into extension, and a coiling action brings you into flexion. Let this be soft, juicy, and relatively subtle rather than a gross, mechanical exercise. Once you get into a rhythm, allow your tongue and tail to guide you into free-form movement improvisation – undulating like a snake, moving in circles, or wagging side to side. Feel free to layer in the various sounding techniques from our previous chapter as you see fit, or enjoy a few rounds of lion's breath (simhasana) as you dance your tongue and tail.

Trust your body to move in ways that feel good, and simply stay curious. In your own time, find your way back to stillness to observe the impact of this practice. If you'd like, further integrate this experience by practicing alternate nostril breathing, seeing if you can guide it from the freedom of your tail (subtly let your tail wag to the closed channel's side of the body and then swish across to the other side when your breath phase commands).

Rib fanning

This is one of my favorite Franklin Method (Franklin 2002, pp.16–17) techniques to help free the thoracic spine, ribs, and respiratory diaphragm. Students have called it magical. It's best to stand for this technique, and we'll do one side at a time for a vivid before-and-after comparison. Figure 6.2 will help get you started.

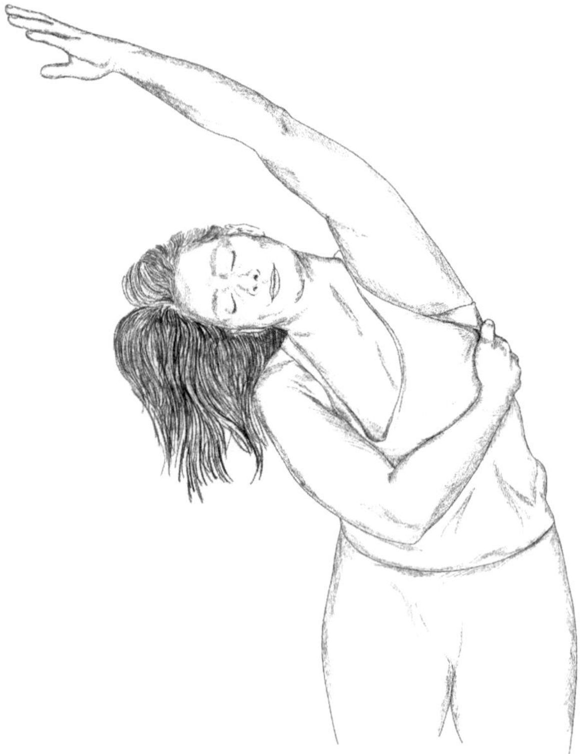

Figure 6.2: Rib fanning

Reach one arm up toward the ceiling, letting your elbow stay slightly bent if that serves you. Pat your underarm and side ribs vigorously with your other hand while leaning into a little more of a side bend, fanning those ribs open. Imagine your ribs like gills drawing in more breath energy, and then release into a side bend in the other direction, allowing your patting hand to just tuck under your arm and your other arm to hang passively to the floor. Let yourself have a moment here to bounce and rest, like you're getting all the stagnant breath squished out of that lung. Repeat this process a few times, fanning the ribs open as you reach up, and then letting the arm hang and lend its weight to the release of the diaphragm and lung. You can add a slight rolling action during the reach and pat – curl into yourself to come forward, and then roll back into a small backbend as you tap and breathe.

Once you're complete, brush down the arm and ribs of the side you're focused on, and then rest in standing stillness. Compare the two sides of your body in terms of posture, breath volume, and pelvic floor. After you've satisfied your curiosity to compare, be sure to give the other side of your body equal care and attention.

Heart to hips

We can help students feel connected to their center, a kind of flexible corset that dynamically relates the ribcage to the pelvis; this relationship can enhance pelvic function (Wiebe 2014). Please do these standing first, although you can also then translate these images into other positions once they're familiar and easy to hold in your attention. The second strategy can be particularly useful for folks who habitually find themselves in an increased lumbar curvature or anterior pelvic tilt.

Rib and pelvic angles with breathing

Find the inferior angle of your ribs in the front, tracing upward and into your midline at the xyphoid process at the base of your sternum. Be gentle here; we're simply highlighting this contour for our brain's attention rather than massaging or using much pressure. Feel this inverted V shape as a pliable arrow pointing upwards toward your heart.

Now visualize or palpate your pelvic outlet, tracing from pubic bone back and outward to each of your sit bones. This V has a slight incline with the arrow image pointing up and forward in space.

Once you can feel or sense the connection of these two V shapes in your body, we'll add breath awareness. Bring your hands back to the rib angle, settling your broad palms across your lowest ribs. Let your legs have a slight bend, and as you take a full volume inhalation, feel what happens under your hands. As the rib angle widens, so too does your pelvic outlet and the pelvic floor. As your exhalation ascends, you may be able to feel the congruence of the pelvic and rib angles gathering and narrowing. Spend a few breaths enjoying this relationship through the breath excursion and then rest.

Xyphoid to pubic bone

Bring the fingertips of one hand to your xyphoid process at the base of your sternum. Use a feather-light touch. Use your other hand to locate the pubic symphysis – and discern whether you prefer your touch at the superior edge or its anterior surface. While holding these two midline points in your body's awareness, imagine an illuminated elastic cord connecting them. Move about, walk, and explore balancing on one leg and shifting your weight in different directions to feel how this dynamic support always comes with you. Move from your center.

You can alter the strength of your "elastic band" in your imagery – if you tend to feel too tense or rigid in your movement, perhaps make it a more pliable thread of awareness. If you tend toward laxity or feeling disconnected, make your metaphorical band thicker and more robust.

Hip integrity

As the hips are so closely connected to the pelvic floor, know that there's a myriad of ways to release or improve their function as a team. First, we must find our femur heads so we can sense their support.

Find your femur heads

Standing, make an L shape with your hands by forming a 90-degree angle with your thumbs and index fingers. Now place your index fingers on the outsides of your hips at the greater trochanters. Allow your hands to wrap around the contours of your body, directing the tips of your thumbs into each hip crease. Bend your legs and wiggle a little side to side to feel the hip creases deepen, and allow your thumbs to descend into that space just medial to the large tendon you'll feel. Stand back up slowly, and sense two to three inches below or deep to your thumbs to imagine your round, smooth femur heads pressing up into the acetabula. Welcome to your hip joints! For many folks, the hip joints are more medial, or closer together toward midline, than they would have suspected.

Free your hips

The next practice primarily targets the glutes, piriformis, and hamstrings, but can have an impact on other surrounding muscles, including the lower back. A standing one-sided technique, we can again access a contrasting kinesthetic experience before we do the second side. We also get to train our balance dynamically here, which can further impact the tone of the pelvic floor. The contrast available through a unilateral exercise can help us identify benefits more concretely and can also help when pelvic function presents differently on one side to the other.

Stand up and make gentle fists with both hands. Use your closed hands to begin pummeling your buttocks and the lower back, around your sit bones, and back again. See if you can feel your hip muscles vibrating freely with the rhythm of your touch. If you can't yet set your bum free, this will be your practice for a few days before adding the next part on; you can also stay standing on both feet if shifting your weight or balancing on one leg causes any distress or discomfort.

Once you've found some juicy freedom in the buttocks, shift your weight onto one leg, letting your other leg trail to the side with your big toe touching the ground. Use your hand on that side to reach behind for your sit bone, taking hold of the flesh from under the gluteal fold to lift it up. Make sure the effort of your hand lifting your posterior hip muscles does not force you into an anterior pelvic tilt. Let your lower back muscles flow like melting chocolate down through the sacrum and tail while you continue with the next steps.

Drawing the buttock up and away from the sit bone, slowly rotate that leg in and out from the hip socket. You can do this with your big toe still contacting the floor; just let it pivot. If you want to continue to explore balancing, let the same moving leg swirl into a figure eight in front of your weight-bearing leg: rotate in and adduct your leg across midline, and then externally rotate as you abduct the femur out to the side – all the while, lifting your buttock. Lastly, you can explore a few leg swings front to back, sweeping your foot across and off the floor as low or high as you wish. Shake that leg out and release your hand when satisfied. Come back to standing on both feet, and brush down the waist, hip, and leg of the moving, butt-lifted side. Return upright to feel and compare the two sides.

Shake your arms out or rest your hands as needed. Feel free to walk around and continue to observe the outcomes. When you're ready, please repeat these instructions with the other hip and leg.

Stand your ground

The way our feet sense and relate to the ground can impact the liveliness of support through our midline, including the pelvic floor, breathing, and overall postural engagement (Myers 2009, pp.179–202). Working with the feet can also induce pleasurable relaxation, affording a sense of safety that further influences movement efficiency.

Enliven your feet

You're welcome to sit comfortably for this next portion. You don't need to use any oils, but I do recommend taking the socks off to get a good grip and to be able to observe the color of your skin before and after. Bring one leg up into a cross-legged or figure four position so you can reach your foot easily. Take the foot in both hands, giving gentle squeezes throughout the whole area. We'll move through three techniques to mobilize and awaken the arches of your foot.

First, we'll clear the "gutters." Observe the top surface of your foot, and palpate from the toes moving upwards toward your ankle. You may feel the thick tendinous bands under your skin. Bring your fingertips to the space between your first and second toes. Follow that groove slowly and smoothly up through the top of your foot. If it feels gravely, tender, or rough, feel free to repeat this gutter clearing or spend a few breaths in specific places with tolerable pressure. Complete this process for all four metatarsal grooves, locating each one with the space between your toes.

Next, we'll swivel and spread our toes and the metatarsal arch at the forefoot. Take hold of your first two toes and criss-cross them around each other in both directions. Move on to the next two toes and repeat until you've touched each one. You may also find benefit from swiveling non-consecutive toes, for example grasp and swirl your second and fourth toes together. Finish by spreading all five toes wide apart with your hands supporting them.

Our last technique targets the tarsal and talar joints and can help facilitate better force absorption in relation to walking. Hold your heel bone, or calcaneus, steady with one hand. Place your other hand across the ball of your foot or arch. Spiral your hands in opposite directions slowly, like you are wringing out your foot. Repeat this wringing action a few times, changing hands if you like, and then squeeze or brush your whole foot to complete the massage.

Take a moment to stand up, noticing how your foot meets the floor. You can observe how the arches feel, as well as how they look in terms of height. Has the skin tone or color changed post-massage compared with your other foot? Take a short walk around to compare your gait side to side, and then when you're ready, come back to your seat. Enjoy taking your time to give this care to your other foot, and then repeat the standing and walking observation.

Is a "neutral" pelvis necessary?

In yoga asana, we have often obsessed about finding a neutral pelvic position, neither too anteriorly nor posteriorly tilted. But what's best for clients? Is there such a thing as a perfect neutral place?

Some research shows a neutral pelvis may best generate pelvic-floor engagement (Capson, Mclean, Nashed 2009) while another study claims that one's habituated pelvic posture may be best (Capson, Nashed, Mclean 2011), perhaps because of its neuromuscular familiarity. Either way, posture represents a dynamic inquiry to facilitate appropriate tissue response. Giving students an inquiry of moving between anterior and posterior tilt, as well as other planes of action, may allow their body to recalibrate to what feels most neutral in standing. Let's try it.

Standing up, let your legs bend a bit. Place your hands atop your iliac crests and visualize the pelvic bones we investigated in Chapter 4. Your iliac crests are the upper rim of the basin, spiraling down into the pubic symphysis and then redirecting back and outward into the sit bones. Your tail is like a curved rudder in the center back of the pelvis, below your sacrum.

Begin moving smoothly through your anterior and posterior pelvic tilt. Now explore the frontal plane, hiking one side of your pelvis up into your palm and then the other. Alternate this action side to side a few times. Last, move through a few small circles, like drawing in the sand at your feet with a long swishy tail. Let your movements become 50% smaller. Take incrementally smaller movements until you arrive at a dynamic stillness that feels centered.

Drop your hands at your sides and breathe here for a moment, acknowledging any change in sensation and pelvic position from before. Movement increases the amount of sensory input we receive, which can help us feel what will work best for us when returning to stillness.

A posterior pelvic tilt can feel safe for people who experience prolapse, heaviness, and pressure, or for those who've learned to grip and contract everything to prevent leaks. Instead of insisting that they find neutral, we can incrementally encourage them to explore letting go of habitual guarding, building strength slowly in new postures and in new contexts. They might feel safer exploring the anterior tilt position and pelvic-floor expansion in a non-weight-bearing context first, for example, and then bringing it into tabletop, seated, standing, and movement. Of course, we could also assess the quality of regional muscle engagement (or lack thereof) to develop more robust support and balanced recruitment around the pelvic bowl with a customized strengthening practice.

Lastly, when we allow ourselves to be dynamically supported by our bones, our organs and surrounding muscular activity can find a more efficient relationship. The front rim of the pelvic inlet, formed by the superior pubic rami, can provide some support to the pelvic organs, potentially lessening the load on the pelvic-floor tissues. Envision and feel this support now.

Inner earth and space, a standing flow

For this vinyasa, we'll explore resourcing support from the ground and dexterous strength of our feet and ankles to connect and reach upward through our midline (Hartley 1995, pp.69–73). This requires engaging both stable dorsiflexion and rising into balance. The arms provide counterbalance and reflect core support we'll revisit in Chapter 10 with the developmental pattern of navel radiation. It's interesting to note, too, pelvic support increases reflexively in anticipation of limb movements (Hodges, Sapsford, Pengel 2007; Sjödahl *et al.* 2009).

You can complete a movement on each phase of the breath or explore moving on one and remaining still on the alternate breath phase. Depending on your client's pressure management skill, you can select the breath coordination that affords them the deepest sense of congruence and integrity. Move slowly, perhaps taking several breaths to explore each shape until it becomes known. For best results, practice this barefoot. This whole sequence is shown in Figure 6.3.

a. Start in standing with your arms at your sides. Let go of mountain pose (tadasana) "instructions" and embellishments and let yourself be natural, standing like a human. Feel your breath moving fluidly before you let the exhale carry you into the next action.

b. Yield through all your limbs, including your spine head to tail, to allow your legs to bend, bowing slightly to your center of gravity and the earth. This is a preparatory movement that allows you to feel the ground and gravity, drawing support from your legs and deep center.

c. Press the floor away to begin straightening your legs, tracing up through your midline with the fingertips lightly touching. Continue this upward connection until you feel a natural lengthening of your spine and arms into the space around you. If your body agrees, go ahead and rise up onto the balls of your feet, feeling your heels leave the ground as you reach for the sky.

d. Gradually bring your heels back to the ground, and let your body recoil with a slight return into flexion through your legs and spine as your arms sweep down to your sides.

e. Continue sweeping your arms behind you as a counterbalance as you feel your feet broad against the floor. Press the floor away again and extend your legs and spine. Slowly let your center of gravity shift forward in space, feeling one long line of connection from the crown of your head down through the heart, the pelvic bowl, and into the ground. This is like a ski-jumping position, where we're focusing on a hinge from our ankles into dorsiflexion. Feel your heart beaming forward and toes spreading instead of gripping. Trust this place.

f. Allow your weight to shift back in space, returning to center over your arches and femur heads. Draw your arms forward into anjali mudra (prayer hands), palms together in front of your heart. Let this gesture of the palms coming to midline support you in feeling a sense of knitting together through the abdomen, a settling in your body as you've completed one round of this flow sequence.

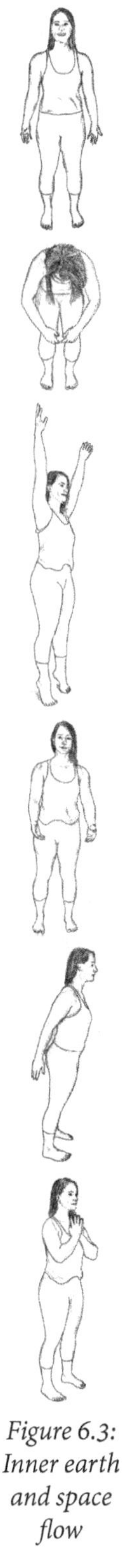

Figure 6.3: Inner earth and space flow

Closing practice – constructive rest position (CRP)

Our closing practice for this chapter will be CRP. Many somatic disciplines use this posture in their own way, and physical therapists at times call it the "hook lying" position (Dowd 2012, pp.6–12; Farhi and Stuart 2017, pp.46–51).

Here, we decompress the spine and unload the pelvic organs from the pelvic floor, feel the feedback of the floor against our back body, and maintain a low level of conscious tone in our legs to track them parallel to each other. While some teachers automatically ask students to prop their knees together by letting the legs turn in, I usually recommend trying it with parallel legs first.

Find a place where you can lie down and be undisturbed for at least five minutes. You might use your bed, your mat, or the living room rug to give your body firm softness to rest back into, allowing your legs to remain bent with the soles of your feet grounded.

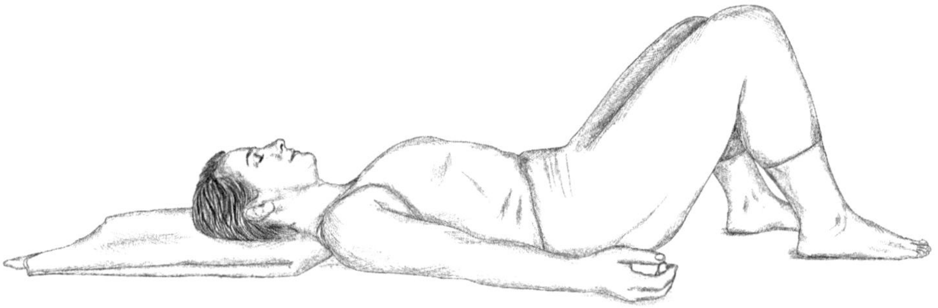

Figure 6.4: Constructive rest position

Once you've organized yourself, let your attention shift into the back of your body. Feel your face and jaw melt. Let your head grow heavy. Continue this melting process down into your neck, shoulders, arms, and entire trunk. Give your weight to the ground. Trust that your breathing will do what it needs or wants to – you get to let go of any control and rest.

Now bring your awareness to your knees, like the peaks of mountain tops. Imagine they receive the warmth of the midday sun, melting into an alpine stream flowing down over your thighs. Let your thighs soften and join this river flowing over your femurs, sliding down into your hip creases. The river's current continues to descend through your hip sockets – let your femur heads sink down into this fluid support. Right femur head dropping. Left femur head dropping. Both femur heads settling. How heavy can you let your bones be? Feel your pelvis broad against the ground as you fully relax into the pristine pool at the base of this river. Can you imagine this river sweeping through your pelvic bowl, filling its expanse? See and feel a calm, peaceful lake spreading out across your sit bones, dissolving your lower back, and flowing out through your tail. Let it pool across the floor under you. Rest deeply.

Let yourself linger in the sensations and insights you've gained from this chapter. Identify which techniques felt the most relevant to your situation, and reflect on why that might be. What created the most tangible changes in your body?

Consider also what you might see or hear from a client that could guide you in selecting from these practices. What might you observe in their posture or movement that would show you what they need? Perhaps they express how worry takes up residence in their neck and shoulders, and wish to release that area. Or you may observe pronation and the beginnings of bunions and thus be drawn to work with their feet to help them connect their foundation into greater pelvic awareness and support.

We'll circle back to physical assessment and teaching applications. In the following chapter, we'll introduce different qualities we might encounter in the pelvic muscles and overview the main categories of pelvic conditions to give us more context for future clinical reasoning.

CHAPTER 7

Insight Into Pelvic-Health Conditions

People deserve to feel seen, heard, and understood. One survey showed 45% of patients found pelvic therapy on their own, with another 45% reporting their doctor shared pelvic-floor therapy as what seemed to be a "last resort" (Cozean 2020). Demonstrating knowledge and competency shows students we care and builds rapport. Knowing the implications of their diagnosis can help us allay their concerns and facilitates clinical reasoning. Speaking this language requires due diligence on our part and supports effective communication with providers on interdisciplinary teams. We may be able to improve primary care referrals for pelvic care, as well.

A full explanation of the myriad different pelvic conditions that exist goes well beyond the scope of this book. Consider this an entry-level, generalist approach to understanding pelvic-health conditions, whereas you could continue your study and further specialize with any one condition or goal. This warrants that we collaborate with pelvic-floor specialists and mentors to obtain an accurate diagnosis and ongoing guidance.

In this chapter, we'll cover four main categories of pelvic-health conditions: bladder and bowel function, pelvic pain, sexual health, and pelvic organ prolapse (POP) (Messelink *et al.* 2005). We'll outline risk factors, considerations, and potentially useful themes for each. We'll also briefly discuss the role of scar tissue. This will give parameters within which to critically consider how to select and deliver practices for students presenting with these conditions.

Even when a condition is incurable or permanent from the medical perspective, we work together with students to manage and do our best to improve their presenting symptoms and overall body image, movement capacity, and quality of life. We're not attempting to diagnose or determine root cause – we instead want to know enough about these conditions and other comorbidities to provide better care. This also allows us to make an appropriate referral when necessary. Toward the end of this chapter, you'll find a list of referral indicators to help build this discernment. We function within a paradigm of wholeness, with respect for the limits of our scope.

People may experience multiple types of symptoms or conditions at once, so we'll begin to illustrate how these conditions may overlap. Also, with the prevalence of sexual assault and abuse, we must be aware of the very real possibility that our students may identify as survivors. Please consider how dissociation can serve as an intelligent response to pain, suffering, or a violation of one's consent or safety. Coming home to one's body, especially the pelvis after it has been a source or site of confusion, shame, assault, or abuse, can feel frightening or unsafe. Tethering one's attention to the present moment through practice, and learning to objectively, compassionately witness narratives and sensations, may support students in gradually restoring a sense of safety.

If being present with bodily sensations feels entirely new or overwhelms a student due to known or unknown trauma history, we may suggest first that the student establishes care and a sense of inner resourcing with a qualified mental-health professional or trauma specialist.

Labels, language, and shifting perceptions

When receiving a label or diagnosis, people could have any number of reactions. Some may feel relief, finally validated that what they've experienced with their pelvic health has a name. Others may feel shocked, disheartened, or even depressed, as though giving their experience a name is a lifelong sentence of brokenness and suffering. Women may feel like they can't trust their body after being given a diagnosis, which can lead to avoidance of the very activities that may help them heal or keep them connected to their sense of purpose and joy. Our role as a neutral witness allows their unique experience to be validated.

Common misperceptions abound, too – that pelvic conditions mean they can no longer pursue fitness activities they enjoy or complete necessary actions of daily living, like lifting their children. As they watch the fluctuations of mind activity and their maturing body, the essence of who they are remains unscathed. Yoga connects them to an unchanging, loving quality of presence.

As a client-education strategy, we can dialogue together about their health history step by step, defining diagnostic terms, and discuss lifestyle and movement habits according to what we know from existing evidence and what we discover through assessment. We can honor the emotions present for the student and the social implications of how a diagnosis impacts them, and support them in finding a more empowered relationship to their condition. Regardless of diagnosis, we ought to do our best to help minimize mental-emotional drivers of and outcomes from pelvic symptoms (Bogner *et al.* 2011; Felde, Bjelland, Hunskaar 2012; Vrijens *et al.* 2015). Language and imagery matter. Each therapeutic alliance will speak its own dialect of embodied experience, communicating qualities of practice and change over time.

In client sessions, I often ask a student to rate or describe their somatic experience. First, I might ask them to discern whether their sensations feel the same or different as a starting point; contrast can help facilitate interoceptive awareness. I then ask them to quantify whether they view those changes as better or worse than before and to do their best to describe how they feel different. Because of the brain's negativity bias, we're often quite skilled at describing sensations we don't like, such as pain. I view my role, in part, as a translator – helping people find words to describe positive somatic experiences, which may help reinforce the new qualitative state of being.

Pelvic-floor patterns

Pelvic-floor disorders rarely have a singular cause and instead likely relate to a variety of factors including but not limited to anatomy, genetics, physiology, lifestyle, and reproductive aspects of one's life (Delancey *et al.* 2008). Another important factor to consider is the state of a student's PFM, as they play a role in symptom presentation and need to be assessed to guide treatment. To simplify, we'll address three key patterns: normal functioning, overactive or non-relaxing, and underactive or "weak" (Messelink *et al.* 2005).

The first pelvic-floor pattern I want to reinforce is the normal, functional one. A healthy pelvic floor can relax and contract when warranted and can modulate the force or contractibility appropriate to the changing, dynamic contexts of exercise, yoga postures, breathing, and tasks of daily living. Basically, the pelvic floor can contribute to movement efficiency, endure lower loads over time, and support higher loads (strength) over short-term lengths of time. The pelvic floor and perineum also need to be able to relax and descend, demonstrated during childbirth and bowel movements, for example. Lastly, the PFM must be able to relax when no demand is present until a new demand warrants a change, and then ideally respond with the timing of breath and synergistically with other core muscles (Prosko 2017).

The pelvic-floor team can also exist in a state of excess or overactivity. A non-relaxing pelvic floor can lead to urinary and bowel issues, painful sex, and low back pain (Faubion, Shuster, Bharucha 2012). One of my first tip-offs that I tended toward a non-relaxing pelvic floor came years ago with the realization that I couldn't pass gas while running. It took slowing to a walk, and sometimes lifting one hip, to release wind. I'm happy to report that I can now easily fart while flying over rugged terrain! Anecdotally, most people I've supported have tended toward this overactive, non-relaxing state. These students may report tension or "tightness" in their hips, or we may suspect that's the case after watching how they move and breathe.

Lastly, an underactive or weak pelvic floor can exist, sometimes described as an absence of sensation or movement upon voluntary contraction. Weakness can be driven by many factors, including as a result of over-recruitment that disallows movement through full functional range and poor motor-recruitment timing that masquerades as weakness. Both cesarean and vaginal births can create changes in connective tissue and core system inefficiencies. Age can play a role in declining PFM function or atrophy, yet yoga and other integrative approaches show promise that we may be able to prevent, reduce, or delay associated symptoms (Burrell 2014; Cramer *et al.* 2012; Lyons 2019).

While we're on the topic of hormonal health, yoga may also be an accessible and safe treatment for menstrual disorders. We're still learning about underlying mechanisms, and more rigorous research is needed to better understand how yoga supports period health (Oates 2017). We can better embrace the rites of passage represented by menarche and menopause when informed, active, and prepared.

Sometimes, a combination of overactive and underactive engagement and inappropriate timing with other muscles occurs, which can create asymmetry originating in the pelvis that can perpetuate compensations elsewhere. For example, for many years, my right side held an overactive, tense state, which allowed my left side to be "sleepy" or delayed in its response and limited in its strength. Interestingly, signs and symptoms such as one-sided pelvic pain, IT band syndrome and other imbalances in recruitment during running, and girth measurement discrepancies in my thighs were all apparent. Resolving these imbalances required a deep investigation and reintegration of my midline, including the psoas major and pelvic floor, and examining my hip and pelvic joint function. The two halves of my pelvis benefitted from customized imagery to improve functional coordination. The frequency and severity of my pain also diminished greatly. This tendency toward asymmetry still garners my ongoing attention, albeit less than before and more easily remedied. It's important to note while asymmetry may be helpful to address, it does not bear out in the literature as a direct cause of pain (Palsson *et al.* 2019). Know that a therapeutic plan for asana may include different postures, imagery, repetitions, or durations for one side of the body in these instances.

In cases of incontinence, or leaking any amount of urine, gas, or stool, it's often assumed that the pelvic floor is weak and needs to be strengthened. A study by Smith, Coppieters, and Hodges (2008) shows incontinence may be linked to overactive PFM. If muscles chronically contract, they have no additional capacity to contain a leak against the force of coughs, sneezes, or raucous laughter. As an aside, we also still tend to generalize and blame weight for back pain and pelvic issues. While that *may* play a role, one study (Smith, Russell, Hodges 2006) shows incontinence and breathing patterns are more strongly associated with back pain than body mass index (BMI) and activity level. Let's focus on function more than judging size.

We cannot effectively strengthen muscles that don't know how to relax and be moved through their full range of motion. This deep core tension pattern could be due to stress, breathing patterns, emotional states, past traumas, and other factors, and demonstrates the need for a proper evaluation from a pelvic-floor physical therapist before assigning any active engagement of the PFM, as this could exacerbate symptoms. It also gives justification for including whole-body systemic and localized pelvic relaxation cueing in each woman's home practice. Even if a student indeed needs activation and strengthening, their exercises will likely be more effective through minimizing effort and tension first, and returning to relaxation at the end of each practice session. Learning to deeply relax may get our voluntary over-recruitment or unconscious guarding out of the way, allowing a more natural way of breathing, moving, and being to restore itself.

Culturally, we employ language that illustrates the non-relaxing or over-recruited pelvic floor. Consider the phrases "uptight," "tight ass," and "anal retentive," as well as the consciousness that may be associated with this unforgiving, rigid quality deep within our core.

In contrast, a truly weak or under-recruited pelvic floor may demonstrate a state of disconnection, even apathy or avoidance, or a habit of collapsing into gravity without any rebound or resilience upward into the crown of the head or the surrounding environment. Regardless of where we start on the spectrum of overactive and underactive, yoga therapy provides pathways to increasing conscious awareness and may help modulate function in the associated muscles through systemic self-regulation, intelligent application of asana, and the use of props and self-touch for feedback.

Lastly, a worked muscle may be more willing to relax completely. Driven or body-conscious students may desire or be attached to a more active practice. Having satisfied more gross sensations of effort and heat, they may more readily give into restorative shapes or more subtle practices from which we discern they'd benefit. Including whole-body active yoga postures, a walking regimen, or other fitness programming as your scope allows might provide a sense of satisfaction and potentially lead to deeper relaxation when offered.

We'll discuss localized PFM strategies and context for their application in the next chapter. For now, let's examine the four categories of pelvic conditions you'll likely come across when working with groups and individuals.

Categories of pelvic conditions

Bladder and bowel health

Bladder and bowel function includes the ability to contain urine, feces, and gas voluntarily, involuntarily, and without leaking (continence), and the ability to void easily and completely when necessary. The PFM, in conjunction with bladder and bowel impulses, need to coordinate the retention and release of waste on command. Difficulty with starting a urine stream or initiating a bowel movement, the sensation of incomplete voiding or evacuation, and constipation may be improved with pelvic-floor physical-therapy interventions.

Constipation can drive urgency, frequency, and leaks as the rectum and bladder utilize similar innervation. Hard, compacted stool can irritate these nerves and create a quality of reactivity in the signals to the bladder (Maeda *et al.* 2017).

Urinary incontinence (UI) affects both men and women, although far more women experience the condition. From a data analysis of over 17,000 participants, Markland *et al.* (2011) found that 51% of women experienced UI, whereas only 14% of men reported UI. Stress incontinence affects more women; urge incontinence seems more prevalent for men. Moreover, several different types of incontinence exist, which are defined below.

- **Stress urinary incontinence (SUI):** Leaking due to a momentary increase of stress or pressure, like a cough, sneeze, or jump; may indicate that pressure management and breathing need attention.
- **Urge urinary incontinence (UUI):** The sensation to void comes on strongly and/or suddenly; may be associated with frequency or voiding more often than every two to three hours during waking or more than one or two times overnight (known as nocturia).
- **Mixed urinary incontinence (MUI):** A combination of stress and urge or frequency.
- **Functional incontinence:** Caused by functional deficits that impact continence, like gait impairments, arthritic hands that make buttons and zippers difficult, or cognitive challenges.
- **Fecal incontinence:** Leaking of gas or stool; can relate to PFM function, consistency of stool and digestive issues, and other factors.

Risk factors for incontinence include gender, age, parity, birth injury, current habit of smoking, and comorbidities like diabetes and neurological conditions (Danforth *et al.* 2006). Other conditions like overactive bladder syndrome and interstitial cystitis often present with incontinence-like symptoms, yet have very different causation and warrant different treatment. Urge suppression and delayed voiding should not be encouraged for students with coexisting pelvic pain; those strategies can be better customized by clinicians. Emerging studies support a yoga-therapy approach to managing incontinence, including in accessible group contexts (Huang *et al.* 2018).

Lastly (and perhaps less embraced in casual conversation as poo is often still more taboo than pee issues) is the distressing prevalence of fecal incontinence. This can include unwanted leaking of either stool or gas, which affects approximately one in eight people (Ng *et al.* 2015). When there's a tendency toward loose stools, addressing dietary causes and nervous-system regulation may help solidify the contents of the bowel, making it easier to contain. Coexisting digestive disturbances and conditions may respond favorably to mindfulness-based treatment like yoga therapy (Zomorodi, Abdi, Rasulzadeh-Tabatabaee 2014). The shame and embarrassment that can accompany fecal incontinence can lead women to believe constant contracting will help prevent leaking, when in fact the same principles apply here – non-relaxing muscles can't contract any more. An approach that addresses relaxation and coordination could restore function and, in turn, continence. It is best to seek a clinical evaluation so the right treatment can be selected.

Pelvic pain

Chronic pelvic pain (CPP) affects up to 26% of women worldwide (Ahangari 2014). We know pain is complex, and there are many biopsychosocial factors that contribute to the experience of pain. In CPP, there's often not just one cause, and conventional treatment focuses on symptom management and quality-of-life measures. Psychological factors may increase one's risk for pelvic pain, and living with persistent pain creates its own host of emotional distress, worry, and fatigue (O'Sullivan 2015). Because of the complexity of many pelvic pain conditions, it may be best to work with a multidisciplinary team.

Pain warrants a whole-person approach and can include pain education, down-regulation of one's nervous system, desensitization through self-touch, redefining sex and intimacy (and expectations therein), and a restored or bolstered focus on social support, meaning, and joy. Some examples of pelvic pain conditions include dyspareunia (pain with sexual intercourse), endometriosis, fibroids, symptoms associated with irritable bowel syndrome (IBS), and painful bladder syndrome. Pelvic girdle pain can be associated with musculoskeletal imbalances, inflammation, and hernia, and sometimes emerges during pregnancy or postpartum. In a sample of patients with lumbopelvic pain, women with strong urinary urge and central sensitization were around three times more likely to have PFM tenderness upon palpation, a sign of PFM dysfunction (Keizer *et al.* 2019; Vandyken *et al.* 2020). Localized tenderness usually points toward an overactive PFM state that would benefit from down-training.

As yoga therapists, we may be able to help women, and their medical providers, gain insight into the complexity of their pain experience. Through a holistic assessment using the panchamaya model, we may uncover physical, psycho-emotional, social, energetic, and spiritual factors related to a woman's symptoms and the level of distress they cause. Some evidence shows adverse childhood experiences may correlate with adult onset of CPP (Schrepf *et al.* 2018). We can also inquire about the timing of their pain and whether it seems influenced by their menstrual cycle, specific movements or positions, contexts, relationships, or places, even certain foods or beverages. Even if they first aren't sure how to answer, posing the question can invite them to observe their lives and identify patterns they may not have noticed before.

Pelvic pain can guide one's practice. While we might assume asymmetrical asana creates shearing or loads the pelvis in ways that cause pain for mechanical reasons, research suggests pain is more complex. It's plausible that tissues and physiological systems have become sensitized to certain positions or movements rather than the reductionist view that blames mechanical forces (Palsson *et al.* 2019). We, of course, also need to assess *how* these postures are performed. We might begin with and return to a bilateral stance, gradually exploring the movements a woman has identified that cause pain in small doses or as regressed variations, thus perhaps decreasing pain sensitization and restoring hope and function. We can offer novel input into the pain system that may help increase their trust in movement, influence sensitized tissues, and thereby decrease their pain responses.

With pelvic pain, less is often more. Learning to generate continuity and sequence force from the ground into the legs, and upward through the body's midline, can instill a sense of safety, harmony, and strength in standing postures. Restorative practices can also calm the "alarm system," which can gradually widen the student's window of tolerance for physical activity. Studies continue to accumulate showing the benefit of yoga interventions for reduced pelvic pain and improved quality of life (Russell *et al.* 2019; Saxena *et al.* 2017).

Determining comorbidities or coexisting symptoms may help us customize a yoga-therapy plan and decide whether a medical consult is needed. Pain is a protector and calls for attentive listening and compassion. With endometriosis, for example, clients may experience low back or pelvic pain, as well as other symptoms, and it can take up to seven to ten years to confirm diagnosis (Johnston, Reid, Hunter 2015). Knowing these patterns and the interactions between diagnoses and systems increases the safety and quality of care we deliver.

Contraindications with pelvic pain include but are not limited to urge suppression or bladder training protocols, unless prescribed by their clinical pelvic-floor therapist, and Kegels or voluntary use of the bandhas may also be cautioned against. Education, stress management, and relaxation are recommended as first-line treatment for pain conditions such as interstitial cystitis and painful bladder syndrome (Miller 2018).

Pranayama techniques need to be used appropriately, and unfortunately there's no standardized protocol as we know pain is such a complex phenomenon. Balancing or pacifying pranayama may be useful in these contexts and may provide a real-time coping strategy for clients during flare-ups when they may be afraid to do their usual physical activities or movement practices.

On the other hand, students presenting with depressive states or diagnosed depression alongside their pelvic pain could benefit from a more uplifting, energizing breath practice. Often, it can be useful to first meet the student where they're at – including where their ANS is most familiar with functioning – and gradually cultivate range or contrast as tolerated. For example, a client with anxiety may first need a practice that's stimulating in nature, to discharge the excess sympathetic arousal that feels familiar, whereas a "calming practice" may initially aggravate their symptoms. It really depends, and we need to assess and reassess our students.

In movement practice, focusing on neutral sensations or holding both pain and comfortable sensations in one's awareness simultaneously can help students reduce fixation on and catastrophization of their pain and lead them toward an embodied experience of equanimity and self-compassion. Rather than full-range movements or prolonged holds of any one position, consider gentle pendulation between different movements, allowing the person to recalibrate their motor control, attention, and trust with incremental steps toward regaining function. Lastly, restorative postures can yield the weight of the burden of one's pelvic pain by accessing deep relaxation, instilling restfulness and hope.

Sexual health

Investing in a loving relationship with one's self will likely yield a return within our other relationships – and perhaps especially so when it comes to connection, intimacy, and satisfaction sexually, whether partnered or alone. We circle back again to the foundations of presence, embodiment, and allowing ourselves to play and experiment in an arena we may have been directly shamed out of exploring when we were young. Or maybe we're discovering how cultural messaging and past experiences placed obstacles in our path toward owning our sexual identity.

Sexuality truly is a complex and beautiful BPSS phenomenon. Sexual health means integrating all aspects of the individual and expresses the dynamic interplay between body systems and the very personal roles of context and perception (Bortolami *et al.* 2015). Sex is an activity of daily living, and many people may express relief when their sexuality is acknowledged by care providers (Rosenbaum 2021).

When specializing in pelvic health, it's essential that we normalize and equip ourselves to at least recognize and screen for sexual-health needs. Each yoga-therapy client could be invited to define what sexuality means to them, personally. Certain aspects of sexual health sit well within our scope, such as addressing self and body image, physical activity and comfort, pelvic awareness, and cultivating ANS regulation, resilience, and social engagement skills. Mindfulness has been shown to be incredibly effective in addressing women's desire and other sexual concerns (Brotto 2018).

Female sexual dysfunction impacts 41% of premenopausal women globally (McCool-Myers *et al.* 2018), and in menopausal and older women, estimates range from between 33% and 51% prevalence (Eden and Wylie 2009). More research and further standardization of sexual-health terms and conditions needs to be done. We're beginning to understand why we experience sexual response the way we do, thanks in large part to a landmark contribution called the "Dual Control Model" (Janssen and Bancroft 2006).

I first learned about this model in the amazing book *Come As You Are*, in which the author unpacks how important it is to know one's self sexually from both sides of the motivation psychology coin – meaning there's what we want that tempts us to seek it, as well as what we don't want that we do our best to avoid experiencing. Movement *toward* and movement *away from* make up our motivation. Libido or sexual desire isn't just about being able to get turned on; we also need to understand what turns us off. She provides the latest science that supports the variability of sexual expression, compassionately reminding us we're all normal (Nagoski 2015).

Self-inquiry, dialogue, and journaling can support yoga-therapy clients in better understanding their behavior, and the embodied strategies and practices we can teach clients can help them recognize and then shift out of a defensive, avoidant, or dysregulated state that keeps the brakes on, gradually helping them awaken their senses to the pleasure available to them in each moment.

Fully expressed sexuality requires an agile nervous system. An intimate encounter moves through different stages, initially requiring a certain level of attentiveness to register safety and connection. Then, moderate sympathetic activation brings us into arousal and toward orgasm. Ultimately, the activation again discharges, settling us into a post-sex peaceful state. Yoga practices help us experience and toggle between these different states of relaxation, activation, and discharge or neutralizing the charge accumulated during practice. Yoga helps us *pay attention.*

Mindful practices of self-touch, starting with body regions other than the pelvis or genitals, might help people discover increased self-regulation and relaxation, learning what types of touch feel good and then being empowered to make requests of a partner. Mudras, as well as gentle tapping, squeezing, or brushing of the limbs, can stimulate different somatic and energetic responses; remember, touch is highly subjective. What feels pleasant for one person may be agitating for another. Allow your client to express preferences without judgment and let them determine the best way forward with self-touch.

Yoga therapy supports self-awareness, nervous-system regulation, stress management, and healthy body image – all of which may support a person's intimate health. To serve clients with sexual-function concerns more directly, team with a sex-positive mental-health therapist, sex educator, or sex therapist, or seek relevant training to further specialize in this arena.

There's also great likelihood of overlapping pelvic conditions. One study looked at connections between women seeking gynecologic and urogynecologic care for pelvic-floor dysfunction and their sexual health. One finding that fascinated me involved whether or not prolapse symptoms worsened sexual function. Regardless of prolapse stage, they found that women *with self-reported prolapse symptoms* were much more likely to report sexual concerns and concluded that women with *asymptomatic prolapse* were not at increased risk of sexual dysfunction. In other words, the group that weren't aware of or experiencing prolapse-related symptoms were also unlikely to report sexual concerns (Handa *et al.* 2008).

Our first-hand experiences, and our perception of our body's function or relative dysfunction, may create a mental-emotional load that impedes our sexual expression and satisfaction. While our physical body may exhibit changes (which may lead to diagnostic labels), we can still be free to explore and enjoy sexual pleasure. A primary conclusion of this study called for clinicians (and I'd add our role as yoga therapists focused on pelvic health) to better understand these patterns and strongly suggested that we proactively screen for sexual-function concerns in students presenting with incontinence or prolapse. Let's learn more about prolapse next.

Pelvic organ prolapse (POP)

Grasping my handheld mirror, I ventured into the bathroom. It had been two weeks since delivering our second daughter, and I was ready to examine how my body had been changed from another pregnancy, my first vaginal birth, and the minor tear I'd had sutured by my homebirth midwife. I felt a mixture of curiosity and trepidation, wondering how the vivid, intense sensations of early post-birth days would manifest visually.

While my sutures had mostly receded internally and were hidden from view,

I found it surprising and unnerving how visible my urethra and urethral tube had become. The opening, or vestibule, of my vagina remained much wider than pre-delivery (very normal), and it felt like my organs overall were still riding lower than I'd long felt and known them to be (also normal this soon after delivering). I admit I felt shocked seeing my urethra protruding loud and proud, and quickly texted a girlfriend of mine who also works with women and pelvic health to relay what I saw. She put me at ease, sharing how common this is for women after a vaginal birth, as well as how my healing had only just begun. In fact, during a visit shortly after that, she shared pictures from her own birth. Ah, to be affirmed that this is all in the realm of normal.

I wondered how many women can access wise peers to inform and encourage them in the early postpartum window compared with what I suspect more often happens – that women don't look, don't ask, and don't share, out of avoidance, ignorance, or embarrassment. Or if they do look, they may become horrified and suffer silently, spiraling alone. I'm encouraged by the network I've cultivated and trust this is part of the future we're creating together by doing this work.

I continued to observe my body as the ascension improved weekly, although never quite returning to pre-delivery appearance. Luckily, the hospital-based midwife I saw for my insurance-covered six-week clearance reiterated how normal everything looked and how my uterine position felt high and well supported, and she encouraged me to trust the ongoing healing that needed to continue. If I remained symptom free, she didn't think physical therapy would be warranted and did not give me a label of prolapse even though my fears and worry led me to that initial assumption.

Armed with knowledge and feeling adamant that women deserve postpartum care, I asked for a referral anyway and received an internal assessment and trigger-point release therapy around five months later. As I gradually returned to exercise, I documented any fullness, urgency, leaking, or dragging sensations to keep myself in check. After implementing a targeted approach to hip stability and postural retraining at ten months, I started to feel a difference – mainly measured by the absence of hypervigilant attention and a neutrality of sensation in my vulva. I still felt nerve sensations and cyclical heaviness monthly that frustrated me.

Another six-week round of diligent strengthening and graded exposure to impact helped me run comfortably again at 18 months. Also, time does heal (usually) when we're patient. I consider the entire first year (or two!) after delivering to be the postpartum window as tissues remodel and we reinvent our relationship to fitness, sexuality, and more.

I'm impressed by the care I received from the hospital midwife at six weeks – to not pathologize changes too early. Colleagues and clients of mine have shared stories in which they weren't treated with such discernment, receiving alarming prolapse diagnoses at only days or weeks after delivering or being told their concerns don't warrant a referral and were to be expected. If prenatal and postpartum pelvic therapy became standard practice, we could better support new mothers, prevent birth injuries, honor the massive rite of delivering a child, and provide systematic, customized care for full recovery.

Vaginal wall changes and the staged prolapse diagnosis system have spurred debate as many women with stage I prolapse remain asymptomatic. Assessment methods and language may need to be revised in the future as we learn more about women's experiences and continue to standardize clinical assessment of POP (Haylen *et al.* 2016). Prolapse is very common, with up to 50% of adult women displaying some amount of prolapse upon physical examination. Thankfully, only a fraction of them report experiencing symptoms (Iglesia and Smithling 2017).

Prolapse is primarily a support and pressure-management issue, being defined as a descent or displacement of pelvic organs, which may include them being visible at or beyond the openings of the pelvic floor. Quite literally it means "falling out of place." The descent of organs can happen in different places, sometimes in multiple areas simultaneously. Cystocele refers to a bladder prolapse, while an enterocele or rectocele affects the posterior pelvic structures of the small intestine and rectum, respectively. Finally, a woman may also experience a uterine or cervical prolapse.

Urinary or fecal problems may also exist due to a prolapse, so an examination with a specialist is warranted when incomplete emptying or trouble starting to void or eliminate exist. Let's not assume to know the cause of a woman's incontinence when it may very well be multifactorial. Another consideration with prolapse includes preventing or managing constipation, as the volume and consistency of the stool, as well as any habit of straining, will further stress the PFM and connective tissues.

Within our scope as yoga therapists, we're well equipped to support women with awareness of their pelvic sensations and discerning how their lifestyle and physical activities influence prolapse symptoms. We can offer modifications and provide guidance on adapting their practice. Bring awareness to whether symptoms seem impacted by the menstrual cycle. Knowing how to regress and progress exercises helps women stay active, rather than creating fear by telling them to avoid activities they love or must continue due to occupation, householding, or caregiving. Maintaining an active lifestyle may help reduce symptoms or prevent an increased stage of prolapse from developing.

Breathing awareness can facilitate pressure management during exercise and yoga practices. To have a feeling of something "falling out" of one's body may create a guardedness and thus a shallow or restricted quality of breathing. This would perpetuate increased tension in the core system; recognize that prolapse doesn't always equate to a weak pelvic floor. Women with prolapse may also present as overactive in their pelvic floor and be well served by restoring the full, calm excursion of three-dimensional breathing. Also, although we don't have strong evidence for this approach yet, it may make sense to focus on gentle inversions and low-pressure activities, such as supine or sidelying practices, supported bridge, and variations of a restorative posture called legs up the wall (viparita karani), gradually reintroducing progressive loads as tolerated (Prosko 2017).

With the psychosocial aspects of yoga philosophy, we can support women in updating their goals and expectations to develop patience and self-compassion for the changes they experience across their lifespan. For some women, adjusting their mindset and identity may prove to be the most challenging but fruitful lesson to instill through compassionate self-awareness.

As a pressure-management subtopic, hemorrhoids can also occur. They frequently relate to toileting habits and chronic constipation, and often stem from an overactive pelvic floor, specifically rigidity and a non-relaxing quality in the deep layers of the posterior pelvic floor that surround and interdigitate with the fibers of the anal sphincters. Learning how to relax while voiding, maintaining a diet and lifestyle that support easeful poops, strengthening regional, global muscles to reduce the perceived need for tension in the posterior pelvic floor, and clinically addressing PFM trigger points may help. Breathing awareness provides continuous pressure management all day, which may also support prevention and improvement of symptoms.

Lastly, discussing perceived stressors may identify areas where more support is needed (childcare, finances, or social community) before one can truly embody more ease.

Scar tissue considerations and self-touch

With surgery or other wound-healing processes, we can anticipate the possibility of scar tissue forming. Episiotomies, natural tearing, cervical procedures, cesarean births, hysterectomies, and other abdominal surgeries can all impact connective tissue, muscles, organs, and nerves in the pelvic region. These events alter tissues and cause separation; embodiment means restoring the somatic connection to and function of the area that had been disrupted. Many things contribute to tissue healing, including biomechanical, biochemical, respiratory, genetic, nutritional, and emotional factors. Socioeconomic status can also affect access to resources for rest, nutrition, social support, and stress management, further impacting scar healing and recovery.

As the layers of one's body may then feel foreign, unknown, or numb, a kind of reacquainting can take place through consciousness, movement, breath, and touch. We may refer our students to (vetted) skillful manual therapists like pelvic-floor specialists, sexological bodyworkers, or massage professionals with advanced visceral training. Establishing another therapeutic alliance may further support a student's ability to voice concerns and navigate consent, promoting a conscious healing of the narrative surrounding the physical event they wish to heal, as well.

We first must respect the initial wound healing and wait for physician clearance or guidance for movement and self-touch practices. Early wound healing creates a necessary stiffness around the site to approximate tissues and restore integrity – *the scar serves a purpose.* Our skin and the volume of flesh beneath it need our care and patience. Like a beautiful tapestry needing repair, the "threads" of a scar may pucker, gather, or pull differently across the blanket of our skin. The patchwork thickening at the site of intrusion or injury is a normal response and does not necessarily indicate a need for massage or remediation, provided we can happily go about our lives asymptomatically.

Once a student has received medical clearance, we might begin by simply guiding attention into the region and eventually directly to the scar. When they can land their awareness with minimal emotional charge, evidenced through subjective feedback and other cues about their nervous system state like their breathing pattern and facial expressions, we may invite them to begin a self-touch practice. We're not prescribing that they touch with the purpose of changing or "doing something" to their scar. Rather, we're inviting consciousness and a compassionate invitation back to wholeness, reclaiming any part of their body that felt forgotten, separated, or judged.

Resting one's hands near or around the site can be a first step (for example, see Figure 7.1), and then cupping or holding the site itself can offer a progression. As they hold awareness with the warmth of their own touch, we can guide the breath excursion or use imagery to facilitate more ease, acceptance, freedom of movement, or comfort. Global movement health may also gently free stuck areas surrounding scars.

When women seem to have addressed it all – dialing in their nutrition, rest, breathing, baseline physical activity, and psycho-emotional factors – and yet still have symptoms, scar tissue remediation could be a missing link (Koch 2020). When I speak to students, they've usually never received hands-on care for their scars. Even if they get regular massage, cesarean scars and the pelvic region typically remain untouched and unaddressed by conventional bodywork.

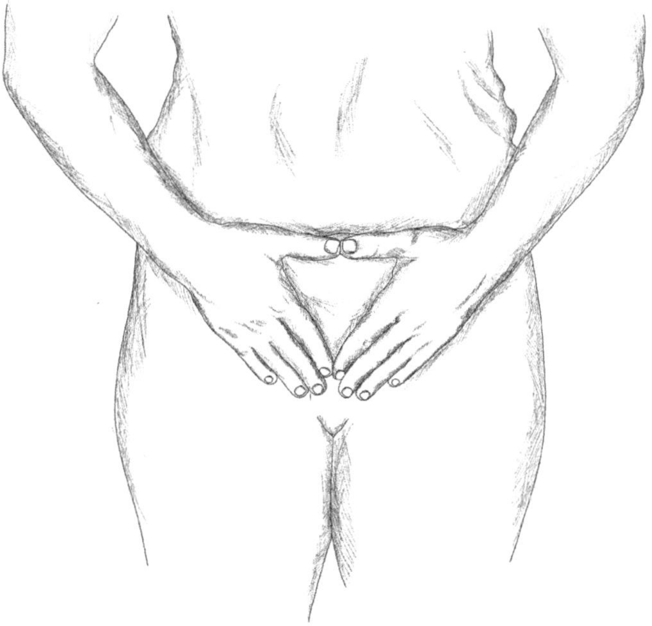

Figure 7.1: Trimurti/yoni mudra (embracing life transitions/womb of creation gesture)

Self-touch, as a practice of embodied svadhyaya, or self-study, can provide an inroad for this gentle homecoming, which might help a woman feel ready for deeper hands-on or hands-in work from a qualified provider. The ayurvedic practice of a warm, oiled massage before bathing can also provide a whole-body approach to awakening and moisturizing the skin, improving circulation, and enhancing feelings of wellbeing and relaxation.

Referral indicators

When students arrive in our office or Zoom room, they generally show up ready and willing to participate. Sometimes, especially during a flare-up of acute pain or with significant emotion present, we may find the need to dramatically change course or even stop the session and ask the student to seek medical care.

Here's a list of key questions that can help you discern whether to make a medical referral before continuing your usual course of yoga-therapy care. A medical evaluation may then warrant changes be made to their yoga-therapy protocol.

Has your student experienced sudden or complete, unexplained loss of bladder or bowel control?

Does your student experience constant or unrelenting pain that wakes them or disrupts their sleep?

Has your client had an unexplained and significant weight gain or weight loss recently?

Have they noticed concerning changes in the texture, amount, color, or smell of their discharge?

Has your student reported blood in their urine or stool?

Does your student experience fevers, night sweats, or other constitutional symptoms?

Has your student expressed thoughts of harming themselves or others?

While we may include questions like these in our new-client screening process, having them on an intake form alone proves insufficient. Conditions change and symptoms fluctuate, so throughout the duration of a student relationship, we can keep these items in the backdrop of our mind. Embodiment and compassionate self-study through yoga therapy can serve as a great complement to medical and mental healthcare, as well as one's work with a pelvic specialist. I'm grateful pelvic-floor consultations can now be delivered online.

At some point, a concern may arise that sits well outside our scope. In cases of intense emotional triggers that linger or affect a student's daily functioning, and with the possibility of trauma and transference, the most ethical choice would be to acquire a mental-health specialist or another qualified clinician to join the team or take over care until the student feels stable in their daily life and can differentiate the roles of their unique providers.

When countertransference, or our own ability to remain professionally objective and compassionately present, interferes with the therapeutic relationship, we're ethically bound to do our own inner work with a qualified mentor or support person outside of the teacher-student relationship. We are responsible for our perceptions, responses, and projections.

Lastly, if your pelvic yoga-therapy passion leads you to work with sexual trauma or assault survivors, having a mental-health support person on your care team can assist you in digesting the stories and potential vicarious trauma accumulated by serving in this capacity. Take good care of yourself so that your teaching can remain potent and sustainable.

Self-compassion meditation

To close our discussion on pelvic-health conditions, let's drop back into practice with self-compassion meditation. Cultivating kindness and nonjudgmental awareness is gaining traction in the literature (Neff and Germer 2013) and has long been a key principle in effective spiritual practices. First, establish comfort in a restorative posture (see Figure 7.2).

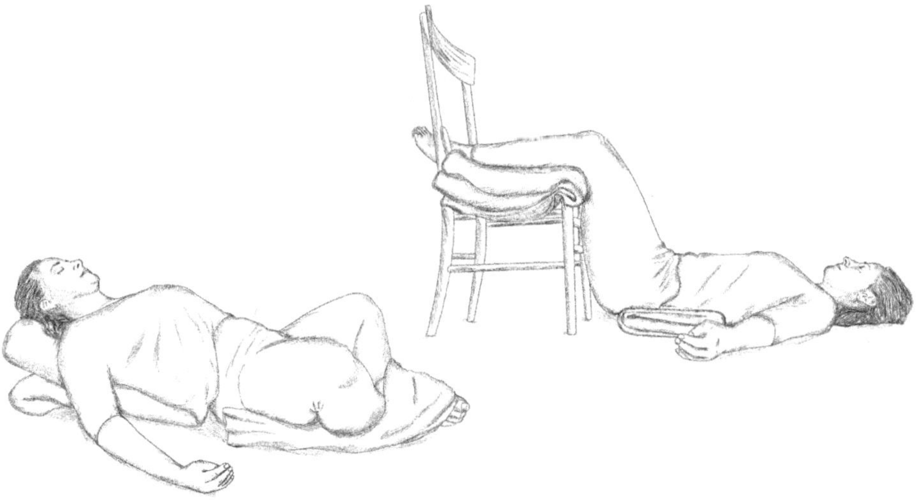

Figure 7.2: Restorative postures

Using the above figure as inspiration, choose either reclining bound angle (supta baddha konasana) or legs up the chair. Reclining bound angle can increase circulation and awareness into the womb space and pelvis, and offers a sublime sense of surrender through the chest and front of the shoulder girdle. Give yourself plenty of support under both elbows and the outer knees. Some women may find this pose revealing or vulnerable. In that case, you might cover and wrap the lower half of your body with a blanket, tucking it in around the outer hips. Further, you could simply allow your legs to drape over a bolster or rolled blanket in parallel alignment.

If you'd prefer a mild inversion, you might find comfort in this variation of legs up the wall. I like to offer legs up the chair, even legs up the couch, when the geometry suits your leg length well, and use props to give a sense of containment and security. You can do this by looping a yoga strap around the thighs after placing a yoga block between them. This can help melt excess muscle recruitment and promote deeper relaxation, as the femurs track directly down into the hip sockets, resting into the firm-yet-yielding boundary of the props. Invite yourself to settle into stillness.

Become aware of your body, the rhythm and quality of your breathing, and the sensations you feel. Welcome it all in with radical acceptance, not asking anything to change. Just observe without an agenda. What is it like to simply be present to yourself in this way? Invite yourself to melt into pure attentive presence.

When you're ready, bring awareness into the heart space. Rest your attention down between the lungs, settling into the heart. How would it feel to appreciate your body, to be held in your own loving awareness? What does it feel like to offer yourself this kindness? Allow the warmth of self-compassion and positive regard to expand and fill your heart, and then imagine it streaming downward to fill your entire pelvic bowl. Can you feel the volume of space within your center relaxing, opening to your sincere appreciation? Rest here, anchored in the sweetness of being with yourself, as you are. Notice and enjoy how your mind, breathing, and body sensations respond to this gift of self-compassion and loving kindness.

CHAPTER 8

What About Mula Bandha and Kegels?

Smoldering under the surface, covered by cultural conditioning, misinformation, doubt, shame, and disgust, the embers of healing ignite when command and compassion are restored from within. We see our students as whole and capable. They're the definitive expert on their embodied experiences. As yoga therapists, may we pray to remember this before each session or class we offer.

Only she can feel the sensations her body creates and the clues they give. Her voice speaks the truth of experience and advocates for her care, dignity, and satisfaction. Only she can breathe more wholly and move attentively, imagine more completely, and sense what is current and what calls her forth – the possibility of reclamation.

Through therapeutic alliance, we provide catalyzing benefits, like the power of connection. The medicine of kindness. The truth of science, portals of self-inquiry. We witness the art made manifest by guiding first-hand embodied practice. Together, these elements create and maintain vital health. We don't heal people; we facilitate and witness their journey to healing themselves.

We've been taught to seek the quick fix culturally, haven't we? We codify and commoditize "the solution" as something external, something we "do to" someone to fix them, often ignoring the innate wisdom of the human body and its desire for attention.

In this chapter, we'll define Kegel and mula bandha and summarize the common misperceptions and possible benefits of these practices. You'll also gain insight around what pelvic-floor engagement entails and how to bring nuance to pelvic-awareness cues. Finally, we'll explore a few simple practices aimed at improving pelvic awareness and coordination. No cookie-cutter, standardized approach will work for every student, so adding depth and detail to your embodied understanding can support discernment and creativity.

Context is queen

Some practitioners hold that teaching pelvic-floor engagement, and specifically Kegels, should stay in the domain of clinicians or be taught only by pelvic-floor specialists with internal palpation for direct feedback. This *might* represent a best-case scenario to some folks – but we know that not everyone has access to a skilled, qualified clinician. If they acquire a telehealth relationship with a pelvic-floor specialist, they'd then be limited by distance and technology, leaving the internal manual-therapy component of treatment and education void. This means observation, dialogue, and cueing becomes paramount.

Access issues aside, not everyone needs or wants a relationship with a clinician. Some women don't feel willing to receive internal assessment and treatment. Frankly, they don't need to give or have a reason. If they don't want clinical care, they still deserve to get the information and practical experience they need to be able to get well. Also, sometimes a pelvic-floor symptom has behavioral roots or can be caused or exacerbated by lifestyle habits or global movement patterns. These students may need very little instruction on localized pelvic-floor engagement, and instead may need to cultivate a more sustainable rhythm in their daily life, foster acceptance and compassion, or tune up their whole body's wellbeing to benefit their pelvic health. Pelvic yoga therapy may suit these women well by delivering sound information, guiding effective practices, and crafting personalized strategies that address the whole person.

When we teach a public group class, it's important to recognize that we rarely have intimate knowledge of every student's history. Even when we know our students well, pelvic-health details may not be shared as readily as symptoms like a headache or lower back pain. Therefore, I suggest we refrain from teaching strong engagement or specific pelvic-floor training strategies in public group contexts and reserve these detailed instructions for the private yoga-therapy client.

What we can offer in group environments includes increasing general awareness and providing inquiries that help students self-assess their posture, movement habits, and pelvic-floor baseline. We might choose cues that reference our concrete and universal pelvic bony anatomy instead of genital terminology that varies or for some may spark a triggering event. Posing a question can go a long way toward helping a student invest their awareness and curiosity, and become more proficient in how they practice on the mat and how they move about in daily life.

Once a client willingly begins to work with us privately, we conduct an intake conversation and formal assessment. We gather up all the clues and observations relevant to create a customized plan. This way, we see the whole picture and determine what will best suit their needs and goals.

Now that we've built some discernment and context for the application of Kegels and mula bandha, let's define them.

What's a Kegel?

Named after the physician who first published a protocol for pelvic-floor exercise in 1950, a Kegel is simply a voluntary contraction of the pelvic floor. More complexity unfolds in the application of Kegels as treatment. Ideally, Kegels become fully customized and can vary for each person depending on speed of contraction, duration of time contractions should be held, amount of repetitions and sets, frequency, degree of maximal voluntary effort, and relaxation intervals. Like any other skeletal muscle, the PFM need consistent training over time (typically around 8–12 weeks) to adapt to the progressive demand of said training. The specificity of this program design requires accurate evaluation and advanced education.

When are Kegels most warranted?

According to a Cochrane review (Dumoulin and Hay-Smith 2010), Kegels (considered here to be PFM training that includes both engagement and relaxation) have been recommended as the first-line treatment for SUI and mixed urinary incontinence (MUI). An updated report (Dumoulin, Cacciari, Hay-Smith 2018) showed PFM training could be significantly more effective for SUI/MUI than no treatment or education alone (without supervised physical training of PFM). For clients presenting with SUI or MUI, and no coexisting pain responses or diagnoses, supervised PFM training and a clinician-designed home program for Kegels may be the best approach.

What could possibly go wrong with a Kegel?

First, when asked to perform Kegels during an examination, 30% of patients did not perform them correctly (Huang and Chang 2021). If women were only given verbal advice on Kegels without receiving education on how to do them correctly, they could exacerbate their symptoms unknowingly, generate frustration and dissatisfaction with care (possibly prompting avoidance of seeking care in the future), or they might be simply wasting their energy.

Second, an isolated muscle contraction does not always translate to better function. We try to parse out individual muscles when movement functions more like a symphony or orchestra (not an individual instrument). As you learned in Chapter 5, each breath provides an opportunity for this harmonious coordinated effort, and our movement practices need to employ and build functional equivalence. It's often insufficient to solely complete localized PFM training. Functional, integrative approaches that include pelvic-health education, global movement efficiency and fitness, breathing, and stress management have proven to be effective for improving quality of life and reducing an array of pelvic symptoms (Baker, Costa, Nygaard 2012; Barbato *et al.* 2014; Bordoni and Zanier 2013; Dugan *et al.* 2013; Hung *et al.* 2010; O'Sullivan *et al.* 2002; Smith *et al.* 2008).

Many people interpret Kegels as a constant practice and focus on repeated or held contraction of the pelvic muscles. Our body remodels around what we consistently do over time, and this constant state of root tension can create neuromuscular, connective tissue, lymph and circulatory, and even psychological impacts. The widespread misperceptions of Kegels being a constant, contraction-focused effort versus a cyclical action, or the theory that more is better, illustrate the klesha of avidya – misinformation, ignorance, and illusion.

For example, we wouldn't walk around repeatedly raising and furrowing our eyebrows… normal social engagement and daily living "train" facial muscles to meet our needs. Of course, if an injury or facial surgery had occurred, some rehabilitative exercise may be warranted during the initial weeks of tissue healing. Similarly, the pelvic floor generally receives sufficient "training" with normal, active living, and when an acute injury is sustained, like a perineal tear during childbirth, there may be a need for direct rehabilitation. Hence, Kegels have their place. Lastly, remember for some people, Kegels will make symptoms worse.

Basic pelvic-health education needs to continue to expand into popular culture, so please share this from the rooftops with your audience! What goes up must come down – a Kegel must include a full relaxation phase after each contraction, as well as a rest period after training events for the best results. Read on to learn about yogic techniques for root awareness.

What's mula bandha?

Traditionally, the practice of mula bandha, or "root lock," was to be done while seated in stillness as a meditative practice – applied most often during advanced pranayama as an extended pause after complete exhalation. Intended to stir, build, and ascend the energy from within the pelvic bowl (specifically the root chakra or muladhara) upward through the chakras sequentially, this energetic seal attempts to enliven and awaken, bringing one's yogic journey into the psychospiritual realms of consciousness. One study showed promising results with mula bandha for improving symptom severity and quality of life in women with mild prolapse (Sweta *et al.* 2018).

This physically static, energetic approach during advanced seated pranayama has since been interpreted to include mula bandha as a continual pelvic-floor engagement during dynamic, breath-based movement during active asana practice. Only quite recently in our western understanding of yoga, particularly found within the Ashtanga lineage, has this subtle energetic practice been widely applied throughout sequences of poses, a style of practice called vinyasa (Hall and Garden 2021; Kaminoff 2010). When used as a static, unvarying, effortful contraction held throughout movement, even if cued as a subtle or submaximal contraction, this approach may increase undue tension, impede breathing, interfere with PFM function, and even alter the natural coupled motions and healthy mechanics of the hip and spine.

If mula bandha was performed in a way that allows the PFM to oscillate functionally with varying force production, using the technique during asana *might* be a beneficial way to increase one's understanding of the support and movement efficiency coming from the deep core system during gross movement patterns and in gravity-varied contexts. Done dynamically with the breath and appropriate to the movement or postural demand of the asana, this interpretation of mula bandha could increase awareness, coordination, and properly timed engagement of the PFM. Then we could also argue whether we're "doing" mula bandha at all, or if we're simply highlighting natural pelvic function with conscious awareness.

Pelvic function (both relative movement or excursion and degree of force needed) depends on the demand of the task in question. Voluntarily, perpetually holding even a partial engagement will override this innate intelligence and adaptability. (We know momentarily contracting the PFM voluntarily can be a sign of PFM health and highly useful when justified, like when we're about to sneeze with a very full bladder!) The bandhas ideally respond spontaneously when we find right relationship to the ground, gravity, and space. Basically, how we move and work with our body will enliven them according to the demand of what we're doing. Approaching asana as a living inquiry means we observe for this natural adaptability.

Ashwini mudra

Another, sometimes lesser-known, yogic practice targeting the pelvic floor is a repeated, rhythmic engagement and release of the sphincters, most often felt or cued from the anus. This dynamic technique may encourage bowel motility and could support the coordination and control of the PFM overall.

Ashwini mudra may encourage energy movement downward, while mula bandha focuses on the energetic accumulation and ascension toward the psychospiritual realms (Desikachar 2018). We might consider body position relative to gravity to neutralize or dampen the apana vayu concentration and instead build buoyancy and levity into one's awareness with this dynamic exercise, perhaps especially for folks experiencing pressure or heaviness, or with known prolapse.

You may have noticed the curious absence of an experiential practice after each of the above techniques. Know that I've consciously chosen to omit descriptions of how to perform Kegels, mula bandha, and ashwini mudra. In part, this stems from the limitations of our scope as yoga therapists and the high likelihood that what we teach may be interpreted or performed differently than intended, as discussed. These all fall under the umbrella of PFM training, which may not be necessary for clients to see positive changes in their pelvic health with yoga therapy.

For more understanding, compare notes from various teachers on the same practice. Better yet, consider developing a strong, collaborative relationship with pelvic therapists in your area. Working with clinicians on your team can help you learn and discuss the nuance involved with these topics and, most importantly, help you to customize your cues and programming for clients when consulting with your multidisciplinary team. I tend to take a whole-body, functional approach to addressing a student's physical needs, weaving in nuanced and personalized pelvic awareness without much attention to voluntary PFM training.

Lastly, take these practices into your personal study for several weeks (or months) to gain familiarity before teaching them. Your felt sense of these subtly different techniques will expand your capacity to cue meaningfully for each client, as well as help you discern through embodied experience what might be useful or contraindicated for your student.

There have also been a multitude of new devices and products aimed at providing women with tangible pelvic-floor feedback in the privacy of their own homes. From yoni eggs (smooth stones for inserting vaginally), to the Perifit gamified device that measures your vaginal contractions and syncs them to your smartphone, to the Innova bike shorts that deliver pelvic-floor training via electrical muscle stimulation (EMS) at home, we can see that the very real concern around pelvic health (and namely continence with some of these products) has driven the market to respond.

If your clients choose to invest in any of these commercial products, my hope would be that they feel supported throughout the process with dialogue and compassionate troubleshooting. Maybe these devices are indicative of an "unshaming" trend where women voice their concerns and questions openly, and know to seek support from a practitioner if the product doesn't work for them, if symptoms worsen, or as a next step in the evolution of their health, fitness, sexuality, and self-study.

What does "good pelvic-floor engagement" mean?

We've already discussed how a pelvic contraction includes both a gathering or closing action and a lift upwards into the body. More nuanced yet, it may be helpful to understand the distinct parts of a pelvic contraction, written here according to vulvar anatomy.

A quality pelvic-floor contraction has three components (Vestal 2019). During a concentric contraction of the PFM, we will feel or see the clitoris nod (the glans of the external clitoral anatomy will bow downward toward the perineum). Also, we'll feel or see the vaginal walls gather together and retreat inside slightly. Lastly, the anus will "wink" or close more tightly during a pelvic-floor contraction. These three zones of awareness may help achieve a more integrated, full engagement of the entire PFM team.

During the release of the contraction, we'll see the opposite: the clitoris comes back up from its nod, the vagina blooms open and descends slightly, and the anus and surrounding tissues relax – like smoothing out the extra wrinkles that appeared during the contraction. All these actions ideally reverse, allowing the entire pelvic floor to relax to its previous quality and location. Sometimes, more complete relaxation occurs after having worked the muscles momentarily.

Beyond this releasing of effort and return to baseline, the pelvic floor may also bear down or descend and lengthen purposefully like during childbirth or bowel movements, or when extracting other objects like a yoni egg or menstrual cup. (With menstrual cups, especially those that create a feeling of suction around the cervix or pelvic organs, you may explore giving a slight counter engagement during extraction so as not to perpetuate descent or dropping of those structures, like with prolapse.) When in doubt about devices like these or whether your pelvic floor "does this right," you can use the self-assessment techniques in the next chapter or, better yet, trust yourself to see a specialist who can help you get clarity.

What might happen instead?

Often, at the outset, people either don't feel "what they're supposed to feel" or they're simply not sure what they feel. There's nothing wrong with the student in this case. Everything we observe can be useful to spur us forward, better customize the cues or chosen practice, and witness the unfolding process of awareness. Here's a few examples of what people may report as they start to become aware of pelvic-muscle activity:

- They don't feel or see anything happen, which might be described as feeling "nothing," the absence of movement, or numbness.
- They get only a partial contraction. (Lift or closure but not both; one of the three aspects of a contraction are missing; asymmetry of function side to side or front to back.)
- Other regional muscles grip, tense, or contract to help during *submaximal* contraction of the PFM. (Extra-pelvic muscle activity, for example in the glutes, lower abdomen, or adductors, is expected and synergistic during attempts of maximal PFM engagement; Messelink *et al.* 2005.)
- They don't feel or see a return to full relaxation or it feels hard to return to complete relaxation after engagement.
- They feel such emotional charge that it's difficult to bring awareness to or sustain attention on their pelvic sensations. In these cases, approach

the practice with compassion and curiosity gradually. Progress could then be marked by the student's ability to complete the experience with reduced intensity or neutral emotional states.

Let's come back to further defining aspects of PFM health.

Five functions of a happy pelvic floor

In the previous chapter, we discussed three common patterns of pelvic-floor function (normal, overactive, underactive), as well as the possibility of contrasting or asymmetrical function of the pelvic floor (differing function from side to side or front to back). It's useful and relevant to know your student's baseline whenever possible from a clinical evaluation and diagnosis, or through interpreting clues from self-assessment and what we observe. This will allow you to establish a target goal together for the first phase of their home practice.

With that said, every pelvic floor needs to be able to function in a variety of ways, which can often be well supported through a personalized yoga-therapy practice. We can move toward comprehensively increased function in five key ways, outlined below and illustrated in Figure 8.1. I've included questions in the list that may help guide conversation with clients. The terminology included for quantifying strength of contraction and PFM relaxation may be helpful for students to articulate what they discover during self-assessment and to standardize communication for interdisciplinary teams (Messelink *et al.* 2005).

Here is the list for assessing function of the PFM.

- **Consciousness:** Can the student land awareness in and sense their pelvic landscape? Can the student self-direct their practice effectively? Does the student have adequate information about pelvic health and function? These three questions exist on a continuum, and we can seek to continually enhance a student's ability to focus, feel, self-guide, and learn about their body and pelvic bowl through yoga therapy.

- **Coordination**: How well can the student breathe with a three-dimensional excursion in the core cylinder, including awareness of the PFM? Can they demonstrate efficient motor coordination and timing in a variety of movement contexts?

- **Endurance:** Defined as the ability of muscles to endure a load or demand over time, to provide continual or repeated contractions over time, or to resist, withstand, or recover from fatigue, injury, or trauma. Does the student exhibit sufficient endurance-based fitness (globally and locally in the PFM) to do what they desire in daily life?

- **Strength:** Defined as the ability of muscles to exert maximal force in the short term. Does the student exhibit adequate whole-body movement strength? And localized pelvic strength? Local-pelvic strength could be measured through internal self-assessment and/or demonstrated by continence during heavy lifting, coughing, and other relatively high-load activities. The student could attempt to quantify their PFM strength with the terms absent, weak, normal, or strong (Messelink *et al.* 2005).
- **Relaxation:** Defined as the muscle's ability to rest completely and consciously, until context changes to warrant activation. Includes ability to reverse Kegel or gentle bearing-down action evidenced by eccentric lengthening of the whole team of pelvic muscles. Can the student feel when the pelvic muscles are tense or not relaxed? Can they consciously let go and relax the PFM when intended? Does the student overall feel calm, grounded, and at ease in their body? The student can also self-assess visually or sense kinesthetically for a "dropping" or "bulging" quality of the pelvic floor as it responds to a full, deep inhalation. Lastly, a student might label their voluntary relaxation of the PFM as absent, partial, or complete (Messelink *et al.* 2005).

Consciousness, or increasing the awareness and felt sense of one's pelvic floor, as well as providing pelvic-health education, offers its gifts to every person willing to embark on this journey. Many students can benefit from guided imagery, anatomical details, gentle and loving self-touch, and other creative ways to invite wisdom and understanding into their pelvic bowl. For students who've become hyperfixated on their pelvis, who have a hard time focusing there, or who experience pain and sensitization, we might introduce this kind of attentive relationship to other parts of the body first, and use some of the same tools like self-touch, affirmation, or guided imagery to dampen the pain response, desensitize certain areas, and calm their concerns. Let's remember that dissociation or difficulties with connecting to pelvic awareness may very well be serving a purpose, and trust our student to set the pace.

When a client presents with an overactive pelvic floor, a smart place to start is often to focus on restoring three-dimensional breath excursions, nervous-system down-regulation (relaxation), and mobility in the hips, lower extremities, pelvic floor, and anywhere else it seems needed based on our physical assessment. For example, they may need thoracic mobility to improve the whole spinal-pelvic relationship in motion, or they may find more freedom in their pelvic bowl after enhancing ankle and foot health to improve how their body receives ground reaction forces. We may assess that certain large muscles need to be strengthened for the pelvic floor to be able to "let go" more appropriately. The bulk of their practice, for the first phase and even later when progressing into more active practices, may remain focused on efficiency and maintaining breath excursion throughout a variety of contexts, closing each practice with a luxurious rest to inhibit the (perhaps longstanding or lifelong) habit of unnecessary holding, guarding, or tension.

Other clients presenting with an underactive pelvic floor may need more active practices, some standing postures, or specific pelvic-floor coordination activities for them to regain command and contractibility of the pelvic floor and surrounding muscles. Of course, these students can also benefit from customized mobility exercises or stretches and a closing relaxation to neutralize the effort of the practice and allow the pelvic floor to return to a calm resting state. They may also need encouragement to increase their daily physical activity or add regular walking to their routine to condition their whole body and train the pelvic floor dynamically, in varied movement contexts.

Much like the five koshas in the panchamaya model provide a road map for us to assess and assist a student in their journey toward health, meaning, and fulfillment as an individual, the five qualities in Figure 8.1 focus on the physical needs of the pelvic floor itself. When muscles have all that they need functionally, it supports the health of the entire system, the whole person.

For many of the clients I've supported, consciousness and relaxation take up the main stage role, with coordination playing a close co-star. Endurance and strength-training goals need more discernment and assessment around both whether they're appropriate for each student and how to apply these goals uniquely for their best results. This is where working hand in hand with a multidisciplinary team can be so wonderful to cross reference each other's plans and reinforce the learning and progress of the student. Collaborative care allows each provider to stay in their zone of genius – clinicians with a targeted, supervised PFM training plan and adjunct therapies, and yoga therapists supporting the whole person with a honed lens toward pelvic health.

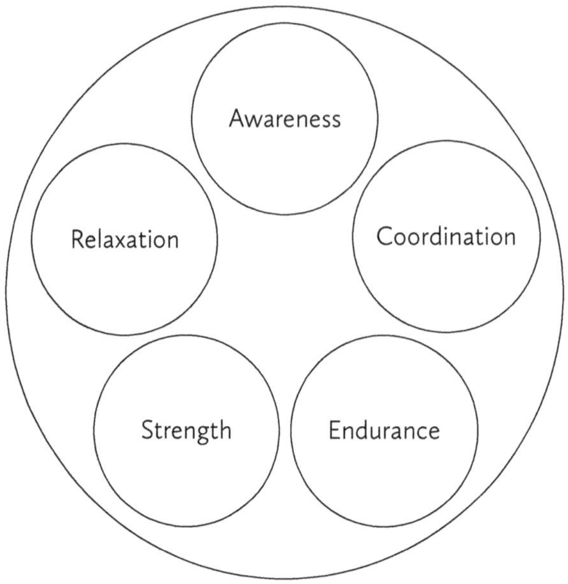

Figure 8.1: Adventures in PFM function

To better illustrate the difference between muscular endurance and muscular strength, let's take running as an example. One student with adequate endurance for low loads or long durations of low demand may be able to walk or hike for miles without any symptoms but experience leaking immediately anytime they attempt to jog or run. The additional ground reaction forces from running pose a higher demand momentarily with each stride – and the PFM are not yet able to withstand that *amount of force*, so they leak. This student could potentially benefit from a strength-based practice and gradual, progressive training into greater impact loads, guided by their symptoms.

Another student may be able to jog or run, not experiencing any leaking at the start. They can handle the increased ground reaction forces at the beginning, but experience leaking after two miles or around 20–25 minutes. Their PFM *cannot endure* those high forces and "fail" in terms of continence as they fatigue. They may benefit from progressive training for running while also targeting isometric and dynamic endurance postures (while maintaining full breath excursions, of course) in their home practice.

Both students above would likely receive continued benefit by including breath awareness, relaxation and down-training, and active recovery in their "running" training program, while using asana to enhance functional relationships in their movement. (A skilled clinician could also help optimize their pelvic-floor function locally.) This is an oversimplified example in some ways, as there can be many different factors in play for a student to be able to run efficiently, free of pelvic symptoms. I hope this example helps you grasp the concepts of endurance and strength, and start to understand how the yoga-therapy practice for these students would need to be different.

Further considerations

In the list below, I use the term Kegel as a catch-all for the various techniques described thus far (Kegel, mula bandha, ashwini mudra, and PFM engagement or training). This isn't an exhaustive list of contraindications and instead gives a few concrete examples of when to avoid actively training the PFM until the student can receive adequate assessment from a pelvic specialist (Dufour *et al.* 2018; Hanno *et al.* 2015; Vandyken *et al.* 2020).

- Do not suggest Kegels to folks with overactive or suspected overactive PFM.
- Avoid suggesting Kegels to students with bladder pain syndrome or interstitial cystitis.
- In general, do not recommend Kegels for students experiencing urgency and frequency without first getting the advice of their pelvic specialist.
- If Kegels cause any pain, distress, or exacerbation of symptoms, instruct your student to stop and seek a clinician's support.

Experiential practices

Let's look now at a handful of practices that may serve *most* women well. With the high prevalence of overactive PFM (Dufour *et al.* 2018) and the ongoing stressors of daily life that perpetuate this non-relaxing quality, we'll focus on restoring baseline awareness and coordination. Not to mention, we know that a muscle needs room to move to contract effectively – so I've made a generalization here that focuses on down-training and relaxation as the foundation for all activity or strengthening to come. Folks with too little PFM activity may still benefit from the practices below, especially the jellyfish practice, as it asks them to gently start enlivening the pelvic tissues in coordination with the breath.

Once you've established a student's capacity to focus their attention and sense their body, they may find they are served by a more localized approach to increase interoception of the PFM. Remember that addressing whole-body health will serve pelvic function, and a global-systemic and local-pelvic approach will likely work hand in hand to best meet your client's needs. Also, if there seems to be confusion or disconnection with these strategies, you may wish to circle back to Chapters 4 and 5, using examples therein as inspiration for your client's practice.

The first two practices provided are intended to be generally safe and useful for most women, most of the time, and for most diagnoses. Relaxation and circumferential, smooth breath excursions can serve everyone's pelvic health.

Voluntary PFM relaxation

This one is simple, in theory. Throughout the day, check in with your body using the baseline awareness exercise detailed in Chapter 1. Notice what you feel and what parts of the body beg your attention and care. Anytime you become aware of tension, give yourself a metaphorical pat on the back – you can't release tension that you don't even know exists!

Once you recognize a holding pattern, move that part of your body, touch, massage, or stretch it gently, and then acknowledge if there's any improvement. You can do this process globally (anywhere in your body that warrants more ease in place of tension) or locally (within the pelvic bowl directly). You're training yourself how to voluntarily override tension and choose relaxation.

When noticing tension within the pelvic muscles or around the bones of the pelvis, you can encourage them through imagery to soften, melt, and dissolve into the seat under you. Feel your sit bones spreading, and release the muscles around your tailbone. Let your seat feel broad, calm, and rooted. Feel how your breathing and the rest of your body likely respond with gratitude, softening as they trust your calm foundation.

Keep in mind that recurring, persistent patterns of tension may point toward musculoskeletal imbalances, motor-recruitment issues or misuse, complex and varied psycho-emotional factors, sensitization or a nervous-system state of stress or threat, breathing habits, or an underlying pathology, so get to the root cause(s) of the tension whenever possible. Muscle tension is an output, and many different inputs can contribute to the pattern either persisting or resolving. Give thanks that you can become aware and create change.

Jellyfish breathing for core cylinder coordination

I adore jellyfish and find they conveniently give an effective image for the fluid action of the PFM, as shown in Figure 8.2. This metaphor could be used to cue the movement of the thoracic diaphragm, as well as the pelvic diaphragm – remember, they work in concert with each other.

Find a comfortable position in which you feel well supported and at ease. Notice your breathing, allowing the inhalation to move the ribs laterally and posteriorly, bringing the breath and its influence downward through the torso. During the inhalation, the jellyfish or irregular dome shape of the pelvic muscles will flatten and descend, spreading the tendrils outward in all directions, free to float apart. As you begin to exhale, the current of the oceanic breath draws the jellyfish upward, restoring its curved dome shape and trailing the tendrils smoothly below it – a sense of calm closure and gathering toward center. Breathe here for a few moments, feeling your entire torso, ribcage, and pelvic bowl moving in harmony.

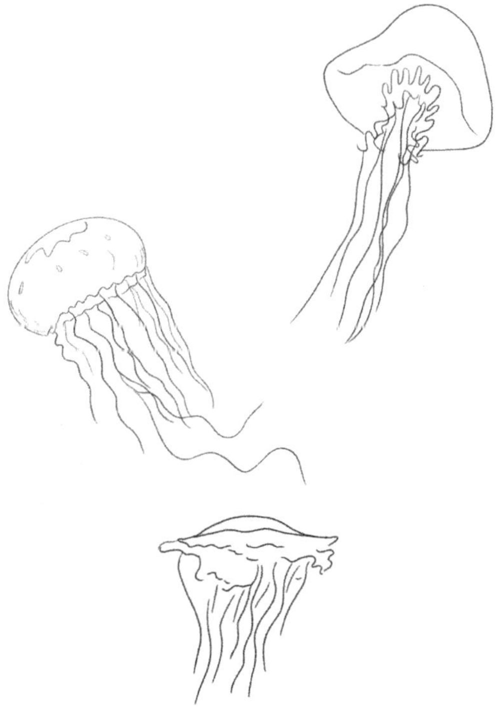

Figure 8.2: Jellyfish

When you're complete or wish to rest, let your breathing return to a quiet, natural rhythm. Rest. Appreciate this magic body you get to experience. You could also add self-touch or the gentle use of props, as described in Chapter 5, to enhance your capacity to feel the pelvic tissues respond. If you find this becomes effortful or forced, drop 50% of your effort, both physical and mental.

Trust that it'll become clearer with practice, and feel free to try this in a variety of positions.

Explore jellyfish breathing the next time you get in a pool. You can hook your arms or chest over a floating support to become weightless, letting your legs trail behind you like the silky tendrils of the jellyfish.

The next two practices will likely be more effective when prefaced with some baseline education around the mechanics of pressure management and need only be applied during a momentary, short-term demand like right before a sneeze or cough. After the high-pressure demand subsides, one can return to coordinated, calm breathing and sensing an overall, voluntary referencing of inner safety and relaxation.

Sneeze pee strategies

FEEL A SNEEZE AND WANT TO SQUEEZE? BUT FIRST – INHALE

When we feel like we're at risk for leaks, it can be tempting to just put our entire pelvic region on hard lockdown. We've hopefully already established how ineffective and counterproductive that can be, so I'll share a different strategy. First, a quick story.

> Sarah started working with me privately when she was just starting her second trimester of her second pregnancy. She'd already been experiencing stress incontinence, as well as pelvic girdle and hip pain. She felt disconnected from her body, her ability to trust herself, and even her baby to a degree – she thought private yoga therapy could help her after trying some of my online group classes. During her first vaginal birth, she had felt "a lot of pain, and a lot of fear." The emotion was still fresh and she had tears in her eyes as she retold her first birth story. She desperately wanted to do all she could to have a different, more peaceful, and satisfying second birth.
>
> The only strategy I taught her early on for the stress incontinence was how to breathe well, even as baby grew and took up prime breathing real estate. We focused her attention and self-touch on the circumference of her ribs, making sure she got expansion in her sides and back, and helped her to focus on allowing the inhale to descend and encourage pelvic-floor relaxation. I asked her to do her best to take this full-volume, 360-degree inhale in the moment before a sneeze or cough, and it worked! She was

very reliably continent throughout her pregnancy with no pelvic-floor training or Kegel strategies. All she needed was deep breaths (and some basic anatomy education and a daily restorative practice). Her hips also stayed relatively content (allowing her sleep to improve, which pregnant women everywhere know is a gift) with simple movements, making sure that she did some circling, tail wagging, and pelvic tilts almost daily.

Months later, when we met for her first postpartum session, she shared with eyes glistening and smile beaming about how sweet, calm, and empowering her birth experience was. She'd been able to communicate well with her partner throughout the intensity of labor and felt proud that she had done good work to recover her sense of agency, her voice, and her trust in her body. It brings me such immense joy to see a woman's spirit intact and thriving, especially in the postpartum window. From there forward, we worked together to resource and nourish her, accommodate her milk-filled breasts with modifications to her favorite restorative postures, and gradually rebuild strength.

Review this rib circumference awareness now, feeling how your inhalation expands your entire trunk, readying the pelvic floor and abdominal wall for the spontaneous condensing, recoiling action of the exhalation. You might support your imagery with self-touch, wrapping your arms around you like a hug to feel your side ribs or placing your hands on the back of your waist laterally near the floating ribs. Instead of focusing on tension, we might first ensure that we've allowed the expansion and relaxation of the PFM with a deep inhalation before the momentary impact of a sneeze.

"THE KNACK"

We've made it to the final practice in this series, and the only one with a voluntary contraction. The "knack" is a well-timed and strong pelvic contraction (PHRC 2019), which may effectively close the orifices within the pelvic floor and can prevent leaks. (While I'm not referring here to the 1979 song "My Sharona" by a band called The Knack, I can't help but imagine how fun it might be to practice pelvic-floor engagement to that sweet bass line.)

I don't recommend this as a long-term strategy. Ideally, we endeavor to restore automatic, reflexive function so we don't need to think about it – it happens on its own. Just apply this right before a momentary increase in IAP or downward force like with sneezing, coughing, blowing your nose, or right before exertion with lifting *only* as needed.

Investigating through advanced imagery

If a client has trouble sensing their pelvic floor, or feeling how it functions dynamically, it can be useful to get more nuanced and specific with our cues to guide their attention in novel ways. Based on what the client shares with you during the initial conversations, or what you discern might relate best to remedying their specific symptoms, you can hand select from the list below, always tailoring the cue to your student. You can also involve them in this process of refining language and pelvic awareness, trialing a few cues to see which one they can best access or which creates the desired result of shifting posture or movement during their practice or symptom management over time.

- Differentiate the closing action from the lifting action, and then put the two together.
- Initiate engagement from the clitoris, the vagina, the anus, or all three together.
- Explore spatial intent, like a slightly anterior trajectory for engagement when addressing cystocele versus a more posterior focus for hemorrhoids.
- Explore the four quadrants statically (sit, stand, lie down) and dynamically (during a wide squat inquiry) to observe patterns.
- Explore contracting from each of the four quadrants independently or moving from front to back, back to front, and side to side to improve dexterity and coordination of PFM.
- Feel your engagement begin superficially and smoothly move deeper sequentially; reverse the pattern to start deep and then sequentially include the superficial layers.

In closing

Remember the self-reflection prompts woven throughout the book? Those questions can help unlock elements of a student's belief system and identity that relate to their pelvic-healing journey. Although we don't explicitly revisit these inquiries here, I trust you value and hold them with as much esteem as these physical strategies. Other key elements like community and social support, home practice and lifestyle, and visioning one's future will be addressed in future chapters to promote continued exploration and synthesis of this experience.

Students learn through inquiry to gently coax the wisdom within their body to reveal itself, while the safe harbor of our presence provides a soft place to land with questions and doubts. We start somewhere useful, designing a customized practice for the person in front of us – and then we stay the course. See what comes. These practices need time to take root and flourish.

We can always reassess and course correct. In this way, we welcome the opportunity to get scientific and look at all the variables in play, and selectively fine-tune *one at a time* to see if it drives a different result. Of course, there's no magic yoga-therapy formula – this is an art and a science glued together by the therapeutic alliance. Every person we meet presents like a one-of-a-kind kaleidoscope of their own needs, history, comorbidities, desires, fears, lifestyle considerations, and relationship to exercise. Kegels, for far too long, attempted to step in and fill the gap for all things pelvic health – now that we know better, we can do better.

As yoga therapists, we focus on function and increasing awareness where the light of consciousness seems dimmed or darkened. We may not definitively know a student's baseline pelvic-floor tone, or qualitative pelvic-floor habits according to a clinical evaluation, and yet our students come to us seeking wisdom. How do we bridge this apparent gap? We practice humbly not knowing. Researching. Sharing with our mentors. Observing. Communicating. Through what you're learning in this book and further integration of your other studies, combined with your personal journey and first-hand experience, I hope there are both more questions arising (as we choose to be forever students if we teach) and some useful answers starting to weave their way into your body, mind, and professional work as we close Part 2 together.

We can help demystify the pelvic floor and open a world of agency, context and discernment, and compassionate playfulness. Let your curiosity guide you forward.

> May we welcome in what we don't yet know.
> May we trust our growing competency and discernment.
> May we thrive together through this teacher-student relationship.

PART 3

HOW DO WE DELIVER PELVIC YOGA THERAPY?

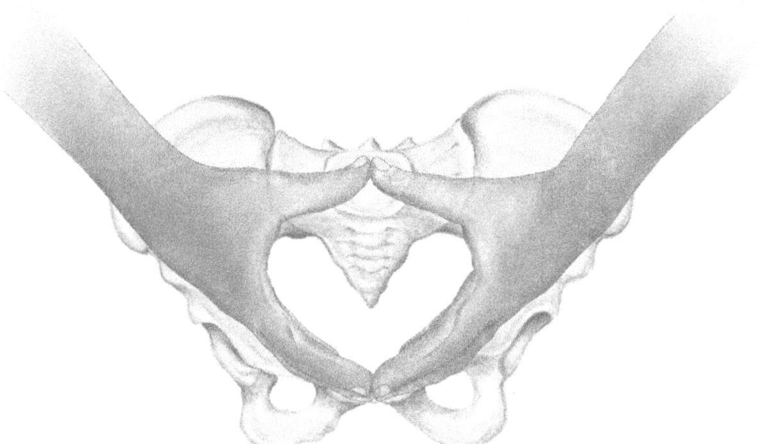

CHAPTER 9

Discovering

One of the hardest lessons for us as humans may be sitting with the unknown. We despise uncertainty and cling to control, deriving comfort from having answers and making plans. Yet this is the only way to see clearly – to surrender assumptions and interrupt patterns, and welcome ourselves to this lived practice with an open mind and tender, willing heart to see where and how our body leads us.

The therapeutic alliance creates a safe container that allows students to begin this loving investigation. They return to foundational practices, eventually coming to realize they've been renewed. The same poses feel different, movements that used to cause pain now feel neutral or induce pleasurable sensations, and the way they view themselves and the world expands. They've changed, and yet, they haven't. We've simply helped them become conscious in their intent and actions, and better understand the functions of their body. Through this comprehensive path of yoga as therapy, students can access inner wisdom that's been there all along.

We return many times to assessment principles, continually refining and co-creating with our student. Delivering yoga therapy requires responsiveness. What may appear to be spontaneous, intuitive wisdom from masterful teachers may be sourced from vast evidence in their somatic memory bank, stored up from countless hours of practice and study, and from working closely with teachers and mentors. They've built discernment by moving through the unknown into action. May we continually rediscover and mature the efficacy of our presence, to wholly witness each sovereign woman that asks for help.

All the content leading up to this chapter serves to provide sound anatomical referencing, context, and discernment – both experiential and intellectual – of yoga as therapy for people with pelvic symptoms. We now step over a threshold and take up our seat as a facilitator of the process of change. Transmission of the yogic way of life must take up residence in the student's lived experience.

They seek our support to end their pelvic suffering and restore thriving. How we customize their plan depends on getting an accurate baseline of the whole person.

What I've found through working with pelvic-health-minded clients is the tricky reality that not everyone can access or feels open to internal examination and clinical diagnosis. Pelvic-floor specialists and yoga therapists alike need to be able to trust what they see, feel, and perceive (as well as decipher what clients disclose verbally) to come to appropriate conclusions. Remember, also, the state of one's pelvic function does not always correlate directly with diagnosis – there's no one-size-fits-all approach to pelvic care. We don't treat conditions through yoga therapy – we support the people experiencing them. My hope is that after reading this chapter, you will feel better equipped to meet your students where they are and intelligently select practices that will make a positive impact on their lives and pelvic health.

We now enter a process of keen attentiveness, ready to discover the individual entrusting us with their care and stories. In this chapter, we'll cover in broad brushstrokes the intake and assessment process, fully recognizing the limitations of teaching this process via written word. This chapter is not comprehensive or exhaustive, as entire books have been created for clinical assessment and client education protocols. Please take what's given here as a template to support you in getting started with clients or refining and standardizing existing best practices. Make these assessment models work for you and the women you serve.

Stages of the intake process

When gathering information from a new client, it can be helpful to have clear, comprehensive systems or forms in place to make it easy for clients to divulge all that may be helpful for us to know about them as their yoga therapist. Two possible assessments include the *Cozean Pelvic Dysfunction Screening Protocol* and *The Primary Care Pelvic Health Screen*. Both can be found in Appendix A. Questionnaires can assist students in disclosing current symptoms and help them self-reflect. Clients may feel embarrassed to share in detail, or they simply may not know what information to share or that certain signs or symptoms could be connected. We can also acknowledge our own growth edge to speak frankly about intimate topics. Thorough intake forms prompt necessary dialogue between student and teacher.

I developed the Pelvic Yoga Therapy Survey for use with group classes and private clients. It not only screens for whether physical symptoms exist, but also can gauge other key aspects related to client satisfaction, like self-efficacy with exercise and home practice, level of stress related to their pelvic health, their ability to relax and resource pleasure, and body image. This survey is included in Appendix A. You can also access the Pro Use Guide to support implementation of this survey on the author's website at www.cheridostal.com.

During session, we practice active listening, mirroring back to the client what they share and asking them to expand on certain parts of their story when we feel it may be useful. Open-ended questions help steer the dialogue toward key topics yet leave plenty of space for the client to self-reflect and answer candidly with what they feel arising as relevant. Consider using questions that begin with who, what, when, where, why, and how, or statements that ask them to "share more" or help you better understand their experience.

Building motivation and buy-in to the therapeutic relationship can be served by mirroring and closed-ended questions. For example, once you've given space to the client's medical and multifaceted personal histories, you can summarize why or how they came to be in your office or clinic. When mirroring, you may also consider reframing what they shared in a negative context (I don't want to keep peeing my pants in public) into a positive goal (I hear your desire to feel continent and trust your body, especially to go about your life in public feeling confident again). Restating goals helps ensure you're on the same page.

Sharing briefly what approach you feel will be most beneficial gives them confidence that you have a starting point, if not a plan, beginning to map in your mind for how you'll help them, and in what timeline. Then, a simple closed-ended question can encourage trust and cultivate program adherence, like asking, "Do you feel ready to dive in with this plan together?" People like knowing where they're going and why – as yoga therapists we can help them develop their tapas, or devotional focus, with intentional dialogue strategies.

Once the intake conversation feels complete, we move into physical assessment and breath observation to collect nonverbal clues from how they move, take direction, and breathe. These pieces of the puzzle often further clarify or strengthen our plans, and we can continue dialogue to gather information about what they feel during movements. Some or all the assessment tools in this chapter could also constitute the student's first home practice or be returned to during symptom recurrences or as a grounding familiarity to maintain results.

Lastly, once you've met with a client, discern whether they've assembled their care team. Any time we feel out of our depth, we're first bound to do no harm, remembering the yoga principle of ahimsa. We can keep the physical assessment simplified or offer a guided meditation or relaxation posture to complete the initial session. This affords time to research on the client's behalf or consult with mentors before designing their home practice. Of course, we can also request physician clearance or a pelvic-floor evaluation before proceeding with additional sessions. (Review the referral indicators in Chapter 7.)

Voice observation

As we talk to our client, we can observe the quality, pace, and pitch of their voice. This doesn't need to become a formalized assessment but may provide us with subtle clues about the state of their nervous system, their personality, and how certain topics may be activating. For example, we may hear higher-pitched, fast-paced speech that sounds constricted when discussing their medical history and then notice a much slower, melodic quality in their voice after moving through a few postures. This could also be reflective of establishing rapport over the course of the session, a sign that the client feels safe in our presence.

There may be moments that instigate a restricted quality or a distinct change in sound, or even create hesitation as if they've momentarily lost their voice. We may see visible tension rising into their neck and shoulders, or a quickening of their breath while they speak about an aspect of their history. When we hear constriction, effort, or higher (than their norm) pitches of sound, we may conjecture that their pelvic floor has heightened in effort as well.

Vocal prosody gives clues about the person's affect or attitude through aspects of communication like rhythm, pace, and intonation. Basically, the same words can mean something very different depending on how they sound, how they are spoken. Remember, social engagement can serve to strengthen the ventral vagal complex of parasympathetic functioning, which can include speaking, eye contact and facial expressions, and listening to human speech (Dana 2020, pp.85–87). Through therapeutic alliance, we hope to witness a client owning their stories and speaking about them with more equanimity and ease. We may hear more easeful resonance, as if their whole body is in support of their authentic expression.

On a more intuitive level, we may register in our own embodiment a feeling of dis-ease and agitation with one client speaking, while another's voice feels warm and easeful. Particularly useful might be when we notice a distinct change in someone's quality of voice or communication during session, and we may gently help them recognize the change within themselves and better understand the underlying source material – or how to return to a more regulated state. When these instinctual observations present as a reliable pattern, we may use that information to guide conversation choices, whether we disclose the observation to the client or not, and perhaps to select affirmations or mantra.

Sample movement assessments

Please explore the assessment strategies below in your own body, reading the commentary after each one to build context and discernment for client assessments and home-practice development. Trust yourself to modify, omit, or add other creative assessments based on your client's history and goals, and how they describe the impact of their symptoms on activities of daily living. Again, this is by no means a comprehensive assessment, so consider what you observe in these movements along with intake and history, pelvic self-assessment data, and what they report during session. Even subtle changes in their facial expressions can indicate importance or prompt us to inquire further. Together, start to identify patterns that can help identify the suspected PFM baseline and overall movement efficiency.

Consider also *how* you might elicit a client's feedback. We practice observing movement qualities visually, we can imagine or trial what we see in our own body for kinesthetic conjecture, and when appropriate we may observe through touch. Let's remember that we cannot feel the student's sensations for them. We need to ask.

Sometimes, what they sense happening hits the mark as far as where we'd expect them to feel effort or stretch sensations based on "textbook" recruitment patterns. What they say might align with what we think we see. Other times, what they share gives invaluable clues about the state of their attention, their mindset about movement, recruitment strategies or compensations they've adopted, cues they may have learned, and whether they enjoy or dislike an activity. Also, note when they express an inability to articulate what they feel or to sense anything at all. Here are a few sample questions to help you gather relevant feedback.

Where did you feel the most sensation in your body during that movement?

What kind of sensation was it?

Can you tell me or touch where you felt the muscular effort of that posture?

How do you feel after, compared with before we did this movement?

While a few of these physical assessments require getting on the floor, you could adapt the principles and movements into other base positions, like seated in a chair or standing, when needed. The first two begin supine with CRP, which you can find in Chapter 6.

Assessment 1: Pelvic tilt from supine

From CRP, feel how your pelvis meets the floor. Notice where you feel pressure or contact, how much curvature you feel in your lumbar spine, and any places of heightened sensation or muscular effort before you begin to move, as seen in Figures 9.1 and 9.2.

Keeping your pelvis on the floor, begin to tilt it forward and back. Imagine your pelvis rolling forward toward your feet and then curling in toward your trunk. Feel how your lumbar curvature changes with each of the movements. Repeat this a handful of times, and then rest in stillness and take note of changes from your baseline.

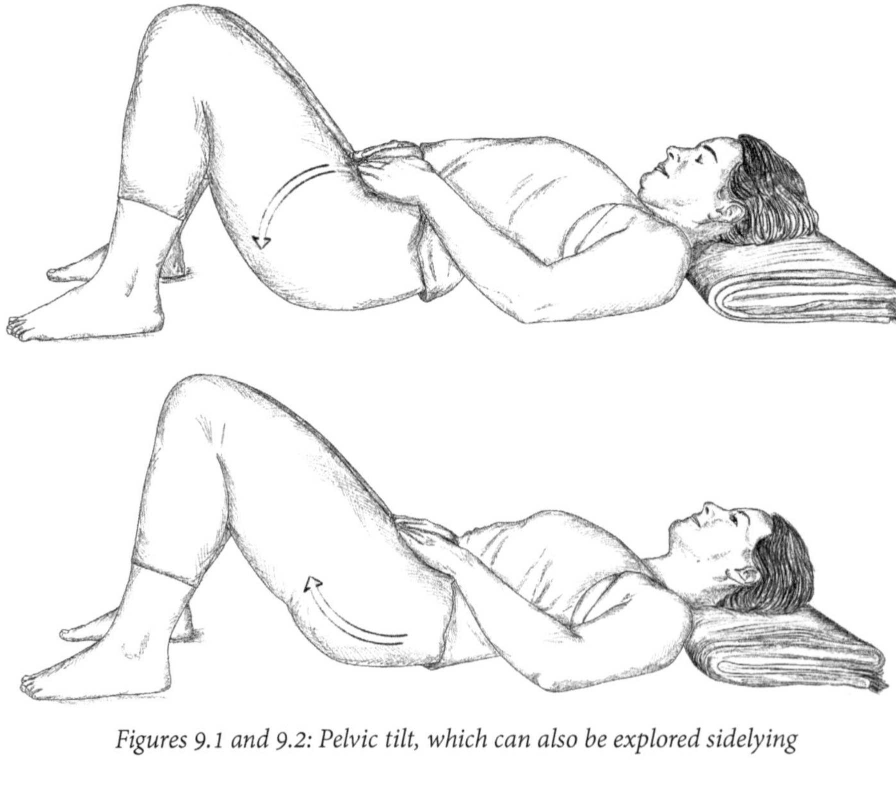

Figures 9.1 and 9.2: Pelvic tilt, which can also be explored sidelying

GOAL

Localized, focused movement of the pelvis.

WHAT WE HOPE TO SEE

- Ability to keep the pelvis grounded on the mat rather than a bridging action that lifts the hips.
- Ability to move smoothly in both directions versus a biased function in one direction.
- Maintenance of midline awareness and the pelvis moving clearly in the sagittal plane.
- Quiet, natural breathing or coordinated breathing with the movement.
- The pelvic tilt movement influences a subtle nodding motion of the skull.

WHAT WE MAY SEE INSTEAD

- Extraneous muscle effort in other parts of the body; using more effort than is needed.
- Gross, mechanical, choppy quality of movement or breathing; undifferentiated joints of lumbopelvic-hip complex (LPH).
- One direction of pelvic tilt receives more time, attention, or range of motion than the other; they move only in one direction and return to neutral absence of the alternate pelvic movement.
- The neck and head are held rigidly in place; absence of the subtle, small nodding response.
- See if what's observed here correlates as a reliable pattern with how they move in Assessment 3, as well as other postures that move the spine or pelvis similarly.

Assessment 2: Single leg march

Start again from CRP, this time bringing your hands or thumbs into each of the hip creases. Flex at the hip joint to approximately 90 degrees to lift one foot off the floor. Lower your foot back to the floor and then repeat that side a few times. Notice what you feel underneath your own hands. Do you feel superficial effort in your groin, hip flexors, or quadriceps, like thick bands of muscle or tendon bulging up into your touch? Do you feel a soft deepening of the hip crease as your leg lifts and the foot leaves the floor?

Pause for a moment with both feet on the floor. Now complete the single leg march into hip flexion on the second side, moving through a few repetitions at least. Do you feel one side behaves differently than the other? Use Figure 9.3 as a guide.

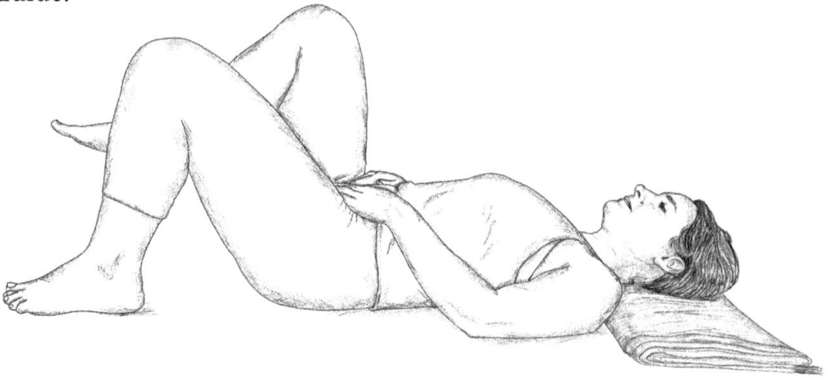

Figure 9.3: Single leg march

GOAL

Efficient stabilization of the pelvis and trunk with hip flexion.

WHAT WE HOPE TO SEE

- Maintenance of midline awareness and the pelvis remains relatively still in all planes.
- Ease and relaxation in most areas of the body – smooth, targeted intent and action at the hip.
- Quiet, natural breathing or coordinated breathing with the movement.
- Deep, soft, relaxed hip creases as the thigh comes vertical to approximately 90 degrees hip flexion; the knee remains bent to minimize leverage and maximize efficiency at the hip.

WHAT WE MAY SEE INSTEAD

- Extraneous muscle effort in other parts of the body; using more effort than is needed.
- The student attempts to straighten the knee or move from a long lever action.
- The pelvis rolls toward one side or hikes up toward the waist as compensation upon the foot lifting.

- Breath holding as a stabilization strategy; doming, coning, bearing down during lifting.
- One side differs greatly from the other in terms of range or quality of motion, or creates visible compensations elsewhere in their body.
- Consider what you see here as a prerequisite for any other supine "core training" or as clues indicating necessary release or repatterning work.
- If this assessment plays out well, consider completing an active straight leg raise from supine, a seated hip flexion observation, or a single leg balance assessment from standing as possible progressions, depending on the client's needs and goals.

Assessment 3: Cat-cow from tabletop

Take a moment to shift into a kneeling table or quadruped position. Use a blanket for cushioning under the knees if desired. First, find what feels like your neutral spinal alignment and spend a few breaths there.

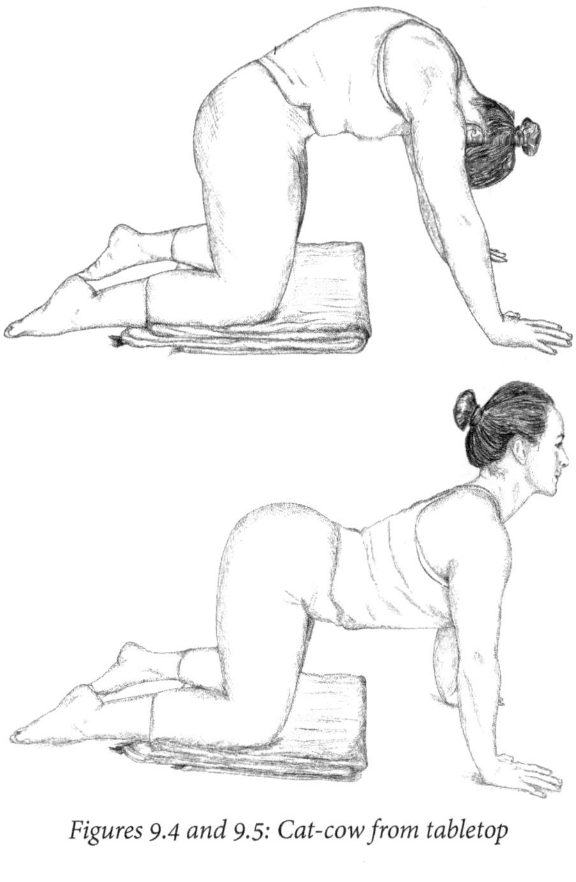

Figures 9.4 and 9.5: Cat-cow from tabletop

After observing this weight-bearing posture in a static context, add movement of the whole spine. Let your eyes look down toward your belly and feel your spine round into flexion. Go the opposite direction into extension and let your eyes scan forward or upward into space. See Figures 9.4 and 9.5. Move back and forth a few times as deeply as you feel comfortable, and then return to what feels like your neutral tabletop position.

GOAL

Coordinated movement of the skull, spine, and pelvis ("head-tail" connection).

WHAT WE HOPE TO SEE

- Easeful transition to table; comfort and ease in active weight bearing.
- Relatively level, organized alignment of the shoulders, hips, and spinal elongation.
- Quiet, natural breathing or coordinated breathing with the movement.
- Smooth, coordinated movement of the entire spine, skull, and pelvis.
- Quality of pelvic movement revolving around the relatively stable femur heads here may hint at the state or coordination of PFM.

WHAT WE MAY SEE INSTEAD

- Reduced, guarded, or inhibited movement of the pelvis or any area of the spine.
- Breath holding as they attempt to coordinate movement; shallow or labored breathing.
- Lack of proprioceptive awareness making the movement choppy, disorganized, or incomplete; could also present as excess lordosis (sway back), forward head posture and/or excess kyphosis in the thoracic area, and other compensations.
- Consider what you see here as prerequisites to repattern before progressing or clues for what you may then observe in standing asanas, table rocking (Chapter 11), and plank pose.

Assessment 4: Half dog at the wall (variation of adho mukha svanasana)

Standing up, place your palms on a wall in front of you at about shoulder height with your elbows bent. Actively press your hands into the wall and step your feet back, folding at the hips to arrive in a shape that feels like 90 degrees. Transition in and out of the pose a few times.

Now find your 90-degree half-dog position (see Figure 9.6) and pause there for a few breaths. When you're ready to come out of the pose, walk your legs forward and return to standing.

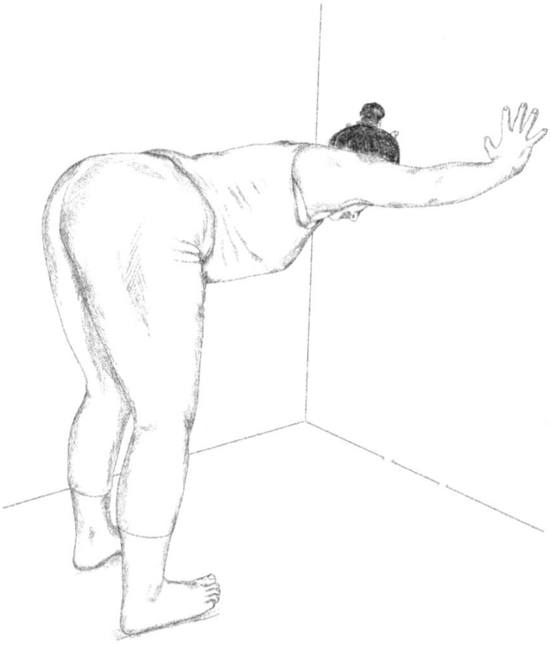

Figure 9.6: Half dog at the wall

GOAL

Coordination of closed-chain movement and axial elongation; assessing hip flexion.

WHAT WE HOPE TO SEE

- Easeful transition to standing; comfort and ease in active weight bearing.
- Active, yielding support of both upper and lower extremities for a smooth

transition in and out of the posture and efficiency and sustainability while holding the posture.

- Quiet, natural breathing or coordinated breathing with the movement.
- Clear, 90 degree hip flexion and axial elongation, possibly indicating coordination of LPH complex, PFM allowing length, and skillful proprioception.

WHAT WE MAY SEE INSTEAD

- Lack of proprioceptive awareness making the movement choppy or disorganized.
- Breath holding as they attempt to coordinate movement; shallow or labored breathing.
- Unyielding lower extremities: moving in and out of the posture with locked knees or rigid ankles, possibly indicating PFM tension.
- Excess lordosis, excess shoulder flexion (sway back); the head may hang lower than the plane of the torso potentially indicating a lack of deep core awareness or support.
- Forward head posture and/or excess kyphosis in the thoracic spine, possibly coupled with posterior pelvic tilt or excess glute engagement, which may indicate PFM guarding or tension.
- Consider what you see here as prerequisites to repattern before progressing or clues for what you may then also observe in standing asanas, table rocking, planks, downward dog, and more.

Assessment 5: Side angle pose (parsvakonasana)

Clients who practice yoga may be familiar with this posture. If so, we could simply state that the next movement we'd like to observe is side angle pose, spending some time on each side as they normally would at home or in a class setting. Remember, sparse cues allow us to see their movement habits more objectively than if we talk them through how to do the posture.

When a client is new to yoga, however, we'll likely need to give them more instruction to complete this assessment. Consider giving a visual demonstration, with a few key concepts like starting in a wide stance and allowing the legs to come into a lunge, and then demonstrating the movement of the spine and hips into side angle pose. Show the second side, too, perhaps silently to allow them to take in visually the kinesthetic essence of the posture. Then ask if they feel ready to try it.

As yoga teachers, we likely know all the trappings of how to embellish this posture, for example arm positions, choosing a drishti or where the eyes gaze, and coming into binds with the arms. For the purposes of observational assessment, I suggest deliberately simplifying the instructions to focus on the lower extremities, observing how the pelvis and spine align. In Figure 9.7, I show the sacral angle with my hand to help you train your eye; showing your student this gesture may change how they perform the posture and create a misleading result. Try the sacrum self-touch for yourself, and then practice *seeing* this relationship in your students.

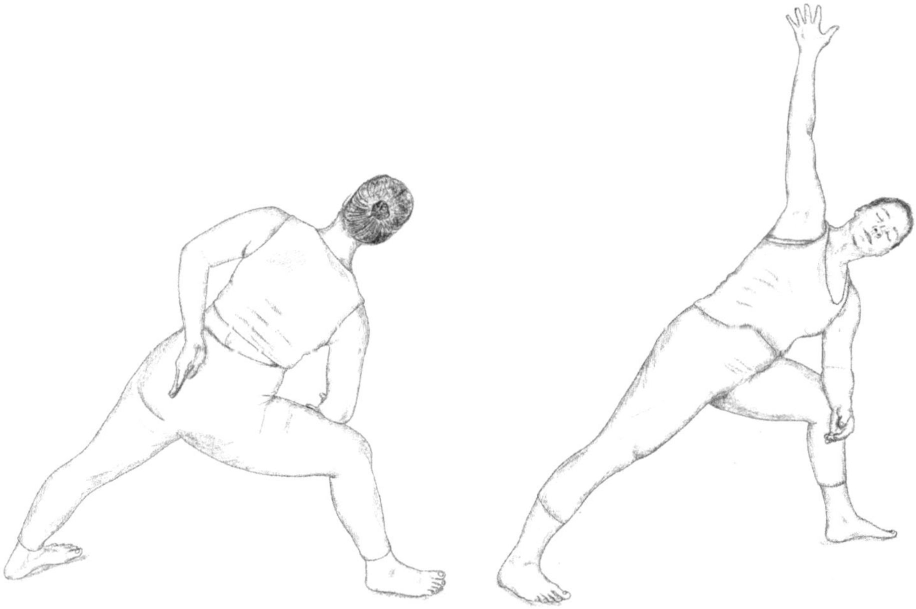

Figure 9.7: Side angle pose

GOAL

Global coordination, aligning the pelvis with axial elongation; stamina of the lower extremities.

WHAT WE HOPE TO SEE

- Easeful transition to a wide asymmetrical stance; comfort in active weight bearing.

- Active, yielding support of the lower extremities for a smooth transition in and out of the posture and sustained comfort while holding the posture; front knee and front foot aligned.
- Quiet, natural breathing or coordinated breathing with the movement.
- Moving from center: do they allow their pelvis to move into the shape of side angle pose?
- Clear axial elongation upon arrival in side angle pose, possibly indicating coordination of the LPH complex and PFM, and skillful proprioception.

WHAT WE MAY SEE INSTEAD

- Lack of proprioception making the movement choppy or disorganized; loss of balance.
- Breath holding as a stabilization strategy or while attempting to coordinate movement; doming, coning, bearing down during the pose; shallow or labored breathing.
- One side differs greatly from the other in terms of range or quality of motion, or creates visible compensations elsewhere in their body.
- Unyielding lower extremities: moving in and out of the posture with locked knees or rigid ankles, excess effort or tension in the limbs, possibly indicating PFM tension.
- The front knee collapsing into adduction and internal rotation, possibly indicating mobility restrictions or a habit of over-rotating the trunk and pelvis away from the front leg.
- A quality of passive weight or "collapse" in the trunk and hips, or a habit of overextending the spine, potentially indicating a lack of deep or anterior core awareness or support.
- The pelvis remains neutral or level with the floor rather than tipping to the diagonal (commonly observed as lateral flexion in the trunk toward the front leg), which may indicate or increase PFM guarding or tension; this could also simply show the way they learned to do this pose, in which case yoga therapy can provide education about pelvic alignment and its relationship to PFM activity as needed.

- Consider what you see here as prerequisites to repattern before progressing or clues for what you may then also observe in other standing asanas and functional movements.

During an initial assessment, we don't want to cue how to do the movement, or what we want to see or have them feel. Let them move independently with minimal guidance. If these same postures or movements later become woven into the home practice, we can give the client in-depth instruction about how to execute the movement and improve functional outcomes. The way the assessments have been written here give a glimpse of how you might cue them simply and objectively.

When working with clients who've had limited experience with yoga asana or physical exercise, some of what we may see as disorganization or compensation may simply indicate a need for kinesthetic learning and instruction – *not necessarily pathology*. When that's the case, trust the power of these simple exercises and layer in pelvic awareness, breathing, and other personalized cues to help them improve the quality of their movement experience.

With yogis, dancers, or athletes on the other hand, these assessments may be oversimplified and not allow us to see or perceive very much detail, as they may have a more practiced threshold of physical function. Select from their repertoire a few more dynamic or complex movements to use in your baseline physical assessment, observing for similar clues or patterns as described. Lastly, be sure efficiency has been established with these movements, using the "what we hope to see" sections as guidance to incrementally progress into the variations you'll meet in Chapter 11.

Breathing assessment

Observe how your client breathes throughout the postural assessments above. Gather information from a variety of contexts to discern any patterns that show up persistently or establish a threshold of their capacity to breathe well. For example, they may breathe easefully resting on the floor in CRP, but when cued to take deep breaths in standing, you observe a shallow, forceful, or paradoxical coordination pattern. Another example could be that the client appears to breathe efficiently in static tabletop but has a hard time coordinating their breath with movement or holds their breath as a strategy to stabilize themselves in the open-chain variation of a spinal balance (lifting the opposite arm and leg from tabletop). This can give you a way to plan exercise progressions and measure change outcomes later.

We can also give the student a moment of silence to relax as we observe where and how their body moves in response to the breath. To show change over time, we can attempt to capture an objective baseline measurement of respiration. One possibility would be counting the number of respirations in one minute. These suggestions are intended as a helpful starting point; a full training on assessment protocols is outside the scope of this book.

Assessing IAP management

The signs listed below can be applied to all physical and pranayama practices you observe and can guide your student during activities of daily living. These indications don't necessarily mean the activity is to be stopped altogether. Instead, they invite us to look more deeply, consider risk and benefit, and facilitate more awareness and efficient movement. For too long, these signs were pathologized, especially when related to postpartum exercise and diastasis recti. The body will only learn how to generate force and restore efficiency through progressive loads and by developing body and breath awareness. In short, we need to move and trust the process of helping our students return to activities they love! When these signs appear, dialogue with your client, reassess the movement or activity in question, and see how efficiency can be improved within or by altering the demand of the activity.

The following are IAP considerations:

- Doming – the abdominal wall broadly protrudes anteriorly.
- Coning – the abdominal wall more narrowly protrudes anteriorly, directly through the linea alba at the midline.
- Breath holding – note the position or at what approximate end range or repetition number when possible, to measure change over time.
- Bearing down or sensations of increased heaviness, pressure, or bulging; leaking of any kind or amount upon exertion.
- Compensation in other areas like neck tension, teeth grinding, or butt clenching (all very common!) may indicate that movement efficiency can be improved.

- Increased symptoms following an activity (usually noticed within about 24 hours).

Proactive self-care practices and compassionate inquiry can restore agency and revitalize awareness. In *Wild Feminine*, Kent encourages us to "learn the territory of [our] own root" (2011, p.45). For the self-assessment inquiries, I've distilled a variety of experiences to create this accessible starting point for a student's direct observation.

Pelvic self-assessment

When women have an intimate working knowledge of their own vulva – what it looks and feels like, they can share important information with us and with their medical providers about how they're doing, voice their concerns and questions more easily, and sometimes get earlier support for changes they witness. Using the pelvic self-assessment as a compassionate self-inquiry extension of their yoga practice, the student can seamlessly navigate an inner consent process that can bolster their capacity to communicate consent with partners and other healthcare providers. (To be clear, this occurs in the privacy of the student's home, not during a yoga-therapy session.) Women can transform the learning of pelvic anatomy from books or apps into first-hand wisdom. They tap into powerful sovereignty when not under anyone else's gaze or guidance, free to follow their own lead.

The pelvic self-assessment process may offer valuable information when working with a clinician is not accessible. If completing this internal assessment isn't a welcomed suggestion for your student, they may still find value in being guided through a baseline experience using the pelvic imagery or sensing strategies covered in Chapters 4 and 5 or by using external, fully clothed self-touch. We can practice detachment and accept their decision at face value, not expecting a reason for why they chose to decline.

As yoga professionals, we each need to sit with our embodied decision-making, also. If we feel hesitant, embarrassed, or afraid to offer the self-assessment option for any reason, it's okay. It may simply be a boundary we leave intact and respect, or it could represent an invitation for growth and reflection.

When a student gives a green-light response to the idea of seeing or touching their own perineum, we can provide them with guidance and instructions to support a positive experience. Your student will complete this take-home assignment independently. For our purposes and scope as yoga therapists, we'll request they focus on two simple intentions: 1) pure appreciation and acceptance for what they see, smell, and feel; 2) observing the quality of pelvic engagement and relaxation.

I've written the self-assessment exercises as instructions to the student in case you want to participate and as an example of how you might describe them to a student for their home practice. The entire process should be comfortable, or at least tolerable, honoring that some physical or emotional discomfort can be a welcome and necessary step in experiencing our intimate geography. Pause and allow yourself to exhale if there's any pain or if you feel your breath become shallow or muscles become tense. Take your time. When there's discomfort, see if you can modify pressure or the location or direction of touch, and let your breathing guide you. Finally, always use gentle touch, and even more so when approaching the top and bottom of the vaginal canal, making sure not to apply deep or firm pressure directly to the urethral or anorectal tissues at the midline.

Always wash your hands thoroughly with warm water and soap before and after this exercise. While sexual activity is often safe and may even provide benefit during pregnancy, it's best to check with your provider before completing an internal self-assessment. Also, wait until about eight weeks postpartum to perform an internal assessment. Be cleared by your provider for wound healing, incisions, or sutures, whether related to labor and delivery, gynecological surgery, or other procedures. Remember, scars serve a purpose, and there's good reason for us to let the tissues heal without interfering.

If you plan to complete this process now, please reference the Pelvic Self-Assessment Worksheet in Appendix A. This form was designed as a client education tool, giving space for them to record observations and questions to bring to their next appointment. Let's begin.

With a mirror

The sovereign act of seeing one's own vulva or genitals has become more normalized but still can present as a bit of a shock when suggested. We see our faces readily any time we pass a mirror or shop window; we gawk at our contours and form when working out all the *other* major muscle groups. Let's not reserve the visual imagery for an annual exam when this sacred territory is ours.

Find a comfortable position, perhaps in bed. I recommend wearing a long skirt or being naked waist down provided you'll be warm enough. Set an intention to allow yourself to rest into this inquiry, accepting and embracing all you see, smell, feel, and notice. Have your knees bent with the feet supported, either aligning the legs parallel or allow the thighs to abduct and move apart, resting into pillows. You can set the mirror against a wall or another prop to keep your hands free.

Notice all the colors, textures, and contours you see, perhaps identifying each part of your vulva by name silently or aloud. You may be able to observe subtle movements that coordinate with your breathing here. Play with different positions, angles, and be open to using touch if that feels supportive. Check in with your breathing and know you can pause anytime.

Next, visually observe your pelvic floor and genitals as you try a few rhythmic repetitions of pelvic engagement and complete rest. A few will suffice; rest when you feel it's time.

This is more an exercise in curiosity than "physical training," although you'll likely feel some increased awareness, maybe changes in sensation, and perhaps warmth in this area as a result. Offer yourself full gratitude for whatever this experience was like today, knowing you can revisit this practice any time.

With internal self-touch

When the above practice feels welcome and familiar, you can add the additional feedback of one clean, well-lubricated finger inserted vaginally. (If this feels inaccessible for any reason, or your student does not have a vagina, they can place their fingers to either side of the perineal body, just medial to their sit bones, for external feedback instead.)

Begin as stated above, getting comfortable and relaxed before you begin. Take some full breaths and feel your body rest into the support under you. This time, while performing a few pelvic-floor contractions and releases, you can have a finger inserted to get more information about what you feel happening. Do you feel both a gathering and a lifting into your body, or do your tissues tend to press or bulge outward, as if trying to slide your finger out? Does your engagement feel absent, weak, or strong? Smooth or choppy? Equal side to side and front to back or uneven?

Concluding the pelvic self-assessment

As you finish the internal self-touch inquiry, rest for a few minutes, and let the experience wash over you. Spend as much time resting as you need before rolling to one side. Once you feel complete, journal about your experience or complete the Pelvic Self-Assessment Worksheet.

It's possible that you or your clients may have been shamed, even disciplined, for genital touch or sexual curiosity as children or young adults. The process described here can elucidate useful data for the student and yoga therapist, as we're about to discuss, but perhaps even more essential is the restoration of agency and loving kindness toward one's pelvic space. Expanding this practice to include gentle, vaginal self-massage may afford increased or different benefits. For details on performing this technique for one's self, read *Wild Feminine* by Tami Lynn Kent. Leslie Howard also includes a brief description of a similar practice in her book, *Pelvic Liberation*.

Students may wish to create a ritual of using the pelvic self-assessment. As their yoga therapist, be mindful to help students not become fixated on getting this "right" or continually reassessing what they imagine is "wrong." If they find these mental or moral judgments intruding rather than receiving the gentle invitation to be in relationship with their pelvic space, we might suggest they let go of this exercise for a time.

How do we interpret or apply these findings in yoga therapy?

While it may feel tempting, we don't necessarily need a firm or definitive conclusion as to whether a client has an underactive or non-relaxing pelvic floor. We may not even receive self-assessment data to use in our intake process if a client declines the suggestion – so how do we know where to begin?

We work with what presents as most prominent or obvious in terms of improving their movement efficiency, trusting their reported experience. We follow their lead. When we meet them where they are, and see improvement, we can trust that as anecdotal evidence that what they're learning is supportive or healing. If we do our best and symptoms persist or worsen, we know there's a missing link that hasn't been adequately addressed yet. They may need a referral, revisions to their yoga-therapy plan, or both.

Here are clues that can help us discern whether we focus on relaxation and down-training or an active, functional, and strengthening approach. Each person is complex and this is solely intended to be a helpful guide – not a diagnostic list.

When a client reports pain or tenderness occurred with self-touch, strong urge sensations, or a partial or absent PFM relaxation from the self-assessment, we may assume they have a baseline non-relaxing or overactive pelvic floor (Vandyken *et al.* 2020; Vestal 2019). For these students, we may also observe generalized excess tension during movement, potentially a habit of posteriorly tucking the pelvis or clenching the gluteal muscles, or guarding as seen as limited mobility or lacking differentiation in the low back and hips. They may report they have stiff or tight hips and hamstrings – see if or how that bears out in active and passive movement assessments. You could be curious, too, about patterns that may coexist for them like jaw tension, abdominal bracing that seems to exceed the demand of a given movement, and shallow breathing. Considering the deep pelvic core is a protective space, high levels of stress, fear, or anxiety could also warrant a down-training, relaxation-based approach.

When a client reports a relatively sedentary lifestyle, we can investigate further about their exercise history and why they stopped moving (or never started), and perhaps assume that they could benefit from a functional, integrated approach to active asana. For these folks, we might see a pattern of deconditioning in their whole body and conjecture that their pelvic floor could be underactive as well. Women in their first one to two years postpartum or transitioning through menopause may report pelvic changes that feel like "weakness," exacerbated by hormonal fluctuations. It's important we consider all factors involved for an individual, as well as life stage (DeLancey *et al.* 2008). We can offer them coping strategies, education, and overall fitness that may improve pelvic support and function.

Finally, when a woman reports a weak or absent attempted PFM engagement from their self-assessment, we might first work to improve awareness and understanding of pelvic function and apply an integrative strengthening approach with the pelvic floor in mind. Even underactive PFM need relaxation, so consider closing active sequences with a neutralizing restorative posture or subtle practice like meditation or pranayama.

While these patterns do show up in pelvic care, they do not give a firm causation for PFM state. Whenever possible, our conclusions can be compared or discussed with the student's other pelvic-health providers.

Lastly, remember to celebrate your client's attention to these details and for sharing boldly with you, and help them identify the things they are doing well for their pelvic health. Any small step toward awareness can be held as hope for the progress to come. Appreciating the whole person in front of you, using all the various assessment strategies and possible observations, will help you discern what type of yoga-therapy plan to co-create.

Assessing all koshas

Now that we've established ways to assess baseline physicality and respiratory function, let's come full circle back through the other subtle koshas to provide a holistic view of the client. Asking insightful questions can elicit information a client may not have thought to share and may unveil powerful psychosocial and spiritual contributors to their symptoms and potential avenues for healing.

When working with a new student, inquire about what brings them joy or relief, or fulfills their sense of purpose. When met with blank stares or a generalized, short written answer on an intake form, become curious about who this person is and in what ways they might wish to live or express themselves that for whatever reason they may not currently be doing. Overwhelm runs rampant in our performative, productivity-obsessed culture. I believe underwhelm is just as common, a kind of perpetual boredom or complacency that numbs us not only to suffering and grief, but also to beauty, intimacy, and joy. If yoga is liberation, our formal practice and the totality of life can be in service to this awakening. Cultivating and directing energy wisely feeds creativity, sexuality, and freedom.

Use these questions on intake forms or in dialogue to identify notable themes of inquiry, illuminating the current state of the vijnanamaya and anandamaya koshas, which relate to values, self-efficacy, relationships, meaning, and purpose.

- What would you like to accomplish by working together?
- How will you know when you've reached your goals? How would your life be different?
- Where do you feel out of integrity with your values?
- What concerns do you have about your sexuality or relationships?
- How motivated do you feel to practice independently? What motivates you?
- What kind of support (time, financial, professional advice, childcare, emotional support, etc.) will you need to feel successful in accomplishing your goals?
- When do you currently feel most connected, fulfilled, or joyful?

Keep in mind that if we're sleuthing deeper into a client's life at large, we want to be able to provide compassionate witnessing and responses at the very least, and a plan to address it at best. If these questions feel outside your scope, trust that instinct and omit or simplify them. Often, when we give inquiries to a client for between sessions, they end up discovering new insight about themselves, their symptoms, and their needs. They become their own "coach." We can trust the process of *facilitating their self-directed growth* rather than trying to provide answers or meaning for them.

Co-create values-based goals

Establishing clear goals together builds client rapport and home-practice compliance, and gives a road map to follow in selecting and reassessing the efficacy of the yoga-therapy plan. This shows the client's needs are understood and may help you articulate how yoga can help. Aligned short-term goals also provide specific and attainable benchmarks toward fulfilling long-term aspirations. This collaborative BPSS process centers the person, elicits their desires and preferences, and informs decision-making (AGS Expert Panel on Person-Centered Care 2016; Prosko 2016).

Sometimes, clients express their goals in a negative context – stating what they wish would stop or what they'd like to avoid, like their pelvic symptoms or more invasive treatment. For example, they may rightfully desire to reduce or eliminate their pelvic pain. They may also know of certain activities of daily living that have historically provoked their pain. Those specific activities, when completed without pain or discomfort, could provide a meaningful measure of success. We can also share observations about how their movement practice has qualitatively evolved, as these subtle changes can happen so gradually they might be easily overlooked. Each nugget of encouragement can spur them on to continue deepening their relationship to themselves and this lifelong practice.

Preventing or reducing suffering only shows us one side of the "motivation equation." Also, creating goals based around pain scales (asking a student to rate their pain from 0 to 10 before and after each session, for example) may prove frustrating for some folks, especially students experiencing chronic or persistent pelvic pain. Sometimes their pain remains, or can flare up without a known reason, even when their overall quality of life or other functional measures improve. These rating scales can still be included in yoga-therapy assessments. We simply want to be mindful of how we use them and how often, especially when dealing with any form of chronic pain or sensitization.

Focusing on pain often serves to perpetuate or fan the flames to increase one's experience of pain – the opposite of our goal with yoga therapy.

The flip side to reducing one's suffering can include finding meaning or feeling more joy. The "motivation equation" cannot only include *movement away from* that which we do not want. Our yoga-therapy plan must also inspire the student *to move toward what they desire*. We can help students figure out their "carrot" of inspiration by examining their values. One of many possible methods to help a student uncover their values would be to ask a question such as, "How would your life be different if these symptoms were completely resolved?" By envisioning how they'd feel or behave without the pelvic-health stress or symptoms they currently experience, they begin to unveil and craft their values-based goals. They may still wish to be free of pain, as we explored above, but the deep longing hidden under that "chief complaint" may be the image of being able to travel comfortably and visit their grandkids, picking them up and feeling strong, and easefully playing with them on the floor. Those relationships and their ability to express love through these physical acts gives them real purpose when completing their daily home practice.

Specific, meaningful goals help us start somewhere useful and show us the way forward. We'll look more closely at big picture bhavana or visualization later in Chapter 12.

Create a plan

We often think about progression being the goal – raising the ceiling on someone's function. We might see more advanced postures or movements as the desired result or measure of success. Our clients may be attached to this conceptually without even realizing they continually seek external validation or performative practices, or may even be addicted to the concept of "more is better" from our capitalist culture. Just as much, if not more, progress can be made and sustained when we address simple, fundamental joint actions and bodily relationships first – raising the ground floor of the student's function, if you will.

As yogis, we know that the riches of this practice can best be unearthed through the process of becoming, studied with enthusiasm and commitment over time. The skill of finding abiding presence and peace in the face of our own suffering sets yoga therapy apart from biomedical, clinical models of treatment that focus more heavily (or solely) on the end outcomes. Both the process and the results matter. Yoga has so much to offer our students by way of learning acceptance, self-compassion, and living with intention and integrity. We don't practice to control the outcome – we practice to be in command of our present-moment experience (or at least our response to the present experience). Yoga asks us to consider our attachments and aversions, as we explored with the kleshas, and it takes humility to detach from making claims or overpromising results and develop trust in the dynamic unknown.

To conclude this process of discovery, consider writing down what you observed and felt while participating in the physical assessment. The more we can articulate somatic experience and sensation, the more we develop our communication skills and clinical reasoning to develop and track the student's home practice and progress. The ability to document kinesthetic information clearly also helps you correspond with other providers and build rapport. You may also wish to contemplate the inquiries presented.

In the next chapter, we're going to drop way down into autonomic regulation and attempt to restore a baseline of relaxation and receptivity. You'll learn why as you continue reading.

CHAPTER 10

Being

Go in and in.
Be the space
between two cells,
the vast, resounding
silence in which
spirit dwells.
Be sugar dissolving
on the tongue of life.
Dive in and in,
as deep as you can dive.
Be infinite, ecstatic truth.
Be love conceived and born in union.
Be exactly what you seek,
the Beloved, singing Yes,
tasting Yes, embracing Yes,
until there is only essence;
the All Of Everything
expressing through you
as you. Go in and in
and turn away from
nothing that you find.

"Go In and In" by Danna Faulds[1]

A grand, resounding "Yes" gives me a quickening in my heart and belly, anticipating the delight of endeavors to come. Desire draws us into the future,

1 From *Go In and In: Poems from the Heart of Yoga* by Danna Faulds. Greenville, VA: Peaceable Kingdom Books, 2002. Reprinted with kind permission of Danna Faulds.

whereas our practice imparts the skills to become and experience joy and revelation happening in the present. The sweetness of lingering at the close of our yoga practice, lounging in the sun, or dissolving into the embrace of a beloved has a quieter calling, still affirmative in its whispers. Our body is with us from first to final breath, and the pleasure of being with ourselves and discovering all life's gifts requires that we regularly attune to this softer request to listen, receive, and unfurl in real time.

Untethering from the cultural expectation of busyness presents a challenge for many. It can feel safer to remain occupied, grasping for external validation, hooked into constant consumption and seeking. When we slow down, we begin to feel. Understandably, we may wish to avoid our discomfort, disappointment, and pain. If you remember from the kleshas, or yogic causes of suffering, aversion and attachment keep us from fully accepting ourselves. Pulled between dislikes and desires, we continually look to change our experience *or* desperately don't want it to change – when, inevitably, we know it will. By welcoming all messengers of emotion and sensation, we watch our experience fluctuate without judgment.

As discussed in Chapter 3, continual dysregulation or up-regulation (chronic over-activation of our sympathetic drive) stands in the way of coordinated, easeful, and efficient movement, breathing, and pelvic function. Author and psoas educator Liz Koch says, "We live in a sympathetic soup" (Koch and Johnson 2019). The addictive nature of social media, concern over world events, endless household and caregiving responsibilities, and preoccupation with our suffering further scatter the tendrils of attention.

Healing begins and integrates from within one's body and lived experience. Potent awareness harnesses this power and supports right action. Being precedes sustainable doing. By resting into santosha, the profound contentment of pure beingness, we remember our wholeness and innate worth.

This chapter explores ways to build the capacity to rest and be still, qualities often assigned to our root chakra. I believe pelvic health is whole-person health. And so, we start by outlining practices that support this slower, attentive way of life and systemic reorganization of the individual. This is deep inner work of restoring a felt sense of safety and enoughness, and may support unlearning patterned behavior, or samskaras, in favor of more conscious, sustainable living.

We exist beyond the boundaries of the physical body, or the limitations we perceive from a pelvic diagnosis. I hope these practices give you at least a glimpse of your expansive self. The somatic inquiries can develop the student's inner referencing to self-assess during asana and exercise, and foster full breath excursion, skills of subtle perception, and ease from which to move as they progress with more active practices in chapters that follow.

> If people express an aversion to stillness, meditation, any of the suggested body positions, or share a history of trauma, please be discerning about the application of what you learn in this chapter. Validate and respect their current limits, while compassionately inviting new ways of being and practicing. You might choose to first trial qualities and themes from this chapter coupled with gentle, dynamic asana to allow the student to track sensation and effort, stay in dialogue with you, and cultivate a sense of trust with learning to slow down. With reliable practice, they may feel more resourced to engage in deeper, longer, or more subtle somatic inquiries and restorative practices, being held by the therapeutic alliance you've co-created.

The importance of practicing baseline perception

To be able to perceive change or progress, we must know what our baseline experience was to begin with, much like the blue dot in our GPS app that shows where we are before giving us directions. We orient to the present as a fundamental skill, a prerequisite for selecting or implementing a yoga-therapy intervention. (We introduced this in Chapters 1 and 3.) Here, we'll give more nuance around how to apply this skill in client sessions.

In Sutra 1.6, we learn that the mind has five distinct, fluctuating modes in which it can operate. With this baseline exercise, we're attempting to objectively perceive ourselves and our sensations with accuracy, what's called pramana, or clear perception (Satchidananda 2008, pp.9–15). Further defined as evidence from the senses, this real-time recognition of embodied experience can only be accessed by the person doing the perceiving. As facilitators of yoga therapy, we accept humbly that we cannot feel what a student feels. We can learn a great deal from how they communicate sensations, including when there's a lack of perception.

Pure observation can bring about a field of equanimity as we watch sensation and perception change, sometimes in a flash, from being observed. For clients who get wrapped up in catastrophic thinking or report their pain as acute and constant, this can illuminate a new possibility to realize their diagnosis or past suffering is, indeed, not permanent. Facilitating interoceptive skill and the capacity to translate the language of the body into verbal dialogue gives us an invaluable tool for discerning whether the practices we've chosen are effective, and when and why to change course, and invites the student to play an active role in their care.

Often, when students feel a positive change, they describe it as the absence of what they felt before. They may state, "I feel less tense now," or, "It hurts less than it did earlier." This is an excellent starting point – they've identified a positive shift. What may reinforce the improvement more, however, is to reframe the language to suit the new, more pleasant experience. For instance, "I feel less pain now" could be restated as "I'm more comfortable and at ease in my body now." We get to help students create a language for embodied pleasure! It can be incredibly motivating for a student to realize that tangible results can be achieved relatively easily and maintained through consistent, independent home practice.

A somatic inquiry gives parameters to guide a student's self-generated investigation (Kaparo 2012, pp.17–35). The three patterns presented here come from embryological development, which has been studied and applied experientially by many somatic educators (Farhi 2015a; Hackney 2002, pp.51–109; Hartley 1995, pp.3–49). These inquiries create the foundation for later developmental patterns that orient us to ground, gravity, and space, and support locomotion and movement efficiency. I've chosen to focus on the earliest imprints with an intention to slow down and source answers from within, and from my firm belief that restorative practices belong in every woman's pelvic healing toolkit.

Developmental pattern 1: Cellular respiration

At the root of health and vitality is respiration that happens internally, almost imperceptibly, at the level of our cells as they imbibe and circulate nourishment and release waste. Our life begins by uniting two cells at conception. Those cells go on to multiply and exist in relationship with each other, following their divine design to become blood, flesh, and bone to bring us into recognizable form. We exist in fluid, as fluid beings in the womb, receiving everything we need through our mother's blood and the beautiful new organ, the placenta, that grows with us.

As we take our first breaths at birth, the air around us transforms from gas to liquid as oxygen passes across the silky membranous interior of the lungs to enter the bloodstream. Traditional Chinese Medicine holds the belief that disharmony and stagnation of energy causes disease and the restoration of this energetic flow nourishes all cells and systems, promoting healing (Traditional Chinese Medicine World Foundation n.d.). Hence, this early pattern of cellular respiration receives support from our fluid system. This receptive, fertile, quiet state can be revisited voluntarily as we embody cellular or internal respiration.

Pattern: Cellular respiration

Core qualities: Innate worthiness, trust, receive, rest

Keywords: Being, yielding, non-form, non-doing, permeable, fluid, shimmer, pulse, vibrate, hum, dissolve, melt, float, coast

Experiencing cellular respiration

You're welcome to explore this inquiry in any position that brings peace, even lying in bed if you like. Finding impeccable comfort may help you perceive this internal ocean of fluid support and cellular life. Use yoga props or blankets to fill spaces between your body and the ground to promote relaxation. My favorite confirmation of comfort is when a student releases an audible sigh of relief as they arrive in the posture.

Sidelying offers access to the thoracic spine, ribcage, and respiratory diaphragm, possibly enhancing breath excursion through the supple volume of one's organs. Place a few layers of blanket under the ribs and waist, and support the head and neck sufficiently. From this sidelying restorative position, we may invite self-touch of the pelvic bones and perineum to enhance awareness.

Now that you're settled, take the next few breaths to let this support wash over you. Feel how your body's contours are held and cushioned, and give your weight to the ground. Rest. Let yourself slow down. Move your awareness inward. Drop below skin, fat, muscle, and bone, drop down into your very existence at the level of the cells. Rest. Rest here in the space between cells, feel them surrounded and buoyed by a kind of gel-like fluidity that holds and nourishes them. Trust that every cell knows what needs doing – there's nothing here for you to "do" – they breathe on your behalf. Your cells shimmer and pulse, vibrating with life as they drink in this moment and nourish you. You are alive. The more deeply you rest and receive, the better your cells can do what needs doing. Let go. Your cells sustain you with their fluid, cyclical rhythm, humming with their aliveness. Imbibing what they need, releasing what's done. Feel yourself dissolve, resting beyond the form of your body, melting. Let yourself stay here for as long as you'd like. Let yourself float, as if time itself has suspended.

As the impulse emerges from within, gradually let your senses come back up to the surface. Notice the temperature of air on your skin, the texture of your clothes or props, the sounds you hear. Slowly rock back and forth until you feel willing to press up to a seated position.

Developmental pattern 2: Navel radiation

Cellular respiration *and* diaphragmatic breathing support the development of all later patterns. The next one we'll explore is called navel radiation. Physical connection to our mother through the umbilical cord orients us to the center through radial symmetry. Tethered to our core, we oscillate between curling around it and unfurling our limbs against the malleable environment of the uterus that houses us all those months.

Still supported by the fluid system, navel radiation connects the responsive core center to our periphery through six energetic pathways that then support structure: the two legs, two arms, and our head and tail. In the womb, we move through a stage (appearing first at five to six weeks gestation, and usually disappearing by around eight weeks) when we indeed have a tail! As an early, pre-spinal stage, the head-to-tail connection remains supple, reflected by the organic support of our digestive system, which we'll explore further in the following section. Navel radiation invites wholeness through fluid form.

The energetic pathways of navel radiation, when explored voluntarily in practice, illuminate where we feel connected or disconnected. Like a garden hose that sat all winter, the first water we run through it in spring might come in spurts as we clear out the muck of its non-use. Our consciousness can likewise clear the channel of each pathway from core to distal end and back again as we trace them through guided imagery, we sense them somatically, or by offering touch support. We know the pattern is becoming more integrated when we can consciously and clearly feel it, which lends cohesion, effortlessness, and flow to how we move.

While cellular respiration is a pattern of being, or "non-doing," navel radiation can be discovered through quiet stillness *and* further integrated as we initiate movement. One example of navel-radiation organizing movement would be opening and closing through a wide squat pattern involving the upper extremities, like a starfish. All six limbs coil around center as we descend into flexion and radiate open, reaching into the space around us through extension as we return to standing. This pattern can also be observed in half moon (ardha chandrasana), with both the expansive volume we feel when reaching into the form and the grace with which we can transition back to the floor through yielding and coiling into ourselves.

Flexor tone, or the imprint of physiological flexion that connects us into our "core strength," modulates the extensor tone we pick up once we're navigating the world outside the womb with gravity. True core stability or strength has an adaptive, receptive quality, whereas it's often misinterpreted as a firmness that becomes too rigid and static, impeding breath and sequential flow through these pathways.

As adults, the assimilation of this pattern can help us feel secure, aware of ourselves in space, and able to return to equilibrium physically, mentally, and emotionally. We even hear it threaded throughout our language with phrases like, "I feel centered." Remember, this return to balance, or re-centering, is a dynamic, adaptive living process, not a fixed point.

Pattern: Navel radiation

Core qualities: Centered, organized, connected

Keywords: Radial symmetry, expand and condense, open and close, pathways, threads, tendrils, radiate, receptive, fluid, core distal, central-peripheral, moving from center

Experiencing navel radiation

We'll explore this pattern in a supported supine position like savasana. Give your secondary curves, or the negative spaces that wouldn't normally touch the ground, something soft to rest into, by placing rolled blankets behind your ankles, knees, neck, and head, for example. You could also place a very deflated soft ball or a few layers of towel under the sacrum to increase comfort. For some students, this can make it easier to locate and perceive their center as mobile, responsive, and receptive to each fluid breath excursion. Consider props as buoys, allowing one to feel supported and suspended by the pontoons of bolsters and pillows.

Feel yourself yield into the support of the earth under you, letting go of the weight of your head, torso, arms, pelvis, and legs. Rest. Let yourself be held here and grow quiet as you draw your awareness inward. Let your attention come down to rest deeply inside your belly. Down into your womb or pelvic bowl. Feel this space within you – does it feel held, rigid? Does it feel free? Can you invite a feeling of responsiveness, softness here, letting your core center be moved by each breath?

Over the next few moments, we'll begin to invite awareness into our six limbs. Do your best not to direct the outcome, instead be open to sensing what comes alive on its own. Feel your navel center, your center of gravity being breathed now. Let your center become receptive, fluid, and alive with the energy of your full presence. Now, let yourself be curious to feel and sense where this energy flows first. Which pathway, or pathways, open to you and become filled, traced with your attentiveness and felt by sensation? Can you follow this pathway to its distal end? Spend some time sensing and noticing if or where it feels disconnected, dull, or numb, and where it tangibly feels touched by your imagination, where you can feel a vital life force flowing through it. Now retrace the pathway all the way back into your deep center, your core. Rest your attention here, letting go of any agenda. There's no right or wrong way to go about this practice.

You may feel complete here after this first invitation, and if so, take a moment to share or write down what you felt and which pathways became available to you first. You may also spend more time here feeling which pathways open to your sensory aliveness next, or even practicing feeling the undulating expansion and condensing of all six limbs – outwardly radiant and reaching into the space around you and then recoiling, drawing back into your center to rest once again. There may be subtle movements you feel inspired to use to express your findings, or you might let it be a meditation, remaining still from an outsider's perspective as you feel moved from within by the orchestrating, organizing energy of navel radiation.

As you finish, offer yourself compassion for whatever you felt or didn't feel. It's all part of the process of becoming attuned to this subtlety through voluntary exploration. Trust yourself, and let this inquiry unfold as you revisit the pattern.

Developmental pattern 3: Mouthing

Jaw tension and teeth clenching often have a southern counterpart, showing up as concurrent tension or a non-relaxing quality in the person's pelvic muscles – as above so below and vice versa. Through embryological development, we see innate connectedness of these deep, internal structures of our core midline. Before we become vertebrates, we have a gut tube. Thus, the organic support we source from exploring the mouthing pattern can enliven harmony within the spine.

In the womb, we practice suckling, finding our fingers, preparing to find our mother's breast upon birth. Our sense of smell and taste intertwined, these senses lead us to nourishment and forge our connection to the world around us and bonding through relationship. As our mouth and tongue become stronger and bodily control improves, we move on to solid foods. Breastfeeding and learning to chew and move a bolus of food around inside the mouth require nasal breathing, which helps develop our palate, jaw, and airway. Nasal breathing also impacts immunity, mental health, and more (Nestor 2020).

Sometimes, this developmental pattern is called mouthing and analing, showing the corresponding sensitivity and expressivity that we can feel throughout our pelvic bowl and demonstrating the intimate connection between what we consume and what must be eliminated. Voluntarily revisiting this pattern with compassionate curiosity can help unlearn personal and cultural shame, inviting the rectum and anus to be normalized and embodied.

Sphincter muscles exist throughout the body and can be found in our eyes, lips, esophagus, and intestines, and around the urethra, vagina, and anus. These gatekeepers often get dubbed "O rings." As a protective mechanism, the PFM register danger or threat, which tends to generate tension to cinch them closed (Both *et al.* 2012). Culturally, we joke about someone being a "tight ass" or anal retentive. We still have a long journey ahead to unravel the pervasive shame that can live here in place of the potential normalcy and even pleasure it can lend to everyday life and intimacy. Let's explore.

Pattern: Mouthing

Core qualities: Juicy, discerning, nourishing, supportive

Keywords: Tongue to tail, digestive system, gut tube, midline, axial support, consumption, assimilation, integration, elimination, swallowing, lubrication, undulating, snakelike, O rings or sphincteric function, beginning to awaken senses to environment

Experiencing mouthing and the organic support of our digestive system

For this last inquiry, we'll rest in a prone restorative (Figure 10.1). You'll need at least a few blankets and perhaps a bolster. Provide the full length of your torso with support from sternum to lower belly, letting your thighs drape off behind your bolster or pillows. Support your forehead with a soft-but-firm prop so your nose takes no pressure and your neck remains comfortable and neutral relative to the torso. Lastly, roll a blanket and place it under your ankles to slightly elevate your feet.

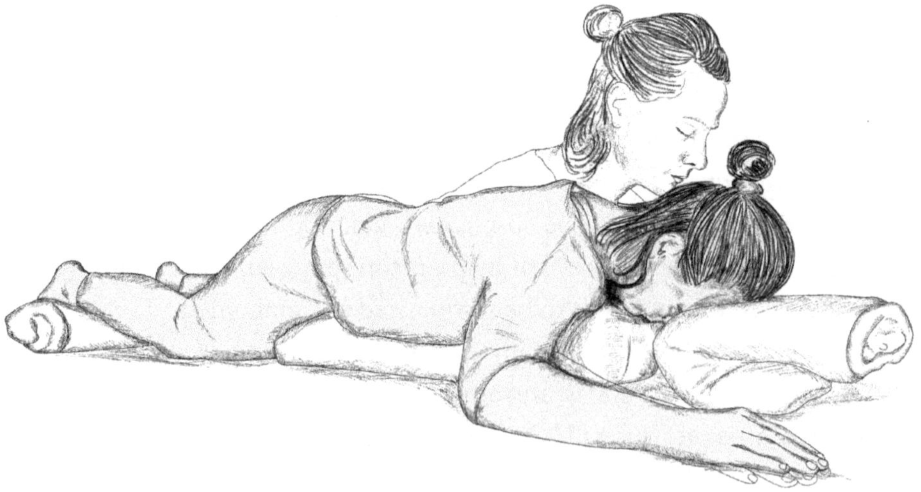

Figure 10.1: Prone savasana

Supplying our soft underbelly with firm but yielding containment may help tonify the digestive organs, restore relaxation to our nervous system, and redirect the breath excursion into the sides and back of our body. This could be a primary practice for clients who feel overwhelmed or depleted, as well as those struggling with constipation. Many years ago, I worked with a woman who arrived at her private session proclaiming she was "totally backed up" and hadn't had a bowel movement for several days. We did a short, potent restorative sequence, including spending time in this prone position. Off she went, at least feeling much calmer from our session. The next day at the grocery store, I bumped into her in the produce section. She high-fived me over a pyramid of oranges, smiling and whispering to me that she "finally went" that morning. Exploring the mouthing pattern (and smart restorative sequencing in general) can illuminate and revitalize our patterns of consumption, digestion, and elimination; it further discriminates and protects us by expelling its contents in the event of, say, food poisoning or a stomach virus. The gut is wise!

You'll arrive into either a neutral spine or a slightly flexed position, yielding the head and tail with your arms and legs a bit lower than your torso. If you feel any strain in your shoulder girdle or upper back, or a tingling sensation in your hands, you can roll a hand towel or blanket and drape a sushi roll of support across the top of your bolster – this will fill the space under your sternum and anterior shoulder and can also provide space for full breasts or a nursing mother's comfort. Once you're settled prone, you may feel your sacrum and pelvis being rocked and your lumbar spine being gently elongated and released by the wave of each breath.

Take a moment for any last adjustments for utter and complete comfort in prone. Offer yourself deep care and positive regard. Trust your props and the earth beneath you, let yourself drop in. Feel the weight of your body being supported and buoyed from underneath, allowing you to float here. Spend a few moments feeling yourself decelerate internally, finding a slower, quieter internal rhythm. Rest.

Now bring attention inside your mouth. Feel your top teeth, bottom teeth, the roof of your mouth. Sense the tip of your tongue, the root of your tongue. Feel your jaw soften, melting your eyes, cheeks, tongue. You may find yourself drooling a bit, which is confirmation of your relaxation response. As you swallow, feel the smooth muscular tube of your esophagus gliding downward. This smooth, strong tube sits right in front of your cervical spine.

Continue journeying downward between your lungs, behind your heart. Guide your awareness through the central tendon of your diaphragm slightly to the left and dive into your stomach. Then flow through the intestines down to the lower right quadrant of your abdomen. Feel your whole belly being massaged with each breath that you accept and release. Rest.

Now follow the large intestine up the right side of your waist, tucked just inside the lower ribs. Sweep your attention across from right to left side, then guide your awareness down the left side of your waist, following the descending colon. Finally, land just inside the left half of your pelvic bowl, then swoop your attention back toward your sacrum, and follow the rectum downward to your anus. Feel your tail being moved by each breath. Can you allow yourself to rest so deeply, relax your pelvic-floor muscles so completely, that your breath moves freely here? Let your thighs be heavy. Feel your glutes melt. Notice any thoughts, sensations, colors, pictures, or feelings that arise as you connect with your tail, your anus, your pelvic floor. You're connected and supported from tongue to tail. You're nourished daily by this system, and by resting, you provide vital and abundant blood flow to your digestive system. Linger here.

You might stay and rest here or explore incrementally lifting the head to elongate and rise toward the smallest possible cobra pose (bhujangasana). Swallow again and feel how the esophagus supports the front of your spine in this gentle extension. Then slowly bring yourself onto one side or press yourself back into a child's pose (balasana) before returning to an upright position. Notice how you feel.

Now that you've explored this early developmental imprint of your soft, muscular gut tube, it might be fun and useful to explore your voice. You're welcome to revisit the breathing and sound inquiries from Chapter 5, chant another familiar mantra, or simply call a friend. As you speak, track what you experience inside your body, observing how the practice may have created a sense of ease in your communication. By freeing the breath and enlivening organ awareness, you may find that your voice feels well supported from the juicy contents of the torso and a clear midline channel. Allow the deeply regulating and rejuvenating effects of this inquiry to liberate your voice and amplify your ability to speak your core truths.

Heel rocking for integration

Pulsing and rhythmic rocking can promote relaxation and enhance circulation. Heel rocking may also illuminate structural pathways for force transfer, creating more congruence from the feet up into the femur heads, pelvis, and spine – an essential connectivity for standing and walking well. If you're feeling at all fuzzy or disoriented from the open-ended nature of the somatic inquiries, this may help you feel more present and ready to transition into other activities.

> From savasana, allow the legs to extend out along the floor; you may place a small rolled towel under the knees if you prefer. With the heels firmly grounded, begin to pump your ankles through dorsi and plantar flexion rhythmically. Find an agile, rebounding pace that requires minimal effort. Feel how the pumping action of the feet sends an impulse up through the leg bones and into the pelvis and spine. Let your breathing be quiet and natural, and feel how your organs and fluids slosh up and down with this pulsation. Keep bouncing, rocking for about one full minute, and then rest in stillness. Observe the effects and then roll to your side.

In client work, inquiries like this can be helpful in overriding physical and mental tension, and may be used as a simple warm-up to increase presence and prepare for movement. If one experiences sacral pressure or discomfort lying on the floor or during heel rocking, consider adding a small layer of cushion like a few layers of fluffy bath towel or a very barely inflated wide ball under the pelvis. Use just enough support to bring comfort and not so much to create an inversion or disrupt the spinal curves.

Inquiries for further self-reflection

Exploring the gentle yet profound medicine of the developmental-pattern somatic inquiries may give rise to new insight, a kind of remembering unearthed by revisiting these universal patterns we each travel through to come into human form. In short, if we get quiet enough, we may start to access our inner wisdom from a more essential, soulful perspective.

Subtle inquiry can be threaded throughout a client's experience during the guided practices or suggested for reflection at home, outside the contact hours with the yoga therapist. You might suggest one or two questions at a time, giving space for the student to journal, meditate, and go on walks while holding these themes lightly as they go about daily life. The continued practice of an accompanying somatic inquiry and restorative posture will provide a physical ground from which to welcome this loving self-interrogation.

What are your beliefs about rest? How well can
you ask for and receive support?

In what or whom do you put your faith? How do
you, or could you, practice surrender?

When do you overextend yourself, if ever? When do you withhold
or shrink back, if ever? Give yourself at least one example of how
you might cultivate a different response to build resilience.

Do you tend to be too rigid with boundaries or too lax? What's one area in
your life right now where you could bring this awareness to work for you?

What have you never told anyone about your pelvis? How would it feel
to speak it aloud, even if spoken privately to yourself as a first step?

What turns you on creatively? Sexually? How do
you invite pleasure into your daily life?

Equanimity can help us close a practice session feeling satisfied. Offer gratitude to both pleasant *and* unpleasant observations to further instill skills of objective witnessing and compassion. Every change can teach us, each sensation informs us. Outcomes guide adaptation or adjustments of the posture we used, what we did to prepare for or integrate the experience, or the duration of time spent.

Take this moment to compare your current state with the baseline perception you felt before completing this chapter. Integrating these subtle practices of being strengthens the foundation from which we move into asana. They're also a balm to return to when we need solace or rest.

May you feel peace fill your belly.
May you feel at peace in your bones.
May you feel peace nourishing every cell that sustains you.

CHAPTER 11

Doing

Developmentally, we begin "movement training" on the floor. Our eyes lead us into rolling, crawling, sitting, and pulling up to standing, inspired by genuine curiosity of our environment and social engagement with caregivers. We meet each milestone by harnessing our connection to the ground, gravity, and the space around us.

By voluntarily revisiting these foundational relationships, one can establish or restore efficiency of movement. Basic actions strengthen the synergistic relationships between pelvic-floor health, hip joint activity, posture, core stability, breathing, and self-expression. We explore in deliberately simplified ways, and begin on the floor to decrease gravity's load and offer support. Then, we translate these skills into increasingly complex movements like walking, squatting, variety in asana practice, dancing, jumping, and running, as desired.

We can help our clients build healthy movement habits from the ground up and find creative ways to enhance motivation by making a game out of regressing to progress. This intentional commitment to integrity and honesty in one's practice weaves in the ethical precepts of the yamas and niyamas, bringing depth and great care to the process. We can only work from where we are now, what's currently available to us. Simple ain't always easy. Going slow strengthens. The exercises in this chapter continue to show up in my practice and teaching because they're scalable and effective, and help us shed the compensations that come with living a modern life.

Each student encounter begins with baseline sensing. We can meet them with suggestions to enhance pelvic awareness and provide adequate, sound education. Awareness comes first. Then, remember a person's PFM baseline will dictate whether you focus on relaxing and lengthening, as with overactive, or bolstering activation and strength when underactive. When both states exist with asymmetrical function (or when you're not sure about baseline PFM state), you may wish to first focus on mobility, length, and relaxation overall, as well as potentially addressing the asymmetry. For most students, close the practice with a period of rest, targeting PFM relaxation to ensure coordination and ease become integrated as the "new norm." Whenever possible, consult with the client's clinical pelvic care team.

The postures and sequences highlighted in this chapter aim to illustrate key concepts like what happens within the pelvic floor with spinal movements and varied actions of the hip joints, and how to regress or progress weight-bearing loads for the pelvis (particularly important for those with prolapse). None of these practices need to cause strong discomfort or pain, compensatory tension, or breath holding – our goal is movement efficiency in all contexts. Move slowly, with smooth, fluid breath awareness and continual inner referencing through interoception. Rather than teaching a posture the "correct" way, witness *how* your body or your student's body performs the movement as a baseline, and then adjust or add intent, action, or cues based on what you feel will most likely benefit overall efficiency.

Cycles of movement

Each breath and every movement oscillates, whether explored dynamically in motion or held as an isometric event. From finite to full range, our cells pulse, and effort varies and fluctuates across joint surfaces, and between different nerves and muscle fibers, to create a regenerative experience that supports healing and longevity. As you practice what may feel like familiar or "mechanical" forms, let these shapes come alive.

While some static or passive stretching may be useful, consider first how you can move the referenced muscle through its active range, both contracting and relaxing it fully a few times before going into an intended "stretch." Remember the vital role of our nervous system, and consider how "tight" muscles likely need to be moved, to receive nourishment and circulation to restore more effective innervation and reset their resting state.

You could embrace this chapter's content as a complete practice from start to finish or take the sections as shorter practices. Consider weaving in spontaneous movement, circles, and figure eights as a warm-up, or to integrate what you're enjoying or discovering. I've chosen not to describe this process here, as it could be quite lengthy to discuss the act of improvisation – and because there's no "right way" to do it. As comfort, efficiency, and awareness grow, allow new movement vocabulary to emerge in celebration (Hackney 2002, pp.34–36).

Embracing the floor

You may wish to revisit CRP from Chapter 6 or take a few moments to become centered and calm. Know you can also always return to the five movement "assessments" in Chapter 9 as a baseline practice for simplicity, to reassess, or if any variations presented here give you pause.

If one has yet to find ease with the single leg march (Assessment 2), know there are many ways to build efficiency and strength with this baseline action of supine hip flexion. For example, you could float both feet off the floor or press your palms into your knees to add resistance as an isometric hold there, or explore tapping the big toes to the mat first unilaterally, alternating sides, and then bilaterally to investigate higher loads. Take your time and select a variation of supine "core stabilization" that suits the baseline and desired outcomes. When moving both legs into hip flexion from supine feels easeful, move into the next two exercises.

90-90 barrel rolling

In this adaptation of supine "core training," we explore how well one can coordinate the core cylinder and limbs as a cohesive unit. Rolling requires that we activate enough to maintain congruence between upper and lower extremities through the core center, and at the same time, learn to yield into the floor to feel steady and stable – too much effort and we may likely topple over. Consider also how the organization of navel radiation can create a sense of cohesion between the limbs and core center during this movement inquiry. Let's try it.

From supine, bring your bent arms and bent legs into a parallel 90-degree orientation above your trunk, what some may call an upside-down table or reverse quadruped. Breathing well here with no excess compensatory tension is your first inquiry and a prerequisite for moving on to the next step.

When efficiency and breathing feel established, begin to roll your body to one side as seen in Figure 11.1, coming to a diagonal facing the ceiling across the room – not coming all the way onto your side. Find the in between place, neither on your back nor completely on your side, and breathe. You may feel and visually check that your hips and shoulders remain square to each other, with your spine neutral and elongated. Your grounded side will yield, creating a relationship to the floor, while you explore reaching across into the diagonal with your top limbs. Lastly, very slowly bring yourself onto your back while maintaining the barrel or core cylinder relationship. Pause and rest, and then set up for the other side.

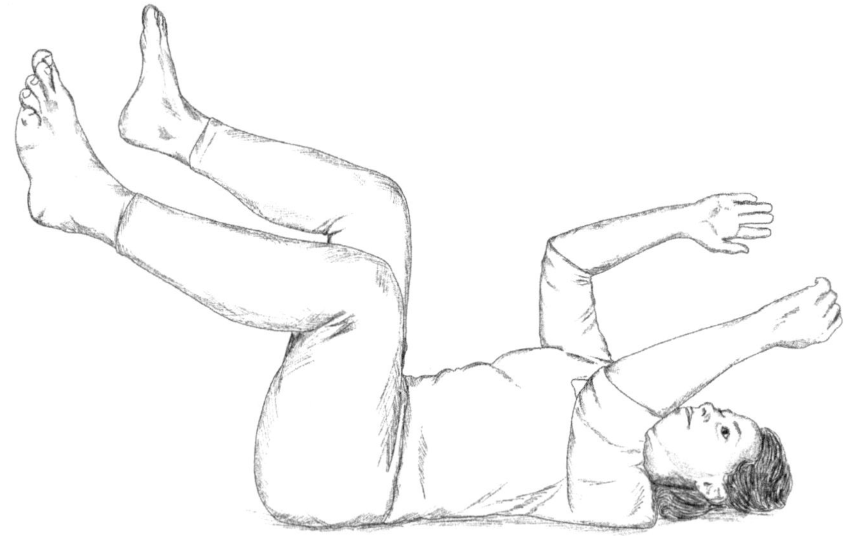

Figure 11.1: 90-90 barrel rolling

Transverse plane butterfly

This next inquiry will examine dynamic coordination of the legs, pelvic floor, trunk stabilizers, and breathing. We'll remain supine with both shoulders and hips, and the back floating ribs, broadly grounded. You may observe how the arms remain at rest alongside the body or can be used as subtle counter leverage if needed initially – then, as the coordination becomes more familiar, arm effort can be reduced or eliminated.

From CRP, bring both feet off the floor with the knees as bent as possible. Spend a few moments in stillness, sensing the pelvic diamond, and feel the PFM relaxing. Maintain your natural lumbar curve.

Slowly allow the knees to move away from each other toward either side of the room and then bring them back to parallel. You may coordinate breathing with the action of the legs and play also with moving slowly enough to take a few breaths to open and another few breaths to return inward. Working slowly can build awareness and may also help one feel the action's impact on pelvic-floor activity, merged with the subtle excursions of how the breath influences the PFM.

Work here bilaterally first like in Figure 11.2, moving the legs in tandem through abduction and external rotation, and then adduction and internal rotation back to parallel. Balancing loads into the pelvis bilaterally often feels easier to coordinate.

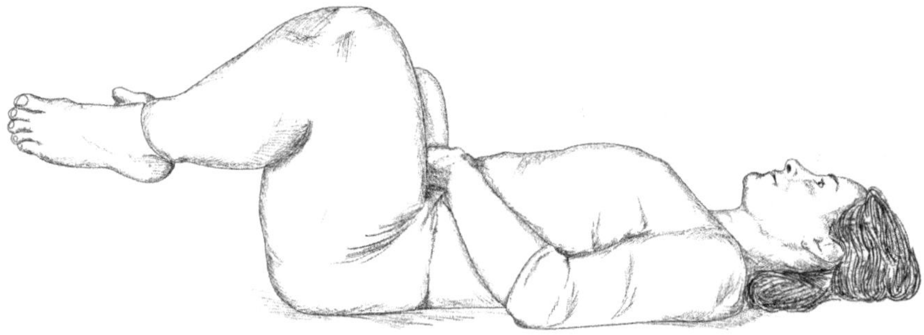

Figure 11.2: Transverse plane butterfly

To progress, you can explore incremental unilateral movements of one leg while the other remains parallel. As one thigh goes away from midline, the leverage increases and the need for counterbalancing and transverse plane stability across the obliques will become heightened. If the pelvis begins to roll toward the side that's opening, scale back the range of motion until midline alignment can be maintained. You could also increase the neuromuscular training effect by elevating the pelvis slightly with support from soft, inflated balls. This less-stable surface and elevated fulcrum requires a deeper level of coordination and strength.

For folks with overactive tendencies, suggest they visualize the relaxed widening of the diamond. They may enjoy resting in happy baby pose (ananda balasana), supporting the knees. Trace an arc with the knees back to parallel, rather than activating the PFM.

With an underactive PFM, encourage sounds and breath strategies that support engagement, cue the closing from drawing the sit bones magnetically together, or ask that they feel and visualize the diamond narrowing.

Prone leg lift

In our society of plentiful sitting and potentially sedentary lifestyles, we may find that a student's glutes or the awareness of them has all but left the building. Sometimes called "mom butt," the flat appearance of one's backside can indicate postural habits (like clenching and posterior tilt "tucking"), as well as a lack of movement contexts required to build and shape the buttocks – namely, stairs, climbing hills, squats, and lunges. Motherhood doesn't guarantee the disappearance of one's booty, nor does this phenomenon only occur in women who bear children.

Howard's book *Pelvic Liberation* (2017) includes an aptly titled section, "Poses to be a Smart Ass," addressing the missing connection to the powerhouse primary movers of hip extension. A bit of humor invites the spirit of play into asana practice and serves to break the ice when asking a student to do something like grab their own cheeks to self-assess.

When we observe or suspect functional deficits in one's hip strength or gait cycle, or find during asana a lack of awareness or engagement in the glutes, it may be helpful to get the lights turned back on with targeted recruitment. It's also very common to see one side recruit more easily than the other; an imbalance easily missed when we always do asana, like bridge (setu bhanda sarvangasana), in bilateral ways, hence the unilateral self-assessment with prone leg lifts first. Focus attention and additional volume of training on the "weaker" side to potentially restore balance.

This prone leg lift can be used as a quick self-assessment before other asana or as an exercise itself. Work toward getting a clear "signal" to each glute, possibly asking it to bulge and contract into your palm before lifting the leg, and maintaining its action through the movement. As the leg lowers down, feel the glute gradually lengthen and then fully relax once the leg rests into the floor. ("Turn the lights off" before beginning the next repetition.)

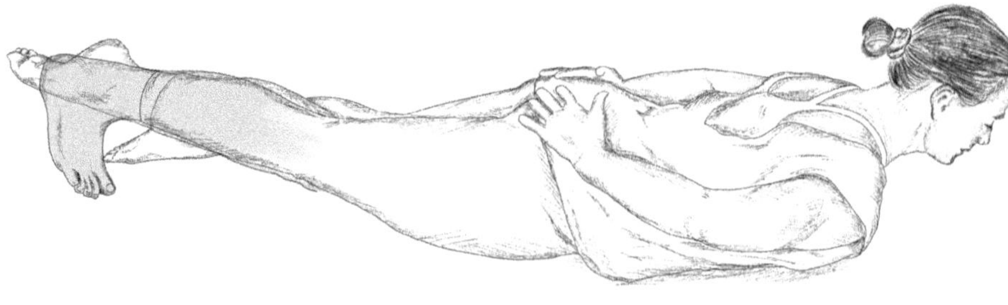

Figure 11.3: Prone leg lift

Let's practice what we see in Figure 11.3. Lying prone with a blanket under the sternum, ribs, and belly, rest the forehead to a folded blanket or the floor. Sweep the arms out to the sides and behind you, placing your palms on the roundest part of the buttocks. Keeping the knee straight, lift one leg away from the floor and hold this hip extension for a full breath. Slowly return the leg to the floor. Repeat that leg a few times to gauge whether you clearly feel the full engagement of the buttock under your hand, if it flickers with a partial contraction, or if it's curiously sleepy in comparison to the other side or the clarity you feel when contracting other muscles.

Rest a moment on the floor and then repeat the inquiry on the second side. Pay close attention to differences from one side to the other, as this can help you customize cues and select postures to facilitate the return of context-appropriate glute power.

If doing this inquiry from prone creates discomfort or postural compensations, adapt this practice to a standing context. Observe the quality of engagement in the glutes during hip extension by sweeping one femur behind the plane of the torso.

Bridge

This movement enjoys common inclusion in yoga classes, workout programs, and even physical-therapy protocols. Like any movement, though, *how* we execute it matters immensely. Bridge can be used to spotlight glute engagement as a progression from the prone leg lift, as a core stabilization inquiry when explored unilaterally, and as a pelvic-floor inquiry. The deep pelvic diaphragm and glutes function together like a team, what's been identified as the "levator ani-fossa ischioanalis-gluteus maximus" or "LFG" complex (Soljanik *et al.* 2007). Shifting attention and weight-bearing load from the balls of the feet into the heels or vice versa can change the recruitment felt by the participant (try it and let me know what you feel).

Let's focus on sensing the relationship between the PFM and a dynamic bridge action, using Figure 11.4 as a guide.

From CRP, feel the pelvic-floor diamond and allow it to be receptive to your breathing. Start to press into your feet and lift the pelvis an inch or two off the floor. Lower down slowly and feel your pelvis rest and PFM relax before beginning again. For each repetition of bridge, invite yourself to take the hips higher, incrementally allowing full hip extension to occur. As you move, notice how and when the pelvic floor participates in active or relaxing phases with the movement. Does it feel like the PFM function in concert with the bridging movement? Can you feel them being moved by the breath within this action, creating an overlapping rhythm of efficiency within the effort?

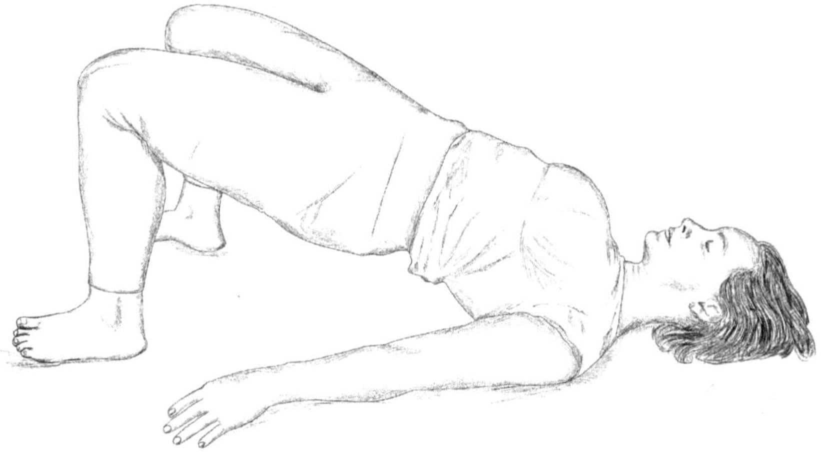

Figure 11.4: Bridge

To enhance the pelvic-floor coordination, we can apply the diamond imagery. As the feet begin to press more firmly, allow the diamond to gather and narrow, possibly moving into a very slight posterior pelvic tilt. Let this action sequence up through the perineal body (the center of the diamond) and spine as you elevate the hips into bridge. Reverse this action, undulating down the spine one vertebra at a time back to the mat, rolling your long, metaphorical tail out along the floor between your feet and feeling the diamond expand and widen. Rest completely into the floor. You could further explore coordination with jellyfish breathing from Chapter 8. Be sure all effort has subsided before beginning the next bridge repetition, especially for students with overactive PFM tendencies.

If you feel any bulging, pressure, or bearing-down sensations during bridge, check in with your breathing and/or reduce range of motion until you can feel a coordinated, synergistic effect from the feet and legs up through the perineum.

To challenge coordination, trunk stability, and glute strength, you may wish to invite in unilateral variations of bridge. For asymmetry, this may better target muscles responsible by not allowing the open-chain side of the pelvis to drop toward the ground in a single-leg bridge. Begin by pressing more firmly through one foot but keep both feet grounded. Then, as efficiency and alignment dictate, the foot can leave the floor. You can play with short isometric holds or move dynamically by generating what's called "hip drive" with a single-leg repeated bridge. This could be used as a strengthening progression for people with underactive PFM or for global fitness conditioning of the regional muscles, which may assist overactive PFM in learning to synchronize and refine their efforts, by receiving the robust support of surrounding muscles. With any reported adverse effects for overactive folks, reduce volume, effort, or range, and spend a greater duration of time with PFM relaxation after strengthening.

Table rocking

Tabletop or all fours is another common base position found in yoga sequencing and exercise. While there's benefit to be gained from static, isometric applications (like a spinal balance with the opposite limbs off the floor) I tend to prefer movement to entrain relationships and efficiency as the context shifts. This subtle rocking between lower and upper extremities can help repattern spinal and pelvic compensations, can restore a reflexive quality of support within the deep core and pelvic floor, and may prepare a student well for increased loads and transitional movements within a vinyasa flow.

Find a quadruped position, allowing your torso and spine to have length and space. You may use a blanket to pad under the knees and shins. Let your breathing move naturally. Envision or feel how the pelvic diamond faces the wall or space behind you – neither tucked under nor tail lifted toward the ceiling. This rear-facing diamond relationship in the pelvis and a lengthened, neutral spine will now be carried throughout the movement of table rocking. We'll move into slight hip flexion, as seen in Figure 11.5.

Shift your weight back toward the feet about 30%, reaching the sit bones behind you, feeling them widen to expand the pelvic floor. Press the floor away to come forward and return to your starting position by reaching through the crown of your head. Move back and forth slowly, feeling your breath in both quiet, natural rhythms and consciously coordinated with the phases of movement. Sit back on your heels or rest in child's pose when you're finished.

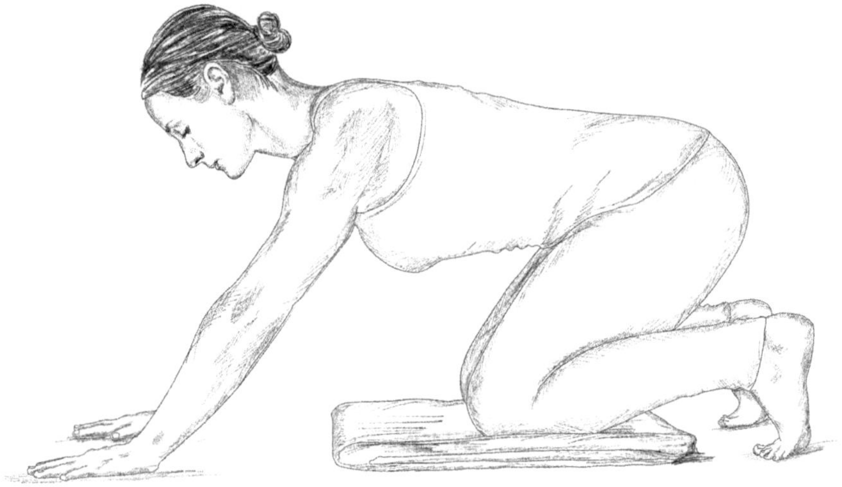

Figure 11.5: Table rocking

This baseline movement of table rocking prepares us for actions like squatting, planks, and downward dog, among others, and gives the hips and shoulders a subtle warm-up. Expand upon this theme by adding lateral shifts of the trunk, circling, or playing with varied positions of one leg to address hip mobility.

Tuck your toes under to bring weight into the balls of both feet. Feel how the soles of your feet and pelvic floor become lengthened and store elastic energy on the way back. Now press the balls of the feet into the floor actively to propel yourself forward. Can you feel in the moment you initiate the lower body push that a wave of support comes up through the perineum and deep abdominals? This variation may help folks learning how ground reaction forces sequence up through the rest of their body to heighten support and connectivity.

Cat-cow initiated with pelvic awareness

Next, let's take a yoga staple – cat-cow from tabletop – and initiate it from the pelvic floor and breathing. Begin in your spacious quadruped position with the pelvic diamond facing behind you. Feel how your breathing moves and influences the PFM. As you exhale, allow the pelvic diamond to shape-shift and become smaller, moving the sit bones toward each other and drawing the tailbone toward the pubic bone. The diamond will rotate in space to face the floor more than the space behind you. You've likely just moved your spine into flexion to accomplish this task.

To flow through neutral alignment and into extension, we'll again focus on how the pelvic floor facilitates the action. Slowly draw the inhalation down and let the tail sweep back away from the pubic bone, and let the diamond widen as the sit bones move apart. You'll feel the whole pelvis swirl around the stable femur heads and the pelvic diamond swivel to face upward behind you, helping your spine come into extension.

View Figures 9.4 and 9.5 to see the shape of these actions. Consider also how the mouthing pattern may lend a supple connectedness between tongue and tail, bringing a flowing quality to your spine.

To enhance segmental, spinal movement, provide novel stimulus, and promote coordination, play with undulating the spine through cat-cow instead of moving the whole spine in flexion and extension. You can lead with either the head or the tail and then follow with each individual vertebra until the whole trunk agrees with the end position, either full flexion or extension. Then, go the other way by choosing a distal end with which to lead and let the rest follow. Moving like a snake here can be useful when a student has lost differentiation, or moves rigidly with excess effort or unconsciously by habit. Doing things differently heightens attention and opens new movement vocabulary!

Consider exploring internal and external rotation of the thighs for both cat-cow and table rocking. You can see both directions of femoral rotation in Figure 11.6. Doing these variations may help a student feel the relationship between actions of the hip joint and pelvic-floor activity. Having the thighs internally rotated may create a wider span across the back of the pelvic bowl, lengthening the PFM, while external rotation may help facilitate their engagement. When in doubt, move between the two and then observe the result.

You could also rotate one leg internally while the other rotates externally to invite contrast and mental agility. Depending on a student's baseline, you may opt to do one and completely omit the other to enhance a chosen outcome.

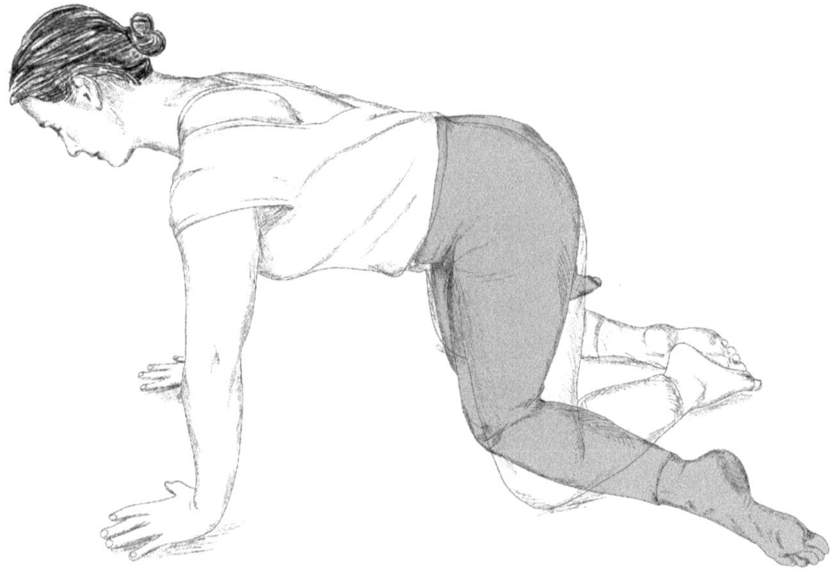

Figure 11.6: Cat-cow with femur rotation

Supported child's pose with side bend

Let's close this floor-based sequence. Grab a few blankets or bath towels, and a bolster or firm pillow. The longer you wish to stay here, the more support you'll want, to reduce load bearing into the knees and provide comfort.

For folks with any knee limitations or discomfort, we'll support the pelvis with the height of a bolster. Straddle the bolster from tabletop, and sit your hips back to one end of the cushion. The knees can be opened a bit to either side. Add a firmly rolled blanket or towel atop the bolster, which will support the chest as you rest. Your arms can wrap around that support, rest into the floor alongside you, or come forward to stack the palms of your hands or fists to create a pillow for your forehead.

As you settle into supported child's pose, you'll likely feel increased pelvic awareness and possibly pressure against the front of your perineum. Adjust your position, or tuck a small roll of towel under the thighs and sit bones to distribute pressure away from the clitoris and pubic bone until you can rest comfortably. Spend several breath cycles here allowing the weight of your body to be held and release fully into the props.

For folks with constipation, this can be a real boon to get things moving. As you sit back into child's pose, slide the end of the bolster snugly up against your hip creases and lower belly, and then let your trunk drape out and down into its support. By intentionally applying pressure to the abdominal viscera, we can also redirect the influence of breathing into the back body and pelvic bowl.

To offer the shoulder girdle more support or take pressure off the chest (especially useful during breastfeeding), place a small roll of bath towel horizontally across the top of the bolster. This strip of cushion will fill the space under the collarbones and fronts of the shoulder girdles, creating a valley in which the chest can rest.

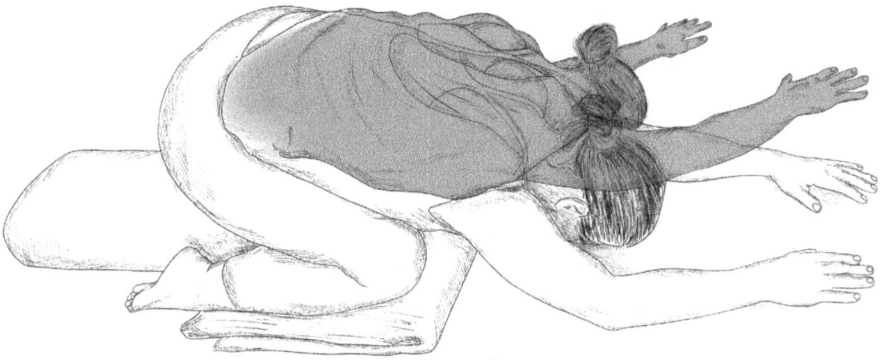

Figure 11.7: Child's pose

When a student presents with a strong tendency toward overworking one side of the PFM, taking a side bend in child's pose (see Figure 11.7) can facilitate breath excursion, and thus relaxation, into that side (Prosko 2017). First, ask them to observe their pelvic baseline. Then instruct them to walk both hands across the mat to reach diagonally away from the overactive side. Rest the trunk into the thighs, and the forehead on the floor or on top of stacked hands. Feel how the ribs and waist open on the opposite side. Inhale deeply to create inner volume, sending the breath down to feel how the pelvic floor expands. Exhale and simply let go, resting. Come back to center and feel the difference.

As an active vinyasa, consider how the pelvic floor could facilitate movement from child's pose into stepping one foot forward to low lunge, all using the ground to sequence force from the feet and legs up through the perineum and axial skeleton. Connecting pelvic awareness to the yield-and-push cycle from the lower extremities can help students find more efficient movement.

Squats: variations on a theme

In daily life, we move at least through a partial squat as we get in and out of chairs and off the commode. To maintain independence and longevity of our squat, we need to practice it, but pelvic symptoms might sway students away from this if it's historically created pain, exacerbated pressure from prolapse, or caused leaks. Women with prolapse are often told explicitly to avoid all squats. This generalized recommendation is misleading and potentially harmful, creating fear of movements a woman needs for daily life. We can educate and customize stance, depth, position, breathing strategy, and pace to find ways for them to trust and train this functional movement again, while managing symptoms.

In this section, we'll look at a few modifications that may help a student regain confidence and comfort in the action of triple flexion – the hips, knees, and ankles moving in coordination. We'll generally move from the least amount to increasing levels of load into the pelvic floor, but please keep in mind that students may have a unique relationship to these movements that doesn't necessarily follow the "logical" progression. Find a way to meet them where they are most comfortable beginning and progress from there.

Squat 1: Unload with "wall baby"

In cases where the client's lower extremities don't allow enough range or afford sufficient strength in weight-bearing squats yet, or when students report leaking, pain, or pressure when squatting upright, we can remove much of gravity's effect by instead inverting this posture. This modification focuses on mobility for the hips, PFM, and ankles and unloads the visceral support requirement, developing skills here that can then be translated gradually into upright exercise.

Find your way to a wall (or near a bed or couch) and lie on your side. See Figure 11.8 for visual reference. Roll from your side onto your back and place the soles of your feet against the solid surface. Confirm visually that your posture feels aligned and centered. Now allow your legs to abduct and externally rotate, moving the thighs away from each other into an inverted variation of happy baby pose.

Find a place where there's balanced support and stretch sensation, and if you feel intensity in the hamstrings or inner thighs, consider scooting away from the wall to reduce the range required of the hips. Spread your toes and feel your feet anchor into the stable surface, and if you'd like, place rolled towels or bolsters under the outsides of your thighs. This support becomes more important the longer, or more passively, you intend to linger here.

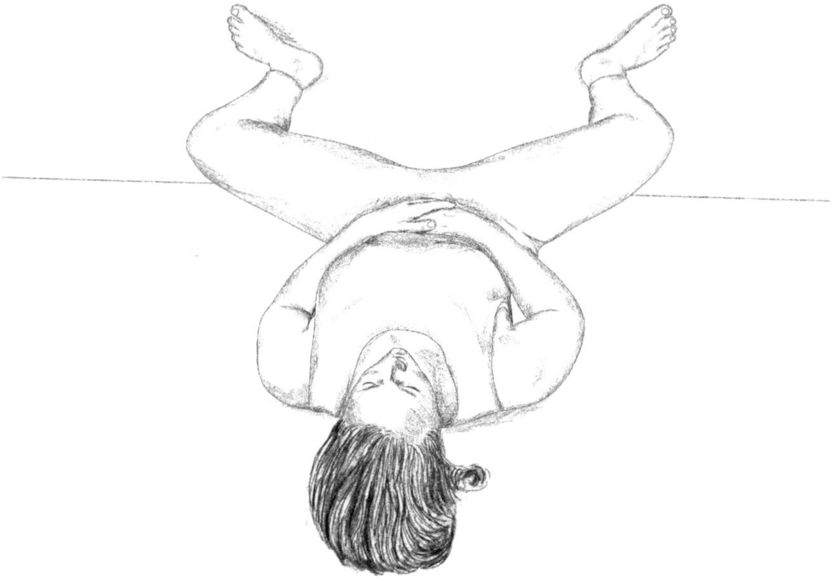

Figure 11.8: Wall baby

If you're intending to build into weight-bearing squats, you can play with subtle engagements. Explore externally rotating the thighs actively, while pressing into your feet with 10–20% effort to simulate a deep squat (mālasana). Feel how your spine wants to participate by elongating with the activation of your feet and legs. Alternatively, you can lie on a blanket to allow your torso to slide along the floor (wood or laminate may work best here) by pressing into your feet more strongly, learning how to exert effort while managing IAP and coordinating PFM support.

Squat 2: Getting vertical

When clients feel ready to attempt squats in an upright posture, using props can increase their chances of feeling contained and supported, as in cases of incontinence and prolapse. As you see in Figure 11.9, we can use a block between and a strap around the thighs to provide feedback during the squat and potentially heighten awareness and support from the PFM. Keep in mind that moving slowly with awareness, using the breath consciously, and modifying the depth of one's squat can all provide ways to mitigate pressure and improve trust, too.

Once they've found baseline function with props, gradually progress away from using them into a free-standing, self-supporting parallel squat. Creating strength in the larger muscles of the hips and legs can help the PFM modulate its activity.

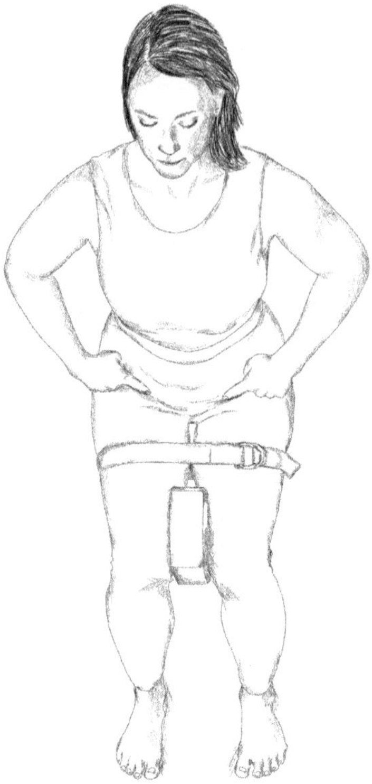

Figure 11.9: Chair squat

Taking the legs out wide (like in our exploration of the bone rhythms in Chapter 4 and as seen in Figure 11.10) can be one of the more accessible ways to help folks feel the sit bones widening and narrowing. However, this wide stance may be challenging if a student leaks with wide stances or feels increased discomfort or disconcerting pelvic pressure. Titrate the width of stance, the duration of time spent here, the depth of range in the squat, and so on to accommodate each student's needs.

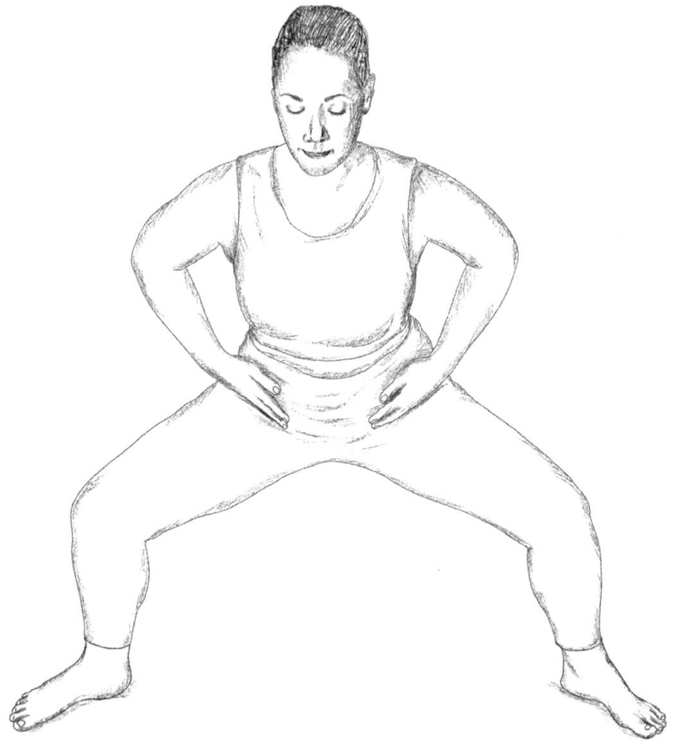

Figure 11.10: Wide squat

Squat 3: Deep squat

Deep squat or what some lovingly call an "ass to grass" squat gets touted as the solution for pelvic-floor tightness. Rightly so, this posture requires great expansion of the PFM, deep hip flexion, and sufficient dorsiflexion in the ankles. For folks with incontinence and prolapse symptoms, however, the increased pressure of the pelvic organs into fully lengthened PFM can feel utterly vulnerable. When that's the case, students can first attempt to move one leg from tabletop toward a low lunge, deep squat-like position. Have them play with sitting back partially into the one-legged variation, using the support of their hands and something to sit on like a bolster. Then repeat on the second side, provided they feel relatively symptom free during and after. (This unilateral prerequisite to deep squat can also be useful when exploring asymmetry in the PFM.)

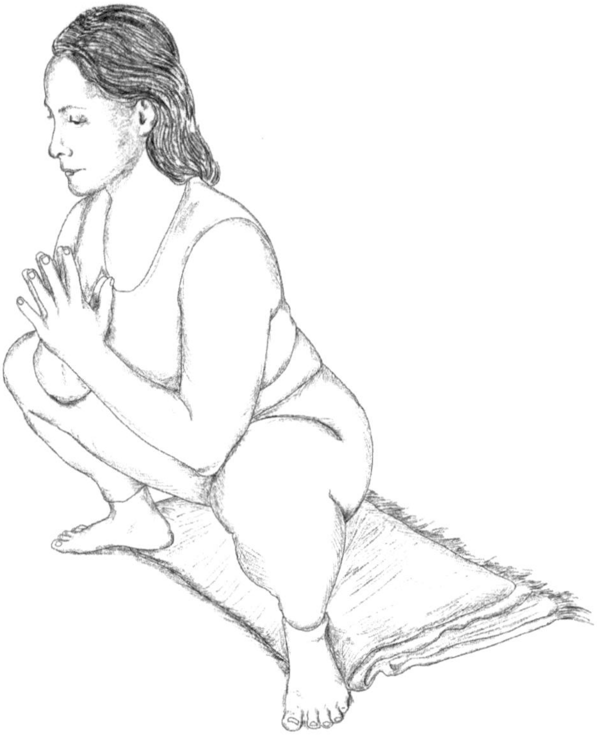

Figure 11.11: Deep squat to ground

When a student feels ready to explore the pose with both legs, we begin by using props. Providing a seat (a bolster or two wide, stacked blocks) can help them learn actions to enhance support, like how they spread and press their feet against the floor or how they can externally rotate the femurs to help engage support through the hips and glutes to float the spine upwards. The reach of the crown may help reduce feelings of pressure and heaviness. See also in Figure 11.11 how I'm using a blanket under my heels – a welcome reprieve for feet that like to pronate or when a student feels distracted by the level of effort or stretch sensation in their lower legs. Spend just a small dose of time here when the posture is new, making sure that their breath keeps moving and little to no symptoms arise.

Standing

You may wish to revisit the inquiries for the feet, finding the femur heads, and standing with dynamic alignment from Chapter 6. Once those exercises feel embodied, we can add on. Of course, myriad standing postures exist in the asana repertoire. My hope, by addressing a few key patterns in wide and narrow stances here, is that you'll feel equipped to transfer the pelvic imagery and alignment principles into other variations, working out what happens anatomically and in response to what may be happening in the PFM.

Wide standing

As we spend much of our waking life in an upright position, I tend to first teach standing postures with a neutral, vertical orientation to the spine. Warrior two (virabhadrasana II) can offer tangible feedback about how we place our feet and legs in a wide stance and whether that creates congruence between the femurs to bridge force efficiently through the pelvic center. This creates an invitation to "unlearn" less helpful cues or striving in favor of seeking more sound alignment and subtle awareness versus depth or intensity.

Wide-stance postures ask the PFM to actively support in an eccentric, or lengthened, state. Keep in mind how we can titrate this load by modifying the width and depth of the stance – smaller at first, and then deeper over time when the student can perform the pose with efficiency and steady breathing, and remain relatively symptom free.

Starting with the pelvis and feet facing forward, place your hands on the iliac crests or anterior superior iliac spines. Let your legs bend a little, and then allow your feet to pivot into the wide lunge. The front leg will need to externally rotate to do this, while the back leg must slightly internally rotate, turning that foot in. Feel how much you must allow these rotations to find integrity with the front, bent leg to align clearly with the foot and into the hip socket. (Any pinching or compression in the hips, pelvis, or up into the low back, or excess tension in the PFM, could be clues that we haven't yet found this integrity. Play with micro-adjustments until you can bend and push off either foot and feel stable and connected, with a centered, calm pelvis and PFM.)

Notice how my hand aims straight down toward the ground in Figure 11.12. This illustrates the verticality of the sacrum and spine in warrior two. You might suggest students try this to enhance interoception and proprioception of their pelvic alignment.

Moving into side angle pose, the whole pelvis must rotate in the frontal plane to reorient to a diagonal position (see Figure 9.7). This fundamental shift often needs to be taught explicitly, as even seasoned practitioners miss this internal cue when attempting to "slide their ribs forward" or "reach with their fingertips" instead. For pelvic, hip, and low-back health, I suggest we orient to and from the center.

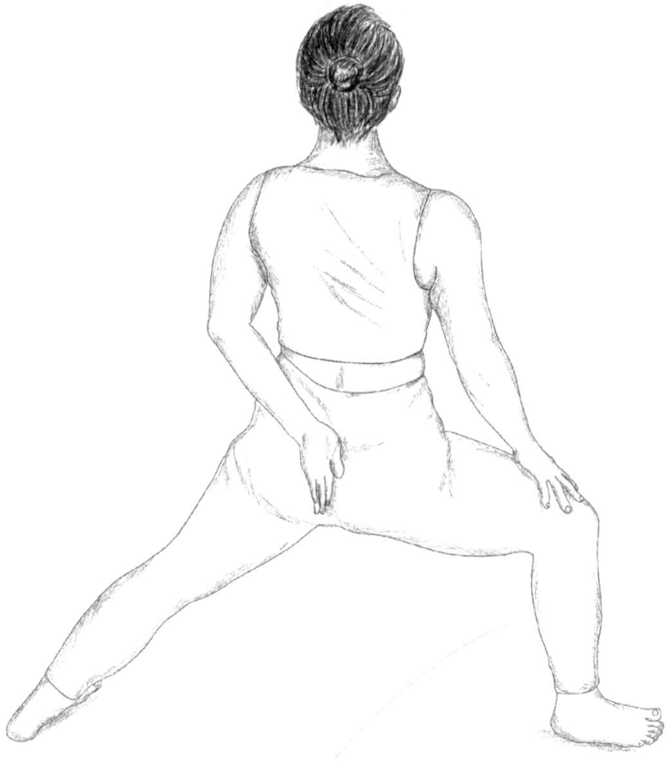

Figure 11.12: Warrior two

After wide, asymmetrical exploration, it can feel neutralizing and stabilizing to come back to center. A wide leg forward bend brings length to the PFM, posterior chain, and inner thighs while unloading the pelvic organs. It also decompresses the spine and can facilitate down-training of the ANS as gravity assists our full, slow exhalations when we're upside down (see Figure 11.13).

Stand with the feet facing forward and hands on the pelvic bowl. Take a small bend in the legs and feel the ilia come forward, rotating the entire pelvis around the stable femur heads in their sockets. Let the sit bones swing back and widen, as the hips "crease" in the front into flexion. Place your hands on the floor or a sturdy chair and breathe slowly here, feeling how the PFM respond and relax with each breath as you let the pelvic organs gently rest into gravity while suspended from the pelvic fascia. When you feel ready to come out, feel your feet. Micro-bend your legs and press down through your feet to come up with active legs, righting your pelvis, spine, and eyes back to the horizon. Step your feet in and notice how you feel.

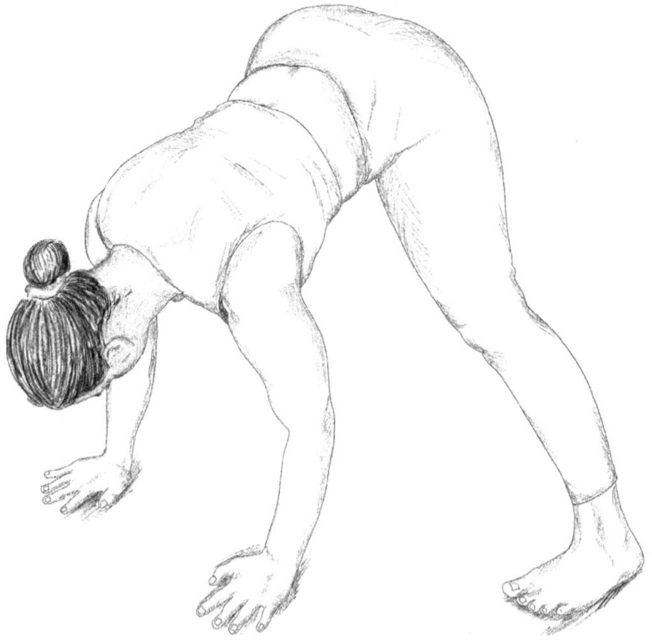

Figure 11.13: Wide leg forward bend

Narrow standing

Working with the legs closer together in parallel or front-facing postures may feel more secure for some pelvic yoga students. Moving in the sagittal plane can also repattern key functional concepts for walking and daily life, and fitness pursuits. We'll explore two postures to demonstrate how the pelvic bones participate. Then you can extrapolate this imagery into other similar asanas like pyramid (parsvottanasana) and warrior one (virabhadrasana I), and exercises like lunges, box step-ups and stairs, as well as walking and jogging.

Start in a normal standing posture. Press down with one foot to bring the opposite leg into a balance, lifting the knee into approximately 90-degrees hip and knee flexion. This is your ninja balance, and it can be a great place to build endurance and efficiency as a prerequisite for more complex balancing postures or running. Try the other side as a baseline experience and then we'll add on.

Notice how my hand touches the lateral aspect of my pelvis in Figure 11.14. The arrow represents the direction of movement of the femur head in the socket as I lift my knee, as well as the "pelvic wheel" motion in response to hip flexion (Franklin 2003). To lift one leg efficiently, that side of the pelvis (in this image, the left pelvic half or innominate bone) must rotate back and down. You can feel this as a lengthening down through your lower back as you lift your knee and as a dropping sensation into the hip crease. Too often, superficial tension accompanies this simple movement. Attempting to keep the pelvis statically "neutral" may create excess effort, when in fact, the pelvis moves slightly for efficiency. When we move, our pelvic bones move. Try the rotation of your palm back while visualizing the pelvic wheel spinning internally a few times on each side now.

When we walk, we need active hip extension to propel us forward, or what can be called "hip drive." (We might explore this hip action in a well-executed bridge pose.) For climbing hills or stairs, the hip moves through a deeper range than in walking on flat surfaces, giving us a prime opportunity to practice hip drive and better train our glutes. We can also functionally practice "knee drive" by imagining a string pulling our knee up (and thus, flexing that hip) to place our foot one step higher. Both these gait actions can be felt and trained with the ninja balance, enhancing everyday movement efficiency through asana.

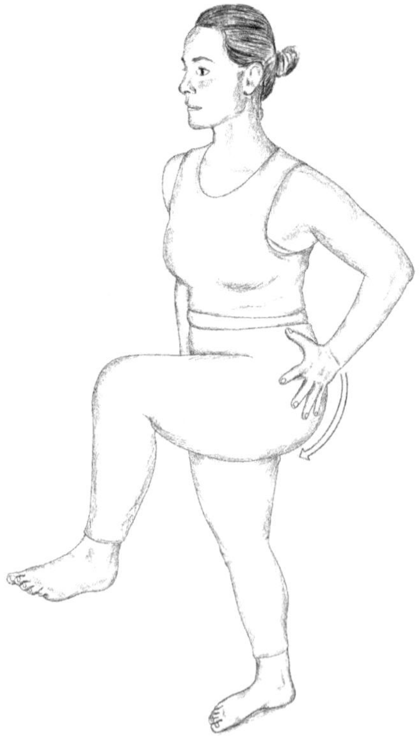

Figure 11.14: Ninja balance

The ninja balance could be considered a functional progression of the supine single leg march exercise we did in Chapter 9. Being able to descend and swirl the femur head in the socket efficiently centers the joint surfaces for optimized movement. See if you can find a similar "deep, soft, squishy" hip-crease quality in your standing ninja balance. Lastly, the pelvic wheel image representing the coupled motion of the hip, pelvis, and lumbar spine can be explored rather easily in supine knees to chest (apansana), too.

People with incontinence registered higher levels of effort in the trunk during balancing postures when compared with people without incontinence (who were more efficient in balancing). As their bladders became moderately full, all participants in the study registered higher levels of effort or tension, possibly making a case for focusing on relaxation, breathing, and efficiency even more when starting to feel bladder signals of fullness (Smith, Coppieters, Hodges 2008).

Practicing transitions can help us organize our changing center of gravity and find an alignment of the legs and feet that supports coherence through the pelvic bowl. From your ninja balance, very slowly bend the standing leg and reach the toes of your open-chain foot behind you, sensing for the mat. Come to the ball of your back foot and feel a long diagonal line of energy connecting the crown of your head through the heart, pelvic bowl, and strong, extended back leg into the back heel. Breathe deeply here to build stamina and then transfer your weight into the front foot to push off and return to ninja balancing. Try the other side, and if needed, place your hands on a wall or kitchen counter for support until this transition feels confident.

In the front lunge (Figure 11.15), we're still working with the pelvic wheel imagery, and you might play with self-touch that encourages the spinning of the pelvic wheel back for the front leg lunging, while the extended back leg's pelvic wheel spins forward to support hip extension. Remember, too, that when we fold into hip flexion, that side of the PFM lengthens or widens as the sit bone moves laterally. You can apply these images as relevant to your PFM baseline or to customize the intent and action of these standing postures for your student.

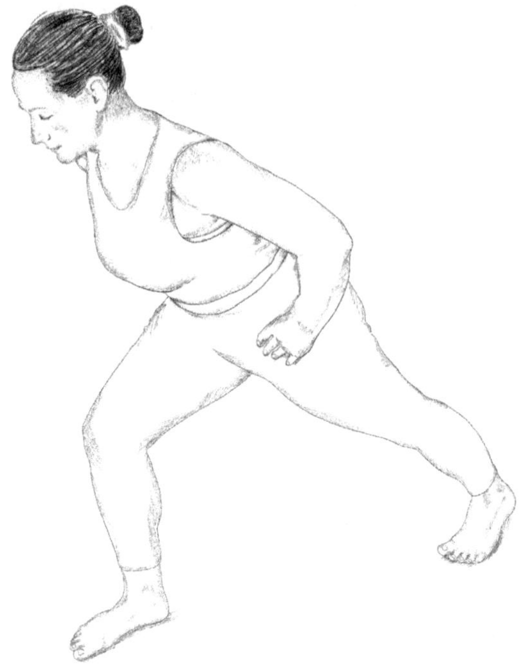

Figure 11.15: Front lunge

Heart womb mudra standing flow

Let's integrate these standing practices with a mudra flow, loosely based on a practice in *Yoni Shakti* (Dinsmore-Tuli 2020). To enhance symbolism and deepen the benefits of this flow, consider learning about the individual mudras (Le Page and Le Page 2014). Enjoy this offering of care and respect to your pelvic bowl and how your arms and hands reflect the internal volume of space created by the breath. Take in the whole sequence by observing Figure 11.16 before you begin.

Begin standing, with your hands together at the heart, in anjali mudra. As you feel your inhalation, let your hands rotate to form a downward-pointing triangle, placing the mudra over your heart with the elbows flared open toward the sides of the room. At the peak of your inhale, enjoy how the elbows may help facilitate lateral rib expansion to increase breath volume. You may also enjoy slight extension of your spine.

Feel how your exhalation creates a gathering sensation through the lungs and ribs, allowing your elbows to return alongside your body as you slide the mudra down to womb level. Let your gaze or a gentle bow of your head bring your attention to the center of your pelvic bowl. You may naturally find your legs bending a bit as you recoil and yield into yourself at the completion of your exhalation.

With your next breath in, blossom your hands forward into the spherical shape of hakini mudra (gesture of wholeness and integration invoking the goddess Hakini, see Figure 13.1). The volume of inhalation and the space within your pelvic bowl are mirrored through the form of your hands.

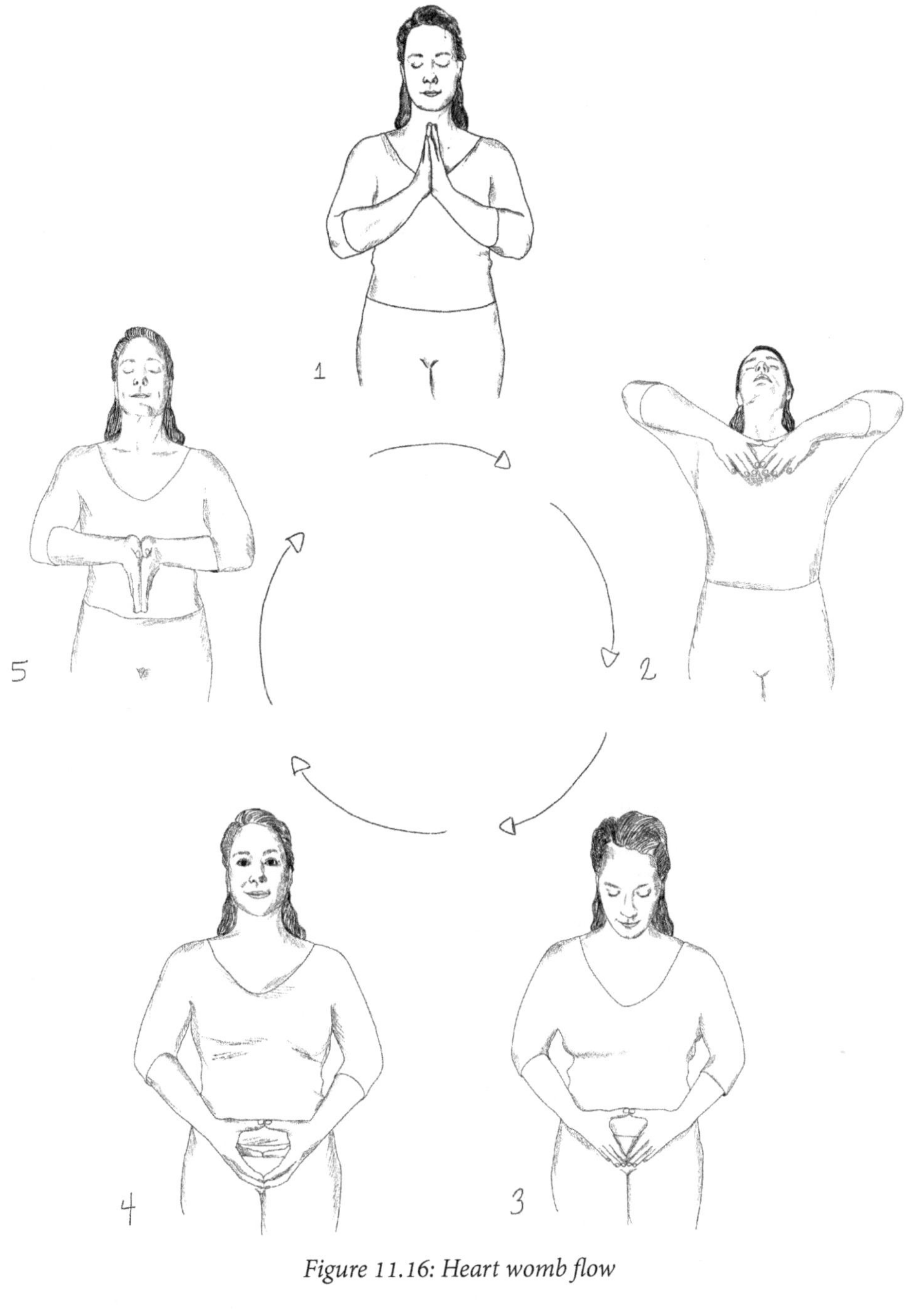

Figure 11.16: Heart womb flow

Lastly, seal the palms together at your midline while you exhale, bringing them back to heart level to complete one round of the heart womb vinyasa. This merging of the palms together might mirror a knitting sensation across the linea alba through a deep transverse engagement of the abdominal wall, providing a sense of security and closure postpartum or anytime we need a more robust connection to our will and resolve. (Let this abdominal action emerge naturally, in response to your complete exhalation rather than pulling your belly in voluntarily.)

Do a few cycles of this looping, breath-based gesture, allowing more energy and loving kindness to accumulate within as you move. Spend a little time appreciating the effects as you conclude, resting with the hands at anjali mudra.

Upgrade your sitting posture

Sitting as a stagnant, unconscious habit might perpetuate a student's tension, fatigue, shallow breathing, and feelings of pelvic pressure and/or pain. Culturally, chairs can be difficult to avoid, so we may as well do our best to make sitting an effective practice. What if sitting could feel comfortable, regenerative, and even enjoyable?

Bringing somatic inquiry into a chair-seated posture can help increase pelvic awareness. It may also help students find a more efficient way to sit at the desk or dinner table, enfolding yoga into their everyday life. Rather than giving static postural cues (for example, "engage your core," or, "sit up straight"), we'll explore micro-movements that may help students recalibrate the way in which they sit. We want to facilitate a "new normal" for their time spent sitting.

Sit in a sturdy chair and observe your baseline posture and pelvic sensations. First, we'll move the pelvic diamond like a swing forward and back with a small pelvic tilt. Feel how your weight will shift onto the back of the sit bones toward the tail as you sweep the diamond forward. Then, swing the pelvic diamond behind you to feel your sit bones widen and tail release back. Do this a few times, building into larger range, and then incrementally move through a 50% smaller range until you return to a dynamic stillness.

Next, we'll move through the frontal plane with sit bone hikes. Shift your weight onto one sit bone, doing your best not to lean your whole torso to that side but remaining upright through the chest and crown of the head. As you root down through one sit bone, feel the other levitate off the chair. Take a breath, hovering, and then set the floating sit bone down slowly. Shift across to the other side, slowly sweeping the "lighter" sit bone up off your seat for a breath. Move slowly to return to the chair. You only need to do a few repetitions of this side-to-side "hip hiking" and then come back to seated and notice what you feel.

This last inquiry I call sit bone walking. You'll incrementally "step" one sit bone forward toward the front edge of your chair and then the other. Alternate sides to "walk forward" a few steps, and then repeat the process to move toward the back of the chair. Go slowly, seeing if you can coordinate the motion smoothly, and attempt to find a similar efficiency on both sides. Return to center and notice how your breathing, posture, and pelvic floor feel now. These micro-movements can awaken and lengthen the pelvic floor, and give you novel awareness of how the pelvis provides a foundation for spinal elongation. Enjoy!

If one side of the hiking or sit bone walking feels awkward or uncoordinated, that likely indicates a window of opportunity for improved function. Do a little more practice with that motion until it becomes as smooth, natural, and efficient as possible.

One small study measured differences in pelvic-floor and abdominal activity, as well as lumbar curvature, in women with SUI compared with those without SUI (Sapsford et al. 2008). Possible takeaways: when sitting, create a clear foundation with the sit bones under you that allows for supple spinal curves, and resist the temptation to engage your abdomen voluntarily. Let it be moved as you relax into the structural support of your bones, breathing calmly and fully.

Returning to the floor

3D hip mobility series

As we return to the reliable support of the ground, we'll look at a variation of supine hand to toe pose (supta padangusthasana) that provides ample opportunity to differentiate movements of the trunk and pelvis from the joystick-like three-dimensional capacity of the femur head in its socket – the hip joint. Rather than having the second leg extended along the floor, we'll use counterbalancing movements of the opposite femur to explore an asymmetrical but bilateral approach. Here, students can learn how to maintain midline awareness and inhibit compensations in the pelvis, spine, and shoulders, targeting each action to the hip. (I learned this approach during my time assisting Donna Farhi with intensives, and it's one I return to over and over.)

Perhaps what I've found most useful as a somatic inquiry is the use of self-feedback at the hip crease, which may help the joint surfaces of the hip better relate to each other to allow smooth, free movement. It can also help inhibit the common tendency to "grip" in the groin and superficial hip flexors, and help teach how to soften and descend the femur head. Lastly, this quality of sinking deeply into the hip crease can assist students in releasing tension around the buttocks and PFM as they release their sacrum broadly into the mat.

Start in CRP, with a cloth yoga strap within reach. Bring the looped strap around the ball of one foot and extend that knee like you're standing on the ceiling. Hold the strap in the opposite hand only so the ipsilateral hand can be free to supply feedback to the hip crease. Each time you slowly exhale, use your hand to nudge the upper thigh's flesh away from your trunk, helping the hip crease deepen and feeling that side of your pelvis supremely grounded. After a few repetitions, you might release the hand's action and allow your strap-supported leg to move into what feels like your complete, comfortable range here in parallel alignment (Figure 11.17).

Next, we'll explore abduction and external rotation. Take the strap into the hand on the same side as the raised leg, and hug your opposite leg into your belly, supporting around the knee with your other hand. (Both feet are now off the floor.) One leg will be extended, supported by the strap, while the other knee remains bent. Follow your inhalation to move the thighs away from each other, opening into a wide angle. Close back to parallel with the exhalation.

After a few repetitions, you might choose to stay in the abducted, externally rotated position as shown in Figure 11.18. A simple test of your midline stability could be to ask yourself, "If the strap were gone, would I end up rolling over to my side?" One goal here is to balance the leverage into the pelvis to prevent this toppling-over effect. Lastly, students sometimes feel their legs falling forward away from their trunk after holding here for a while. When that's the case, you might encourage them to "increase their creases," meaning reestablish the triplanar action, which includes hip flexion here. The thighs can be invited to move in a curvilinear or diagonal way, versus directly to the sides of the room. Come back to center and rest if needed before going to the third variation.

Figure 11.19 shows the final direction of this inquiry, the mutual crossing and internal rotation of the thighs. Take the strap into your contralateral hand across your body. Use the other hand to once again bring touch awareness to the hip crease. Beginning with the strap-supported leg in parallel, rotate the femur head internally in its socket. Visually check the angle of your toes and feel their diagonal trajectory toward your opposite shoulder.

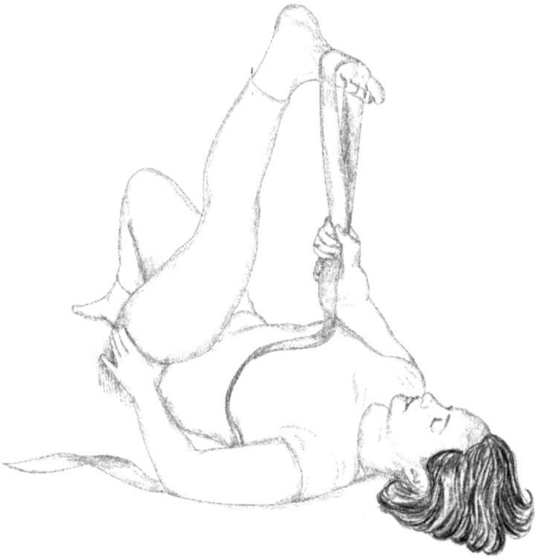

Figure 11.17: Parallel

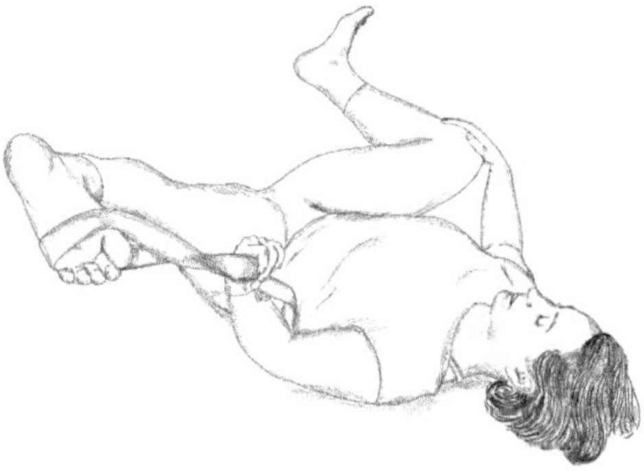

Figure 11.18: Open

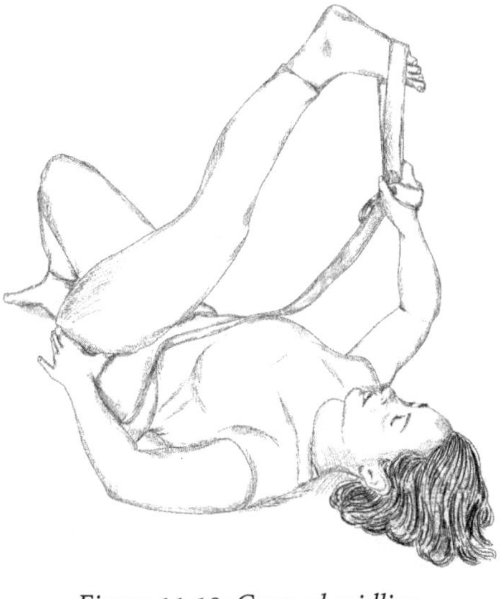

Figure 11.19: Crossed midline

Combine the actions of hip flexion, internal rotation, and adduction to titrate your movement along this path. For many folks (myself included), this is a small motion and can be quite sensational. The bent leg that began in CRP can now internally rotate to gently cross behind the extended leg, equalizing the forces delivered into the pelvis. Breathe smoothly as you explore how to maintain a midline awareness of your tail, sacrum, and spine. After exploring this three-way adventure for one side, pause in CRP to notice what you feel, comparing the two sides of your body.

Sidelying quadriceps lengthening

An option to close this three-dimensional sequence involves bringing the hip into extension. With the strap or your hand around the same foot you've just worked with, bend your knee and start to roll onto your opposite side. (For example, you'd roll onto your left side and hold your right foot for a quadriceps stretch.) Working from sidelying requires that we keep a sense of axial elongation or midline core support, yet it gives us the freedom to not concern ourselves with balancing as in standing or have our range dictated by the plane of the floor as it could be if we laid prone. If being on one's side feels uncomfortable or unstable even after some practice, adapt this to another position.

Spend a few moments feeling the pelvis gently press forward in space. You might choose to press the foot back into your hand with 30% effort or, alternatively, allow your heel to come incrementally closer to that sit bone. You may find it useful to employ a looping image from tailbone to pubic bone and up through the abdomen to support your lumbopelvic junction, and send the lengthening sensation down through the anterior hip and quadriceps, reaching out through your knee.

After resting in CRP to observe outcomes, allow yourself enough time to complete this whole series on the second side.

Savasana with ankle pumps and leg swivels

We return to stillness and take a final, closing rest. This pause restores a baseline of relaxation and ease. After "doing" our practice, we let ourselves "be" and receive the rewards. (Although this could also be the first pose in someone's practice, especially if they tend toward excess PFM tension.)

Keep in mind the restorative postures we've explored in other chapters, as you might like to weave them into your practice here before a final, neutralizing savasana (review Figures 5.3, 7.2, 10.1). You can select a restorative pose based purely on preference or to address specific needs and goals. As we've discovered how prevalent a non-relaxing PFM state may be, the extra care and support may afford a deeper "reset" to a relaxed baseline.

For savasana (Figure 11.20) we offer support to all the spaces, or secondary curves, of the body that arc away from the ground. For example, placing rolled blankets behind the Achilles tendons at the ankles, under the "pits" of the knees, and beneath the head and neck give a firm contact to yield into and can provide a sense of security as the props cradle and contain one's physical form.

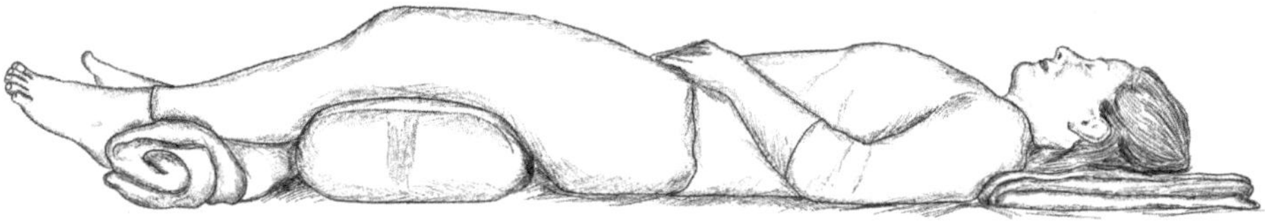

Figure 11.20: Supported savasana

Once you've had a moment to settle in savasana, bring awareness to your feet and lower legs (Prosko 2017). Alternate flexing and pointing both feet with the phases of your breathing. Take your time and really move through all the intricate dexterity in your ankles, feet, arches, and toes. Feel how the front and back muscles of your lower legs alternate between effort and stretch sensations. After a few cycles, let your legs release back into gravity passively.

Now alternate rotations of your legs – the "swiveling." For example, on the inhalation, turn both legs inward consciously, feeling your big toes come closer to one another. Then during the exhalation, roll both legs firmly but gently into complete external rotation. You could do the breathing the opposite way and feel what occurs in the pelvic, hip, and thigh muscles; let go of any preoccupation with getting it right and let it flow. After several cycles, allow your entire body to drop into relaxation. Melt the weight of your legs into the props underneath them. Rest, content in quiet stillness for as long as you need.

Some students have found relief from nighttime urinary frequency and urgency using this sequence after they slide into bed. The gentle breath-based movements seem to provide a form of progressive relaxation to the lower extremities and pelvic bowl that may calm bladder reactivity, helping them fall asleep without extra trips to the bathroom.

Journal about your experiences of trialing these practices, and if it feels useful, identify the few exercises that you feel might be most relevant and beneficial for you to repeat. Trust your body to guide you both by what feels most challenging or new and what brings a sweet, immediate sigh of relief or comfort.

Let what you've learned here inspire new movement inquiries and wise student applications. May this chapter be a springboard for you and your students to soar to new heights of reverent awareness, robust strength, and skillful confidence to lead a joyful, active life.

PART 4

HOW DO WE SOURCE INSPIRATION AND SUSTAIN ACTION?

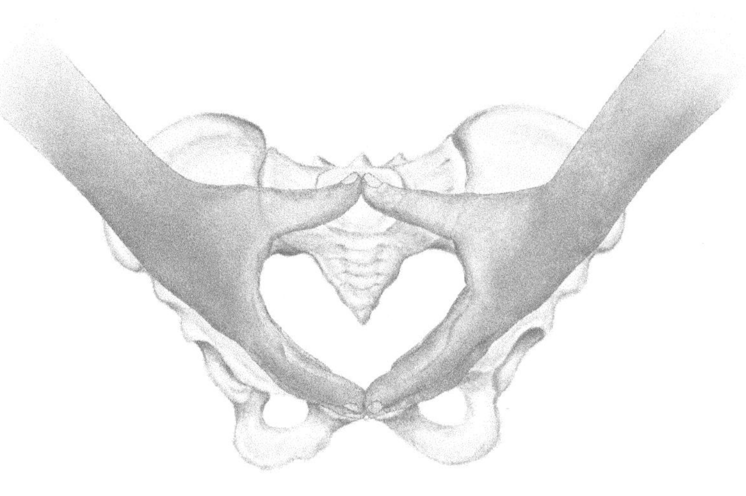

CHAPTER 12

Cultivating Commitment

Inherent in the methodology of delivering yoga therapy, and most somatic disciplines when executed and received well, lives the gift of self-efficacy. We aim to support students in their endeavors so well that they can find relief, navigate the inevitable challenges and questions that arise, and maintain positive results on their own. If the goal of yoga is liberation, at some point students may no longer require our services. When they succeed in this way, we ought to celebrate.

Therapeutic relationships marked by maturing interdependence and mutual benefit bring great sweetness. Some private clients have worked with me for more than a decade – not because they expect me to do the work for them. Our work together has tapped a well of self-inquiry, and they appreciate the ongoing flow of guidance, collaboration, and insight that swells as we meet each other through seasons of life, watching how we've both evolved.

Ask any yoga professional or healthcare provider, and they've likely had students who struggled to comply with the recommendations or program assigned. How do we motivate and inspire agency and consistency in our students? We're already convinced this practice works; we must help students *believe it will work for them.*

Being honest about what it may take for the student to accomplish their goals can help them form realistic expectations and commitment. We need to become candid, fluent communicators of this practice. For students to stay the course and continue to investigate with curiosity requires humility. And yet, this practiced familiarity with "not knowing" leads to self-actualization – they come to know themselves deeply and intimately. In the process, they develop skill and confidence.

Confidence expresses heartfelt trust, like the anchor of peace we feel when we can truly rely on someone or something. The Yoga Sutras call this shraddha, or faith in one's self and the validity of practice (Sovik 2021). Arriving on the mat regularly with enthusiasm brings students results more quickly than chasing distractions or becoming agitated in anticipation of results not yet achieved. Yoga requires patience, devotion, and faith that a goal can be reached.

In this chapter, we dig into the power of intention, active language, and visualization, as well as behavior-change strategies for supporting students in developing self-efficacy and consistent effort. We'll close with a yoga nidra meditation that invites one to dream beyond current symptoms and begins to affirm the potential to be free from pelvic suffering.

Sankalpa: crafting a powerful intention

Staying true to the collaborative process of using yoga therapeutically may allow its benefits to impact the essential, ephemeral aspects of identity, meaning, and purpose. This calls us to value the subjective lived experience of the student equally beside their medical history and other objective measures we attempt to collect. May this also serve as a loving call for discernment for healthcare providers wishing to integrate yoga into their methodology. Asana and breathing practices may lose power when separated from their philosophical frameworks, thus explicit training needs to be obtained to offer yoga with integrity (Sullivan *et al.* 2018b).

The sequence in someone's yoga plan can be objectively "correct" for their symptoms or condition, but may fall flat when presented devoid of personal intent and meaning. For yoga therapy to take root in a person's life, we infuse their story, preferences, and desires into the chosen practice. This may help the student take ownership, and therefore consistent action.

This illustrates, unfortunately, my very first experience seeking pelvic-floor therapy. I received a few exercises that may have helped but felt like I wasn't well listened to and was denied the internal examination and detailed answers I requested. I left that clinic feeling frustrated and invalidated. The therapist didn't do anything wrong, yet the lack of connection and communicating purpose meant I never went back – nor did I do those exercises very consistently, as I felt I had already exhausted their benefit in my personal practice. Luckily, with time, further research, and meeting another caring provider, I did receive the healing support I craved.

As yoga therapists, we mindfully *and* continually put the student in the driver's seat and help them tap desire as fuel for practice. The ritual of practicing yoga can become a small ceremony, an act of spirituality or faith. Suddenly, the mundane and routine take on new meaning as we witness changes in our behavior toward that which we value. Sincere, fervent motivation can be nourished by applying the concept of sankalpa, or intention. Born from two Sanskrit root words, let's define it here (McGonigal 2021).

"san" = connection to the meaning of one's life

"kalpa" = a vow or rule to be followed above all others

Stemming from several wisdom traditions, the concept of intentionality shows humans have tried to source rich meaning for their existence for ages. In some traditions, a sankalpa is to be chosen and practiced diligently over time, whereas in many contemporary asana classes, teachers may ask students to create a new intention at the beginning of each class based on their theme inquiry or planned sequence.

For powerful results with a customized yoga-therapy plan, develop a sequence and sankalpa that work hand in hand. Distill the student's values and needs to concentrate the contents of the home practice. Then, encourage them to stay with that material for a season of time to extract its wisdom. Let its roots run deep. The Yoga Sutras support a discriminating, focused approach. Students gain embodied wisdom from the limbs of yoga practice known as dharana, practicing concentration, and dhyana, achieving the state of meditative absorption. Staying with a set practice controls how many variables get involved and helps you make appropriate changes when warranted.

Determination and thoughts precede behavior. Representing a yogic strategy of the mind and will, exploring intention can make unconscious habits conscious and strengthen resolve. Like drawing a metaphorical line in the sand, write the sankalpa down by hand and keep it visible. This act can create healthy boundaries and shore up our values by getting really clear about the kind of life we desire. Intentional action builds integrity. We begin to make more deliberate choices about whether a behavior will continue as is, cease altogether, or change to better serve us and our goals.

A student's sankalpa may take the form of a behavior they wish to stop – like giving up worrying or eating sugar, for example. When the intent to stop is clear, we can help the student investigate the underlying need, emotion, or desire that habit has served. (Remember from Chapter 3 how we discussed that there's no such thing as a maladaptive strategy? That can apply here, too.)

Instead of eliminating a behavior and perhaps implying its morality, we can bring compassionate inquiry to understanding the purpose it serves. Maybe a student reaches for sugar to soothe a specific emotional state, or to feel pleasure and activate the reward centers of their brain, or to pick up their energy in the waning late afternoon hours at work to stay awake. All these needs could be addressed in new ways with personalized yoga practices, providing a positive replacement. This daily dose of practice in place of the old habit can then be bolstered by a revised intent that more clearly identifies the student's need or deeper longing. One could state, "I'm learning to sustain and respect my energy," instead of, "I will give up sugar." Rather than focusing on the undesired habit, we give the student tools to build a new path that feels more aligned with their values and brings greater nourishment.

Sometimes, sankalpa can be interpreted and applied as spiritual wishful thinking or toxic positivity in the form of generalized affirmations. Some folks may feel discord when comparing current experience with the desired future. The phrase may painfully remind us of what we don't yet feel or believe about ourselves. Framing the intention with present tense, active language can provide a simple, powerful remedy for this disharmony. When the intent feels true (or at least possible or partially true) we may find ourselves embodying that value more tangibly. For example, instead of stating, "I love my body," when we're in the throes of body dysmorphia or self-disgust, one might pivot to a more believable phrase like, "I'm learning to appreciate my body," or, "I practice showing my body loving kindness."

These reframing strategies can also assist students in holding the outcomes of their practice lightly by placing the focus on what they can more likely control in the present. This generates inspiration for change and consistent action.

Self-contract: taking consistent action

How we facilitate goal setting can help people place faith not only in tangible results and outcomes, but also on cultivating the qualities of thought, affect, and behavior that will allow them to weather future challenges or setbacks. For example, if the person sets a goal to never again experience pelvic pain, they may likely become dismayed during a flare-up and assume the practice has failed them. Worse yet, they may quit altogether, believing they've failed and are forever broken.

If we clarify the goal as reducing the intensity, severity, and frequency of their pain episodes, and to cope well when they experience pain, the goal becomes more measurable and actionable. They can learn compassionate witnessing, and how to tend to their needs skillfully as they change. This built-in resilience coaching brings a fresh dose of reality and the empathy needed for a peaceful relationship to ourselves during hard times.

When beginning with a new client, or reassessing in a new season with a long-term client, I often guide them to select three words to use as their "daily non-negotiables." These succinct verbs become a mantra and self-contract, and give them a quick, convenient way to check in with their goals. Each verb links back to an aspect of the practice or specific behavior changes that were identified during the intake and assessment process. In their home-practice notes, this mantra is spelled out with more explicit, detailed instructions.

Let's say a client experiences SUI and tends toward overactive, non-relaxing PFM. Because of a desire to not leak, they've stopped nearly all hydration and tried to clench and hold in all the ways they could to prevent leaking – which rarely helps. In working with you, they learn that relaxation may allow their PFM to function better to prevent leaks, and they now understand the importance of hydration for their bladder (to keep their urine from becoming too concentrated and potentially lead to urgency or irritation) and other body systems to function properly. They also now appreciate and understand how breathing plays a role in PFM relaxation and coordinated function.

For their daily non-negotiables, they choose the words sip, ground, and breathe. First, they understand how many servings of water to drink gradually throughout the day, and "sip" gives them an easy cue to spread out the water intake instead of guzzling. Second, the word "ground" relates to finding a sense of calm and allowing the PFM to learn to relax, practiced with self-touch, awareness, and customized postures. Third, they seek to find breath excursions expanding into the PFM throughout the day, as well as completing their formal pranayama practice for stress management and mental health.

This three-word phrase "sip – ground – breathe" can create top-of-mind awareness and a convenient way to hold themselves accountable. I typically request students check in with themselves after work or before bedtime to confirm whether they've checked each box for that day. When they haven't yet, it can light a motivating fire to fit the practices in (or forgive themselves when there were valid reasons they didn't accomplish all three). As they see their own success growing more consistent, it can give them a sense of pride and momentum to keep going.

Lastly, using verbs to spark behavior gets the student focusing on what they can control instead of the outcome – they become invested in *the process*. Many goal-setting strategies exist to support program adherence, so implement what feels relevant and relatable for your people.

Supporting adherence: giving students "homework"

Keeping it simple supports clarity and perceived convenience, which can enhance compliance. Collaborate with your student to determine the physical location of their props and practice space, what time of day will work best, and how often they will practice. Create a clear map of what's expected and share how or why you feel the practices will benefit them. Show your client how to succeed by resolving as much of this guesswork as possible.

We can also consider how space – be it literal, physical space to move, time and energy in their daily routine, or mental-emotional bandwidth – differs for each student and can be driven by societal privilege and access to resources. When this plays a role, we'd be wise to acknowledge their struggles compassionately, affirm where they do have resources or control despite systemic injustices, and do our best to support access to vital resources that may help them form an effective personal practice.

It can be tempting to want to address all their needs and concerns in the first phase of your work together or give them what feels like a "full practice," like when we plan for group asana classes. The arc of a group class sequence can be pared down to what we believe to be the few, most potent elements for that client at that time. Consider telling a story with three baseline components to their home practice, choosing a beginning, a middle, and an ending. You can always fill in more detail to the story as you develop depth and nuance, play with volume and frequency (how much practice is expected and how often), and explore intensity.

The subjective experience of intensity to build capacity and resilience can be applied in several different ways; we seek to choose the path most suited to the client's needs and goals. For example, capacity might be investigated and built through increasing physical effort and movement vocabulary for goals of fitness, or longer meditations or restorative postures for attentional focus, or it may include the depth to which you're asking your student to inquire within by posing powerful questions for self-study and reflection. The therapeutic relationship can be like a wilderness guide, helping students venture into the unknown territory of source material, psyche, and spirit by trusting they won't get lost. We provide companionship and wayfinding as they make their way home, integrating who they are as they travel.

Understanding regression and progression principles of physical exercise can help you tailor the practices to your client's baseline capacity, keep it interesting with new variations, and keep it challenging enough for them to feel satisfied, yet reduce overwhelm from giving too many elements, details, or cues.

While it's outside the scope of this book to discuss in detail the exercise principles behind how to program, regress, and progress physical activity, they've been woven into the way practices are presented in earlier chapters, and the sample practices in Appendix B. Know that you can make a game of simplifying or challenging any asana or movement according to the client's goal. For example, you can work on increasing the duration of isometric holds of a posture for endurance, adding external resistance to build strength, or enhancing balance and stability by playing with novel patterns or positions, adding arm or head movement, or standing on a squishy mat to challenge the feet and lower extremities. You could take a full-range movement into an inquiry of "incrementalizing" it – moving only 10% of the way, then 20%, and so on to invite more refined modulation of attention, sensation, and effort. Understanding the physics of a body in motion allows us to make the physical practices infinitely customizable, playful, and inspiring.

Beyond the formal practice on the mat or meditation cushion, yoga therapists can play an important role in translating skills gained into other physical pursuits and a student's broader goals for their life. Taking skillful, reliable action on one's own behalf can positively impact daily routine, self-talk, their communication with others, and even initiative and completion of seemingly unrelated projects. Helping students identify and celebrate tangible examples of how they now respond differently to stressors, or experience more ease, can breed motivation to continue developing their formal yoga practice, too. The embodied self that emerges through devoted practice impacts all areas of life – because the person is at the center.

Overcoming obstacles together

Inevitably, students will at some point face a curveball. Whether they experience a pain flare-up, have a change in life circumstance or resources, lose a loved one, or feel creeping thoughts of self-doubt thwarting regular practice, we're poised to offer wisdom through the heart-to-heart connection of therapeutic relationship.

We can dialogue with our students to unravel the tangled yarn ball of confusion, inaction, and frustration, restoring their ability to run one thread smoothly in their hands again – providing a clear path forward. We assist them in regaining focus and bolster their commitment. Accepting that challenges and seasons of wavering motivation are normal and to be expected can help them forge ahead or make necessary adjustments.

Rather than going back to the drawing board and reinventing the wheel (as in completely overhauling their chosen practice, unless that seems warranted), we can consider this an invitation to explore the mind and personal values, or manomaya and vijnanamaya koshas. Habits of thought, core beliefs, and one's sense of meaning, purpose, and identity can determine the value or place of importance a student assigns to their yoga-therapy practice. Instead of changing the practice, we might suggest deeper self-reflection by introducing personally relevant yoga-philosophy concepts or journaling prompts to help them see through the opacity of a perceived barrier to new insight.

We might examine their schedule of yoga-therapy visits and suggest a higher frequency at the onset of a new client relationship or while a student navigates changing circumstances or a new diagnosis. This may not always be accessible due to financial constraints, or a lack of time and energy on the student's part or ours.

Lastly, we could consider how we're supporting a student in their program adherence beyond scheduled appointments. A simple text, email, or handwritten card can be an easy, low-cost way to show we're here for them. Offering a practice reminder, praise, or a relevant quote or poem can sustain their momentum and may make them feel seen and well cared for between sessions.

The power of visualization

We can offer respect to the negativity bias of our mind, its desire to keep us safe, and our embodied responses to safety, threat, and life risk as outlined in Chapter 3. Posing a question for a student to take home as svadhyaya homework can help them develop more discerning witness consciousness and skill in the vijnanamaya kosha.

The willingness to reflect constructively may indicate a readiness to enter a more distinct, meaningful, and lasting practice of visualization and transformation. One such strategy, pratipaksha bhavana, comes from Sutra 2.33 (Satchidananda 2008, pp.127–129).

Vitarka badhane pratipaksha bhavanam.
When disturbed by negative thoughts, cultivate the opposite.

This sutra asks us to notice our wayward, harmful, or self-doubting thoughts and attempt to see the other side, cultivating positive thoughts instead. This requires a steadfast fierceness, a kind of mental-emotional vigilance to bring one train of thought to a full stop and hop on another. By delinking or de-identifying with the habits of mind we feel cause or contribute to suffering, we may begin to see other paths or courses of action. No longer held hostage by our patterned thoughts, we can create new, more beneficial ones. Neuroplasticity both explains this capacity to change our minds and shows that directing the discursive patterns of consciousness influences the pruning and development of neural pathways, changing the brain itself (Dana 2020, p.190).

Some students may need to establish a physical, breath-based practice for some time before introducing bhavana. The grounding skills developed with physical movement, tracking sensation, and understanding how to skillfully guide one's breathing for desired results can provide an anchor into the present, a way to return "home."

Before practicing visualization, get into a regulated or relaxed, present state. From this state of trust, safety, and informed consent, one may be able to conjure more vivid imagery than when feeling a "filter" or perception of despair and isolation (dorsal vagal shutdown) or the tunnel vision and tension of mobilizing our defenses (sympathetic charge). Find comfort first.

The last principle involves shifting from using bhavana as solely a thinking or cognitive exercise (or verbal dialogue) into a somatic, sensory-rich experience. As the student envisions their future free of pelvic symptoms or suffering, for example, we can instruct them to imagine how it feels in their body versus creating a mental picture like watching themselves on a video. We can ask what they see and hear, how their food looks and smells, and what they wear and how it moves with them as they walk down the street.

To further enhance pelvic health, we might suggest they watch what images, sensations, thoughts, and feelings arise when imagining future menstrual cycles, exercise pursuits, creativity, sexual expression, and an improved quality of relationships. Whatever they've felt unable to do or enjoy consistently up until now because of their pelvic symptoms can be used to design inquiries and prompts to facilitate their ability to dream their way toward a more embodied, joyful future.

In the following practice, we'll explore bhavana and anchor it back to a present-tense sankalpa that may support the student in taking targeted, relevant actions in daily life that serve their long-term vision. Enjoy.

Yoga nidra: Dreaming forward with bhavana

As a long-form meditation translated as "psychic sleep," yoga nidra allows us to access deep states of consciousness that can instigate lasting change. We hover between waking and sleeping in a state of attentive relaxation, exploring our inner world. Most often, this practice is guided by a teacher. You may find it easier to record yourself reading the script aloud and then get comfortable to receive the meditation. (Alternatively, you can download an audio recording from https://library.singingdragon.com/redeem using the code YHKCWYB. The first, for pelvic health, relates to what's written here; the second allows pelvic yoga professionals to explore a career-related bhavana.) If this practice is new to you, consider inviting a friend to join you or plan for a conversation after to help integrate your experience.

We'll be using creative visualization to conjure images, sensations, and feelings, and see new possibilities through your future self, free of pelvic suffering and full of thriving, pleasure, and vitality. If you find this challenging to imagine, take heart and know it will become more vivid and potentially easier as you practice this skill. If you have a known mental-health diagnosis that makes exercises like this pose any risk – real or perceived – please consult with your medical and mental-health providers before practicing. Know that you can roll to your side and pause any time.

I know you'll do your best to remain attentive and awake. If you happen to drift off or fall asleep, please offer yourself compassion. It's okay. When you notice this state, guide your attention back to my voice and resume your practice of yoga nidra.

Make yourself comfortable by lying down in savasana with all the support shown in Figure 11.20. Be sure that you'll be warm enough since your core temperature will likely decrease as you rest here in stillness. Feel free to cover your eyes and slide your hands onto the lower belly with the triangular trimurti or yoni mudra gesture if that feels welcome. Offer yourself the gift of making any final adjustments now, so you can be completely comfortable and rest deeply.

Welcome, friend.

We now begin our practice of yoga nidra.

Acknowledge the support you feel under you and the privilege of this time to practice yoga nidra. Notice your breathing and body sensations, without asking anything to change. Gather all the tendrils of your attention inward, offering yourself sincere, potent awareness.

If you'd like, take a few deep, slow, conscious breaths now – expanding the volume of your inhalation and completely surrendering the exhalation slowly. Following the next exhalation all the way to its end in your own time. Now, allow your breathing to rest and grow quiet. Let go.

Feel your body spread into the ground. You are fully supported. Drop deeper into being, choosing stillness. It's okay to settle in more. Give your weight to the earth, dissolving any effort that isn't needed. Let your breath do what it wants, finding a quiet natural rhythm. Welcome yourself into this quiet space.

Welcome home.

Let this restful state open you to possibility. Change is possible. Change includes being honest about what we don't want and the compelling vision of what we most desire. Both require we remember our power, our choice in moving forward.

You likely know what you wish to resolve. The pelvic symptoms. The stress. The suffering, discomfort, conflict, or shame you long to release. Take a moment to reflect on your current or past experiences. Offer them gratitude for teaching you, by the virtue of contrast, what you no longer wish to experience.

Consider how you could mine wisdom from these aspects of your story. What have you learned about yourself or life through this suffering? Trust the first thought or image that arises. One of many gems you carry with you. Consider now the possibility of a thriving future. How might you prevent future suffering of this nature?

Observe your sensations and let your body continue yielding into the floor as you listen for answers to these questions. There's no rush. There's no right or wrong way to go about this. If all that comes is thank you, I'm ready for a change, that's more than enough.

Thank you for trusting yourself. Offer yourself sincere gratitude for all you've endured, all you've overcome, and the gems of insight you've polished through this suffering. The Yoga Sutras teach us that future suffering is to be prevented – you're already gathering the wisdom of how to do that. Change is possible.

It's time to follow our most sincere desires and dream.

Make this sacred vow your intention:

I trust myself to dream.
May I see clearly all that's possible for my pelvic vitality and embodied thriving.

Select a timeframe in the distant future, possibly years or decades forward from this moment in time. Envision this future self that is free from suffering; fulfilled, connected, joyful, and at peace.

How would your health and fitness, relationships, sexuality, emotions, spirit, life's work, and legacy feel if your pelvis was wholly, absolutely, well and vital?

Trust your intuition and bodily sensations to guide you with which of these topics you carry through the visualization, choosing the ones that feel most potent or letting all meander and merge into a complete picture of YOU in the future. What would it feel like to be liberated?

Imagine yourself walking down the street or moving about your home. What do you see and hear? How do your clothes move against your skin? Who is with you? How do you express yourself creatively? Sexually?

Feel this future vividly. Let your body take on this new identity and ease. Trust the threads of imagery, sensation, or narrative that come through for you, and be patient and kind with yourself if nothing clear comes. It will, in time. If you were completely liberated from all past suffering, how would you express that freedom, joy, and fulfillment? How much power could you hold? How much pleasure could you experience? How deep a well of peace might already exist within you?

Ask your future self for ONE word, image, or feeling that most clearly expresses what will nourish and inspire you now. Trust what you receive in whatever form. Let this message drop in, permeating every cell of your body. Distilled to your essence, become this sankalpa.

As we guide awareness around your physical body, fill yourself with this essence. Let your attention move swiftly and easily. Allow each part to come alive, held in loving presence. Feel your whole body – see your body's imprint on the floor under you and the space around you – the volume of your contours taking up physical space. The boundaries of your skin.

Under your skin is a fascial, fatty matrix, soft and supple, intelligent, and nourishing; this fleshy connective tissue covers, warms, protects, and gives you a soft place to land. Muscles – red and richly fed with blood, hungry – they move you. Bones – yielding and alive – they provide a framework of support, solidity you can rely on. Organs – steady, slow and reliable, always communicating with each other and you – you're learning to listen and translate their secrets. They express your vitality.

Continue diving your awareness deeper into the core center of your body – into your cells and the fluid spaces between them – arrive in your pelvis – your center of gravity. Gut instincts and intuition, creativity, and sensuality all reside here.

In your center
Trace from your center to your right foot
Trace from your center to your right hand
From your center to the crown of your head
From your center to the left hand
From your center to the left foot
From your center through your tail, your root downward
Feel the toes on your right foot
The fingers on your right hand
Right toes
Right fingers
Right leg
Right arm
Whole right side flowing back into your core center
Feel the toes on your left foot
The fingers on your left hand
Left toes
Left fingers
Left leg
Left arm
Whole left side flowing back into your core center
Become aware of your pelvic floor

Become aware of the crown of your head
Pelvic floor
Crown of your head
Pelvic floor
Crown of your head
Cervix
Throat
Abdomen
Heart

The pelvis sits at the center of your being; radiant, fluid, and generous, she supports your entire body, carries life, sheds the old, and inspires new creations.

This is your connection to power, pleasure, and peace.

Notice the pause at the end of each quiet exhalation. Every breath reminds us to be present, a small window into the possibilities that await us. The pause creates space.

Each pause helps us remember we have a choice.

Your potential for healing and happiness exist here, now.

Take the word, image, or feeling received from your future self.

Recite it silently as a present tense affirmation.

I am
I am
I am

As you feel your next breath come, let yourself fill up on the inhale. Pause and suspend the full volume of breath within you for just a moment, and when you exhale, let go of this imagery, release this meditation.

Bring your senses back up to surface… Notice the temperature of the air on your skin and the texture of your clothes. Any faint taste or smell. Notice the sounds you hear, let them gently awaken you.

Our practice of yoga nidra is now complete. When you're ready, blink your eyes open and closed a few times. Let the world come to you through your vision. Begin to move in any way that feels kind, circling, stretching, eventually rolling over. Offer yourself appreciation.

Closing

We practice to remember we're whole and worthy as we are, without "doing," earning, or striving. And yet, through this practice, our actions become more skillful on the mat and in life. Each day, we touch back in to our center and meet our most basic needs – to breathe, focus, move, feel, and rest. It can serve our motivation well to respect the ongoing, dynamic nature of our needs as human beings, for they will persist until our last breath. Whether we "feel like" practicing or not, the devotion to tending our hearts and bodies creates a meaningful undertow that carries our practice and life forward.

Ultimately, yoga therapy is a process of befriending one's whole self. The process of yoga happens here and now. We allow the range of our experience to exist *and* to teach us. As Donna Farhi states, "While pain may be the catalyst that brings us to Yoga practice, it is joy that renews our commitment" (Farhi 2003, p.20). We actively build our resolve and witness within ourselves a growing contentment that cannot be swayed or taken from us. No longer constricted by aversions or grasping attachments, we reclaim power from these apparent opposites to forge steadfast devotion. By committing to practice, we commit to ourselves. Pause to connect with your commitment through hridaya mudra (Figure 12.1) for three slow breaths.

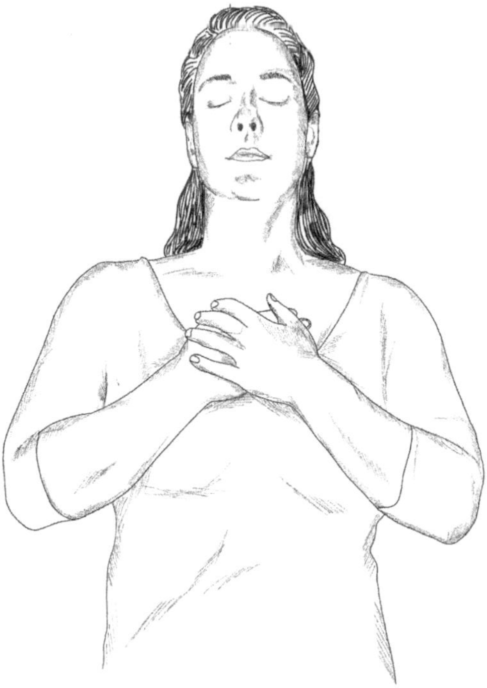

Figure 12.1: Hridaya mudra (heart gesture)

Next, we'll explore how to fortify this essential relationship to one's self with pleasure, belonging, and integration. When we reliably receive these kinds of nourishment, we can begin to feel held and whole in our struggles and unstoppable in our vision.

CHAPTER 13

The Gifts of Belonging

Ancient wisdom teachings and modern integrative approaches to health and wellbeing understand the truth of interconnectedness. The pelvic floor does not function in isolation from the rest of the body, and we do not function separately from collective society. Most of us would find it unlikely that we could fully escape from working, paying bills, and tending to our families and communities. It's rare to find someone completely free of the "householder" role. We are bound to each other.

Supportive relationships may help our clients navigate struggles more compassionately, gain perspective, and break through to increased wellbeing. Burdens and joys become shared. We cannot possibly serve every need students have, but we can support their process of self-inquiry. We can welcome their reflections around intimacy, friendship, and connection in the yoga therapy session, using yoga philosophy to encourage more equitable and fulfilling relationships.

For us yoga professionals, relationships sustain, challenge, and celebrate the work we do. They offer a place to land during our own times of suffering so it doesn't interfere with client care. Mentors and colleagues help us grow and hold us accountable. And the more we evolve and refine our unique methods and niche in pelvic yoga therapy, the more we find our place and prosper.

Imagine your social networks, your family, friends, teachers, and mentors, and broader community woven throughout life like golden threads of a quilt that holds you in integrity, adding warmth and strength to the work you do professionally. Many people and experiences have shaped and led us to this moment.

Belonging can be fraught with challenges like shame and judgment, the initial discomfort of being witnessed in our vulnerability, competition, and social conflict. Yet when we strengthen our resolve to show up in all our messy humanity, true community and kinship can be formed.

In this final chapter, we explore placing and meeting our basic needs within a collective context, ideas for resourcing pleasure and joy, and how to build community. After contemplating your professional place in offering pelvic yoga therapy, we'll close with a mudra meditation. I encourage you to take in this chapter both for your own benefit and through the lens of offering these insights to clients.

Sovereignty and service

Sovereignty is power. Our historical misunderstandings and misuse of power (colonialism and patriarchal structures, and the many examples of abuse in yoga lineages (Dinsmore-Tuli 2020), for example) have led some to believe it's an asset to hold *power over* each other. In the therapeutic relationship, we actively share our power *with the student*, placing them at the center of their own story. In this way, we can adopt the definition of sovereignty as a self-governing state.

When clients initially come to see us, they may need to feel our self-regulated state, connecting perhaps for the first time to another's ventral vagal neural platform of safety through co-regulation (Dana 2020). Yoga therapy is a co-regulatory process that can entrain and strengthen this self-governing capacity. Instilling confidence, embodiment, and self-efficacy in students allows them to contribute their unique creative, generative power to the benefit of society (Hartley 1995, pp.299–304). We all win when someone heals.

In the classic book *Women Who Run with the Wolves,* Dr. Clarissa Pinkola Estés, Ph.D., talks about the wild nature within that we long for and return to when we come into right relationship with ourselves. Her definition of this integrity of self reminds me of the yogic concept that through practice we restore connection to our true nature.

> [This] means to establish one's territory, to find one's pack, to be in one's body with certainty and pride regardless of the body's gifts and limitations, to speak and act on one's behalf, to be aware, alert, to draw on the innate feminine powers of intuition and sensing, to come into one's cycles, to find what one belongs to, to rise with dignity, to retain as much consciousness as possible. (Estés 1995, p.11)

Yoga supports a community-care approach. After all, the word yoga can be translated as union or a pervasive sense of oneness. We owe it to future generations to zoom out from the often-introspective time spent on our mat and see our place in the bigger picture. As interconnected beings, we play an essential role in the health of our families, our communities, and the collective. Even nature herself depends on us to live consciously, respecting and tending the earth like our pelvic center – we are nature. Also, remember the bidirectional nature of wellness – the systems, policies, and organizations we create and manage also need to support personal wellbeing and community care (Jain 2020).

The eight limbs of yoga practice described in the sutras begin with ethical concepts and loving self-interrogation (refer to Chapter 2 for an overview). The yamas ask us to abstain from certain behaviors, while the niyamas welcome observation and self-inquiry around others. Practicing these boundaries helps place us behaviorally within a social framework (Bhavanani 2018). We become aware of how our choices, thoughts, and actions impact others, and seek to build a compassionate framework for living and relating.

While self-responsibility is a desirable trait that can be developed with yoga therapy, over-reliance on one's self that generates fear or disallows relationship and co-regulation may present as a conditioned behavior or a remnant of response to trauma or adverse childhood experiences (Porges 2004; van der Kolk 2014, pp.212–215). We fundamentally need community care. A simple example of community care is how we kindly deliver food to people who have just had a baby, lost a loved one, or recently moved into the neighborhood. Relational resilience allows us to graciously receive without guilt when we need support and freely give when we can. Feeding someone nourishes us in return, as we help meet their basic needs. Aligning our individual actions toward collective wellbeing brings belonging and fulfillment.

Here, we'll pause to chant a full-length verse called the ayur mantra (Farhi 2015b). First introduced to me by one of my teachers, I love this mantra, as it concludes that personal practice in turn can serve the greater good. We ask for abundant nourishment so we can share it with those around us. Consider speaking or singing it aloud, remembering that your voice powerfully connects you to the ventral vagal complex.

Ayur mantra for healing

Om āyur dhehi prāṇaṃ dhehi

Om apānaṃ dhehi vyāhaṃ dhehi

Om cakṣur dhehi śrotraṃ dhehi

Om mano dhehi vācaṃ dhehi

Om ātmānaṃ dhehi pratiṣṭhāṃ dhehi

Om māṃ dhehi mayī dhehi

May my life be nourished. May the upward flow of energy be nourished.

May the downward flow and circulating flow of energy be nourished.

May my sight and hearing be nourished.

May my mind be nourished and my speech nourishing.

May my soul be nourished and may I rest deeply in this nourishment.

Through this nourishment may I bring joy to others.

If you feel like a novice with Sanskrit pronunciation, consider how your heartfelt conviction and sincerity afforded this prayer its power as you silently read, whispered, or sang it aloud. With this intent infused by the resonance of our collective voice, let's continue with practical ways to bring more nourishment into daily living.

Make life your beloved: strategies for joy and pleasure

Presence precedes pleasure. Attentiveness to what we see, smell, taste, hear, and feel opens gateways for sensory aliveness to nourish us. This can include bringing sacred curiosity to mundane acts like toileting, eating, and getting dressed, as well as choosing to engage with arousal and erotic self-expression, the spectrum of emotion, ceremony, ritual, and spiritual practice.

Sometimes, pleasure can feel fleeting, even elusive. Maybe deep, lasting pleasure comes from allowing *what is* with a spirit of radical acceptance. See the beauty in the boring day to day, the discomforts, and the awkwardness of figuring out who we are, why we're here, and how to make life feel like it matters. When we welcome contrast and range, all of life can inspire.

When we're depleted and frazzled, it can feel difficult to carry on, let alone be concerned with our legacy or being of service to others. Burnout is all too common. A key principle in yoga therapy involves making sure our clients establish a resourced state. We may first consider adding nourishment, support, and building their reserves. Our physicality is the vessel through which we experience life, and pleasure is restorative. Here are a few suggestions for slowing down and sourcing more embodied pleasure and connection.

- Give yourself time to turn a meal into a meditation on savoring through your senses. See the colors and textures of your food and smell their aromas. Notice your eagerness or appetite, maybe your mouth is watering in anticipation. Chew each bite a minimum of 20–30 times, observing how texture and taste evolve in your mouth. Set your utensil down at times, allowing yourself to take deep breaths, and settle back in your chair. Let yourself be nourished by more than mere calories alone as you awaken your senses.

- Schedule a date with nature. Go to a new or most-beloved landscape, and if possible, walk barefoot. Feel how the soles of your feet meet the ground. Move slowly. What do you hear and see in the distance? What temperature do you feel on your skin? Some research suggests that the act of stepping on solid ground, or even imagining walking on the earth instead of a concrete sidewalk, can improve diaphragmatic function (Tibbetts and Peper 1996).

- Notice what feels sexy or sensual to you personally. Notice when you feel relaxed and calm, what makes you feel excited or become aroused. Maybe there are ways you dress and adorn yourself, how you move, or being naked and feeling your receptive skin. Attuning to yourself as a sexual being can invite erotic energy to playfully spark unexpected moments of pleasure and nourishment.

- The next time you explore self-pleasure or partnered sex, explore ways to slow down and observe sensation. Let your breathing accompany you.

Trust what you desire, ask for it, and allow new adventures to unfold. If you don't know what you want, allow yourself to be with that question in an unhurried, compassionate way. Your body will guide you.

- In your next conversation with a close friend, use what has been presented about the power of connection. Meet their eyes and hold a soft gaze. Imagine your inner ears opening to receive the melody of their voice. As you speak, track internal sensations and your breathing, and allow yourself to share from the heart sincerely. Hold each other in loving kindness as you co-create what could become a rich, meaningful exchange.

Witnessing each other

For some women (myself included during young adulthood), being witnessed in sisterhood might feel like a foreign concept or may feel incredibly difficult. Unfortunately, comparison, self-deprecation, and harsh judgment are commonly conditioned behaviors among women socially. In short, we may not feel safe with peers.

It took one of the hardest years of my life to allow women to companion me in ways I hadn't even known I was missing. Women to sit with as I cried, to keep watch while I slept upstairs, and to bring me soup – people willingly stepped in when I crumbled under the weight of betrayal and pregnancy loss. That season of vulnerability cracked me open to the lifeblood of women caring for women.

Circling "formally" as peers and equals, and setting clear boundaries for expectations of behavior in social groups, can help us all settle into the truth that we can be loved as we are. We can learn and co-create a new paradigm of unconditional support and "enoughness" that allows us all to thrive and celebrate each other. Gatherings like women's circles and retreats can give a sound container for connection and meaningfully mark the passage of time.

On the verge of getting remarried, I received an invitation to join a women's circle that met by phone. We gathered weekly for four years (other than a handful of exceptions) to discuss challenges and breakthroughs, to celebrate gratefully what was good in life, and to be witnessed. We had different roles but agreed to treat each other as equals and that it wasn't a time to give advice or comment on another's experience. We witnessed silently and gave each woman complete presence to hear her own thoughts spoken aloud, to find her own solutions in her own time.

Although I thought I'd complete my time in that circle much earlier, the timing was serendipitous. When I joined, I envisioned the circle ending as I entered motherhood. I didn't know at the time that two cross-country moves and big professional leaps were in the picture before we'd feel ready to conceive. I'm so grateful that our circle lasted years longer than I anticipated, until after my first daughter was born. They held me through the first handful of very difficult months postpartum.

After that transition, I found my way to in-person circles in our new community. Sitting in my now dear friend's living room, one evening a woman shared about her traumatic labor and delivery, the despair and devastation she felt as a new mother, and how her relationship to herself, her spouse, and her body had changed. I spoke gently and fiercely only a few words, to let her know I'd been there and it was okay to feel however she felt. In this same living room, women's circle was where I shared and digested the news that I'd been invited to write this very book. Circle work reminds us we're not alone and sparks dreams into reality.

Peer circles function with clear expectations and boundaries. A skillful facilitator makes the circle's purpose known and holds all members of the circle equally with loving accountability and inherent value. Author Jean Shinoda Bolen, MD, shares in *The Millionth Circle* that facilitating circles is like learning to improvise with other musicians, stating, "Playing together as equals takes practice and presence" (Bolen 2003, p.46).

In my online program for women's pelvic health, we use three simple agreements to open community calls. I also include these agreements in client intake forms. This creates a solid sense of purpose between members of the group, and becomes a container for how we treat ourselves and each other, which reinforces safety and a sense of belonging. You can read them here; then, consider writing your own.

I honor my capacity for change, growth, and learning.

My choices and habits are rooted in self-compassion.

I agree to co-create a safe, confidential space where I'm safe to explore and promise to offer my full support to others.

When we embody and demonstrate our values in action, in the language we use on our website and business communications, people will know where we stand. Taking a stance on key issues and who we can best serve creates a certain magnetism for clients and collaborations to find their way to us, allowing our business to flourish and purpose to be fulfilled.

Our purpose beckons

As this book offers a generalist approach to specializing in pelvic health, you may wish to further develop your skills to support people with a specific condition or primary goal that drives them to hire you as their teacher. One common path for further specialization could be focusing on a condition you personally have learned to manage well through yoga therapy. First-hand experiences give you invaluable compassion and empathy, and could potentially awaken newfound hope for students on a similar path. I've included a few questions to help you discern your professional path forward.

- What are your guiding values as a yoga professional?
- How do your values and personality support you in serving a specific population?
- What conditions, symptoms, or pelvic-health goals speak to you or tug your heartstrings?
- What problem would you like to help resolve for folks with pelvic-health concerns?
- What gaps do you see in the market currently or in your local or regional area?

Finally, consider adapting the third yoga nidra script to explore your professional dharma through visualization. See yourself several years in the future, or at the end of a long, satisfying career. Allow those feelings, images, and thoughts to guide your present choices and actions for serving others through pelvic yoga therapy.

Closing integration: hakini mudra meditation

Let's pause for one last practice together. This meditation (adapted from Le Page and Le Page 2014) weaves together the imagery of the pelvic diamond, breath awareness, and hakini mudra to encourage the merging of apparent opposites into a unified wholeness. Invite the possibility that everything you've read and are learning through this book will integrate in time – and you are already whole, powerful, and ready to serve others in this moment.

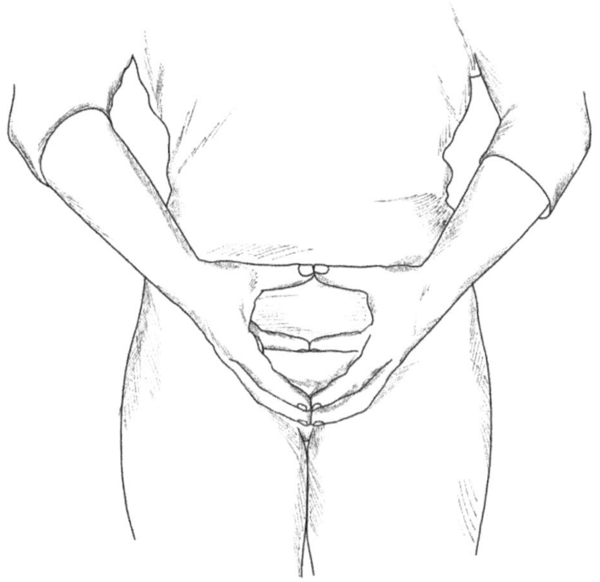

Figure 13.1: Hakini goddess mudra, to harmonize polarities and remember one's wholeness

Sit comfortably on a bolster or a stack of blankets, or in a chair. If possible, let your legs align parallel so your pelvic bowl can feel supremely centered.

Bring your fingertips and thumbtips together, forming a spherical volume of space inside your palms. Rest this mudra in front of your pelvic bowl. Feel your neck and shoulders melt, flowing into and through the circular quality of your hands and arms. Gently bow your head and rest your attention now inside your pelvis.

Envision and feel the diamond shape within your pelvic bowl. Feel the bony ridge creating the front of the diamond, and the fanning deep pelvic diaphragm (levator ani group of muscles) and the coccyx creating the back of the diamond. We'll use the diamond to guide our breath awareness.

Let yourself exhale completely. Take the next three breaths into the front half of the pelvic diamond, feeling it respond with inhalation and exhalation. Then, shift your attention to the posterior and spend three more breaths expanding and condensing the back of the pelvic diamond. Feeling the horizontal seam across the middle of the diamond (between the sit bones, following the transverse perineal muscles through the perineal body), enjoy one integrating breath cycle to merge the front and back halves together.

Repeat this contrasting process with three breath cycles into the right side of the pelvic diamond, and then the following three breaths into the left side of the pelvic diamond. Allow one full breath in and out to merge your attention into the central midline of the pelvic floor, from pubic bone to tailbone.

Now allow your inhalation to fill the entire pelvic diamond, relaxing with your exhalation. With each successive breath cycle, allow the inhalation to fill into the next chakra upwards, giving yourself time to draw energy up from the root all the way into the crown. Let your inhalations activate this ascending imagery and sensation, while the exhalations help you find ease and rest into the charge you're accumulating.

Once you've expanded the imagery to include your whole body, root to crown, feel the space around you as yours – your energetic kinesphere. Sit in the center of this sphere you're envisioning, surrounded by pure awareness. The microcosm of space within your hands mirrors the volume of the inner contours in your pelvis and reflects the symbolic connection you have with the entire world around you, to source and spirit.

After enjoying the fullness of this meditation, let go of the imagery and mudra as an exhalation comes to completion. Rest. Let yourself sit quietly with this aliveness circulating for as long as you'd like. Thank you for practicing with me and for reading this book.

How softly the petals of the heart unfold
when hands, lips, and eyes are open to another,
and the touch, words, and witness prove acceptance.
How deeply penetrates the root of a life well lived,
pulling up the essence of the humble earthen form.
Feel, speak, behold without judgement, allow your source to enter you,
To move freely through the terrain,
and bloom with ease.

Poem entitled "The Petals of the Heart,"
from *Beyond the Leaving* by Gil Hedley (2011)

References

ACOG (2018) *Optimizing Postpartum Care*. Washington, DC: ACOG. Accessed on 23/08/21 at www.acog.org/clinical/clinical-guidance/committee-opinion/articles/2018/05/optimizing-postpartum-care.

AGS Expert Panel on Person-Centered Care (2016) 'Person-centered care: A definition and essential elements. American Geriatrics Society.' *Journal of the American Geriatrics Society 64*, 1, 15–18.

Ahangari, A. (2014) 'Prevalence of chronic pelvic pain among women: An updated review.' *Pain Physician 17*, E141–E147.

Aljuraifani, R., Stafford, R., Hall, L., van den Hoorn, W., and Hodges, P. (2019) 'Task-specific differences in respiration-related activation of deep and superficial pelvic floor muscles.' *Journal of Applied Physiology 126*, 5, 1343–1351.

Anderson, B. (2015) [Video] *Over-cueing the Pelvic Floor. Cue the Breath! Pelvic Floor Follow Up*. Accessed on 23/08/21 at https://youtu.be/dih56AMrTMo.

Anderson, S. (2010) *Alignment Yoga: An Intelligent Approach to Ancient Wisdom*. Wisconsin: Blue Mounds Publishing.

APTA (2020) *ABPTS Certified-Specialists Statistics*. Virginia: APTA. Accessed on 23/08/21 at https://specialization.apta.org/about-abpts/abpts-certified-specialists-statistics.

Association for Hanna Somatic Education Inc (2021) *Truth About Stretching*. Accessed on 23/08/21 at https://hannasomatics.com/the_somatics_difference/truth_about_stretching.

Baker, J., Costa, D., and Nygaard, I. (2012) 'Mindfulness-based stress reduction for treatment of urinary urge incontinence: A pilot study.' *Female Pelvic Medicine and Reconstructive Surgery 18*, 1, 46–49.

Barbato, K., Wiebe, J., Cline, T., and Hellier, S. (2014) 'Web-based treatment for women with stress urinary incontinence.' *Urologic Nursing 34*, 5, 252–257. PMID: 26298935.

Bhavanani, A. (2018) 'Are we Practicing Yoga Therapy or Yogopathy?' *SYTAR 2018 Keynote: IAYT*. Accessed on 23/08/21 at https://cdn.ymaws.com/www.iayt.org/resource/resmgr/docs_sytar2018/presenters/anandabhavanani__finalyogopa.pdf.

Blakeslee, S. and Blakeslee, M. (2007) *The Body Has a Mind of its Own*. New York: Random House.

Bogner, H. R., O'Donnell, A. J., de Vries, H. F., Northington, G. M., and Joo, J. H. (2011) 'The temporal relationship between anxiety disorders and urinary incontinence among community-dwelling adults.' *Journal of Anxiety Disorders 25*, 2, 203–208.

Bolen, J. (2003) *The Millionth Circle: How to Change Ourselves and the World.* Berkeley, CA: Conari Press.

Bordoni, B. and Zanier, E. (2013) 'Anatomic connections of the diaphragm: Influence of respiration on the body system.' *Journal of Multidisciplinary Healthcare 6*, 281–291.

Bortolami, A., Vanti, C., Banchelli, F., Guccione, A., and Pillastrini, P. (2015) 'Relationship between female pelvic floor dysfunction and sexual dysfunction: An observational study.' *The Journal of Sexual Medicine 12*, 5, 1233–1241.

Both, S., van Lunsen, R., Weijenborg, P., and Laan, E. (2012) 'A new device for simultaneous measurement of pelvic floor muscle activity and vaginal blood flow: A test in a nonclinical sample.' *The Journal of Sexual Medicine 9*, 11, 2888–2902.

Bradley, H. and Esformes, J. (2014) 'Breathing pattern disorders and functional movement.' *International Journal of Sports Physical Therapy 9*, 1, 28–39.

Brotto, L. (2018) *Better Sex Through Mindfulness: How Women Can Cultivate Desire.* Vancouver: Greystone Books Ltd.

Brown, B. (2010) *The Power of Vulnerability.* Houston: TED. Accessed on 23/08/21 at www.ted.com/talks/brene_brown_the_power_of_vulnerability?utm_campaign=tedspread&utm_medium=referral&utm_source=tedcomshare.

Brown, R. and Gerbarg, P. (2009) 'Yoga breathing, meditation, and longevity.' *Annals of the New York Academy of Sciences 1172*, 54–62.

Burrell, J. (2014) *10 Ways to Really Rock Your 3rd Age – Powering Up Your Perimenopause and Beyond!* Accessed on 23/08/21 at www.burrelleducation.com/10-ways-to-really-rock-your-3rd-age-powering-up-your-peri-menopause-and-beyond.

Calais-Germain, B. (2003) *The Female Pelvis: Anatomy and Exercises.* Seattle, WA: Eastland Press, Inc.

Calais-Germain, B. (2006, first published 2005) 'Analysis of the Principal Types of Breathing.' In *Anatomy of Breathing.* Seattle, WA: Eastland Press, Inc.

Capobianco, R., Mazzo, M., and Enoka, R. (2019) 'Self-massage prior to stretching improves flexibility in young and middle-aged adults.' *Journal of Sports Sciences 37*, 13, 1543–1550.

Capson, A., Mclean, L., and Nashed, J. (2009) 'The effect of lumbopelvic posture on pelvic floor muscle activation and intravaginal pressure generation in continent women.' Accessed on 23/08/21 at www.ics.org/2009/abstract/473.

Capson, A., Nashed, J., and Mclean, L. (2011) 'The role of lumbopelvic posture in pelvic floor muscle activation in continent women.' *Journal of Electromyography and Kinesiology: Official Journal of the International Society of Electrophysiological Kinesiology 21*, 1, 166–177.

Chaitow, L. (2016) 'Functional movement and breathing dysfunction.' *Journal of Bodywork and Movement Therapies 20*, 3, 455–456.

Cobb, W., Burns, J., Kercher, K., Matthews, B., Norton, H., and Heniford, B. (2005) 'Normal intraabdominal pressure in healthy adults.' *The Journal of Surgical Research 129*, 2, 231–235.

Cozean, N. (2018) *Simple Screening Questionnaire for Pelvic Floor Dysfunction.* Herman and Wallace Pelvic Rehabilitation Institute. Accessed on 23/08/21 at https://hermanwallace.com/blog/simple-screening-questionnaire-for-pelvic-floor-dysfunction.

Cozean, N. (2020, first published 2018) *Do I Have Pelvic Floor Dysfunction? The Pelvic Health Screening Questionnaire.* Laguna Hills, CA: Pelvic Sanity. Accessed on 23/08/21 at www.pelvicsanity.com/post/screening.

Cramer, H., Lauche, R., Langhorst, J., and Dobos, G. (2012) 'Effectiveness of yoga for menopausal symptoms: A systematic review and meta-analysis of randomized controlled trials.' *Evidence-based Complementary and Alternative Medicine: eCAM*, 2012, 863905.

Dana, D. (2020) *Polyvagal Exercises for Safety and Connection: 50 Client-Centered Practices.* New York: W. W. Norton and Company, Inc.

Danforth, K., Townsend, M., Lifford, K., Curhan, G., Resnick, N., and Grodstein, F. (2006) 'Risk factors for urinary incontinence among middle-aged women.' *American Journal of Obstetrics and Gynecology 194*, 2, 339–345.

Delancey, J., Kane Low, L., Miller, J., Patel, D., and Tumbarello, J. (2008) 'Graphic integration of causal factors of pelvic floor disorders: An integrated life span model.' *American Journal of Obstetrics and Gynecology 199*, 6, 610.e1–610.e6105.

Desikachar, K. (2018) [Video] Yoga FAQ, episode 064. *What is the difference between Mulabandha and Asvinimudra?* Representing Krishnamacharya Healing and Yoga Foundation. Accessed on 23/08/21 at www.youtube.com/watch?v=ONWGSVAzPuE.

Desikachar, T. K. V. (1999, first published 1995) *The Heart of Yoga*. Rochester, VT: Inner Traditions International.

Dinsmore-Tuli, U. (2020, first published 2014) 'Preface to the Revised and Updated Edition.' In *Yoni Shakti: A Woman's Guide to Power and Freedom through Yoga and Tantra, 2nd edition*. London: YogaWords.

Dowd, I. (2012, first published 1981) *Taking Root to Fly: Articles on Functional Anatomy*. New York: I. Dowd.

Draper, A. (2021) 'The history of the term pudendum: Opening the discussion on anatomical sex inequality.' *Clinical Anatomy 34*, 2, 315–319.

Dufour, S., Vandyken, B., Forget, M. J., and Vandyken, C. (2018) 'Association between lumbopelvic pain and pelvic floor dysfunction in women: A cross sectional study.' *Musculoskeletal Science and Practice 34*, 47–53.

Dugan, S., Lavender, M., Hebert-Beirne, J., and Brubaker, L. (2013) 'A pelvic floor fitness program for older women with urinary symptoms: A feasibility study.' *PM&R* 5, 672–676.

Dumoulin, C. and Hay-Smith, J. (2010) 'Pelvic floor muscle training versus no treatment, or inactive control treatments for urinary incontinence in women.' *Cochrane Database of Systematic Reviews 1*, CD005654.

Dumoulin, C., Cacciari, L., and Hay-Smith, J. (2018) 'Pelvic floor muscle training versus no treatment, or inactive control treatments for urinary incontinence in women.' *Cochrane Database of Systematic Reviews 10*, CD005654.

Eden, K. and Wylie, K. (2009) 'Quality of sexual life and menopause.' *Women's Health* 5, 4, 385–396.

Estés, C. (1995, first published 1992) *Women Who Run with the Wolves: Myths and Stories of the Wild Woman Archetype*. New York: A Ballantine Book: Random House Publishing Group.

Farhi, D. (2000) *Yoga Mind, Body, Spirit: A Return to Wholeness*. New York: Holt Paperbacks.

Farhi, D. (2003) *Bringing Yoga to Life: The Everyday Practice of Enlightened Living*. San Francisco, CA: HarperCollins Publishers, Inc.

Farhi, D. (2015a) *The Yoga Teacher Training Manual*. [Received as a senior associate while assisting this course in New Zealand.]

Farhi, D. (2015b) [Video] *Mantra for Self Blessing: Ayur Mantra*. Accessed on 23/08/21 at https://youtu.be/Q30-jT7iLCE.

Farhi, D. (2018) *Developing Kinesthetic Acuity*. Accessed on 23/08/21 at https://donnafarhi.co.nz/acuity.

Farhi, D. and Stuart, L. (2017) *Pathways to a Centered Body: Gentle Yoga Therapy for Core Stability, Healing Back Pain, and Moving with Ease.* Rangiora: Embodied Wisdom Publishing.

Faubion, S., Shuster, L., and Bharucha, A. (2012) 'Recognition and management of non-relaxing pelvic floor dysfunction.' *Mayo Clinic Proceedings 87*, 2, 187–193.

Faulds, D. (2002) *Go In and In: Poems from the Heart of Yoga.* Greenville, VA: Peaceable Kingdom Books.

Felde, G., Bjelland, I., and Hunskaar, S. (2012) 'Anxiety and depression associated with incontinence in middle-aged women: A large Norwegian cross-sectional study.' *International Urogynecology Journal 23*, 3, 299–306.

Franklin, E. (2002, first published 2000) *Relax Your Neck, Liberate Your Shoulders: The Ultimate Exercise Program for Tension Relief.* New Jersey: Elysian Editions, Princeton Book Company.

Franklin, E. (2003, first published 2002) *Pelvic Power.* New Jersey: Elysian Editions, Princeton Book Company.

Franklin, E. (2012) *Dynamic Alignment Through Imagery, 2nd edition.* Champaign, IL: Human Kinetics.

Goode, A., Hegedus, E., Sizer, P., Brismee, J., Linberg, A., and Cook, C. (2008) 'Three-dimensional movements of the sacroiliac joint: A systematic review of the literature and assessment of clinical utility.' *The Journal of Manual and Manipulative Therapy 16*, 1, 25–38.

Gross, R. (2020) *The Clitoris, Uncovered: An Intimate History.* Scientific American. Accessed on 23/08/21 at www.scientificamerican.com/article/the-clitoris-uncovered-an-intimate-history.

Hackney, P. (2002, first published 1998) *Making Connections: Total Body Integration through Bartenieff Fundamentals.* New York: Routledge. [Pages 51–109 cover three of six patterns of connectivity – Breath, Core-Distal, and Head-Tail – which are similar in nature to those in Chapter 10.]

Hall, C. and Garden, S. (2021) *Lost in Translation: Is Mulabandha Relevant for Modern Yogis?* Yoga International Online. Accessed on 23/08/21 at https://yogainternational.com/article/view/lost-in-translation-is-mulabandha-relevant-for-modern-yogis.

Handa, V., Cundiff, G., Chang, H., and Helzlsouer, K. (2008) 'Female sexual function and pelvic floor disorders.' *Obstetrics and Gynecology 111*, 5, 1045–1052.

Hanno, P., Erickson, D., Moldwin, R., and Faraday, M. (2015) 'Diagnosis and treatment of interstitial cystitis/bladder pain syndrome. AUA guideline ammendment.' *Journal of Urology 193*, 1545. Accessed on 23/08/21 at www.auanet.org/guidelines/guidelines/interstitial-cystitis-(ic/bps)-guideline.

Hartigan, S. and Smith, A. (2018) 'Disparities in female pelvic floor disorders.' *Current Urology Reports 19*, 2, 16.

Hartley, L. (1995, first published 1989) *Wisdom of the Body Moving: An Introduction to Body-Mind Centering.* Berkeley, CA: North Atlantic Books.

Haylen, B. T., Maher, C. F., Barber, M. D., Camargo, S., *et al.* (2016) 'An International Urogynecological Association (IUGA)/International Continence Society (ICS) joint report on the terminology for female pelvic organ prolapse (POP).' *International Urogynecology Journal 27*, 4, 655–684.

Hedley, G. (2011) 'The Petals of the Heart' from *Beyond the Leaving*. Self-published.

Hjartardottir, S., Nilsson, J., Petersen, C., and Lingman, G. (1997) 'The female pelvic floor: A dome – not a basin.' *Acta Obstetricia et Gynecologica Scandinavica 76*, 567–571.

Hodges, P., Sapsford, R., and Pengel, L. (2007) 'Postural and respiratory functions of the pelvic floor muscles.' *Neurourology and Urodynamics 26*, 3, 362–371.

Howard, L. (2017) *Pelvic Liberation: Using Yoga, Self-Inquiry, and Breath Awareness for Pelvic Health*. Emeryville, CA: Leslie Howard Yoga.

Huang, A., Chesney, M., Schembri, M., and Subak, L. (2018) 'A randomized trial of a group-based therapeutic yoga program for ambulatory women with urinary incontinence.' *The Journal of Urology 199*, 4, e645.

Huang, Y. C. and Chang, K. V. (2021) *Kegel Exercises*. StatPearls Publishing. Accessed on 23/08/21 at www.ncbi.nlm.nih.gov/books/NBK555898.

Hung, H. C., Hsiao, S. M., Chih, S. Y., Lin, H. H., and Tsauo, J. Y. (2010) 'An alternative intervention for urinary incontinence: Retraining diaphragmatic, deep abdominal and pelvic floor muscle coordinated function.' *Manual Therapy 15*, 273–279.

IAYT (2020, first published 2016) *IAYT Code of Ethics and Professional Responsibilities*. Arkansas: International Association of Yoga Therapists. Accessed on 23/08/21 at https://cdn.ymaws.com/www.iayt.org/resource/resmgr/docs_certification_all/2020_updates_scope_ethics/2020-09_code_of_ethics_v2.pdf.

Iglesia, C. and Smithling, K. (2017) 'Pelvic organ prolapse.' *American Family Physician 96*, 3, 179–185.

Jain, A. (2020) 'Commentary: Pain, stigma, and the politics of self-management.' *Pain Medicine 21*, 5, 888–890.

Janssen, E. and Bancroft, J. (2006) 'The Dual Control Model: The Role of Sexual Inhibition and Excitation Sexual Arousal and Behavior.' In E. Janssen (ed.) *The Psychophysiology of Sex*. Indiana University Press. Accessed on 23/08/21 at https://kinseyinstitute.org/pdf/Janssen_Bancroft_2006.pdf.

Johnson, K. (2021) [Podcast: *Sex Birth Trauma*] 'Jaguar bites #1: Yoga, meditation and the nervous system.' Episode 114. Accessed on 23/08/21 at https://podcasts.apple.com/us/podcast/sex-birth-trauma-with-kimberly-ann-johnson/id1286485146?i=1000513289249.

Johnston, J., Reid, H., and Hunter, D. (2015) 'Diagnosing endometriosis in primary care: Clinical update.' *The British Journal of General Practice: Journal of the Royal College of General Practitioners 65*, 631, 101–102.

Kaminoff, L. (2010) [Video] *Bandhas in a Modern Practice: A Historical Perspective*. Accessed on 23/08/21 at www.youtube.com/watch?v=oakh34gY70U.

Kaparo, R. (2012) *Awakening Somatic Intelligence: The Art and Practice of Embodied Mindfulness*. Berkeley, CA: North Atlantic Books.

Keizer, A., Vandyken, B., Vandyken, C., Yardley, D., *et al.* (2019) 'Predictors of pelvic floor muscle dysfunction among women with lumbopelvic pain.' *Physical Therapy 99*, 12, 1703–1711.

Kent, T. (2011) *Wild Feminine: Finding Power, Spirit and Joy in the Female Body*. New York: Simon and Schuster, Inc.

Kepner, J. (2015) 'IAYT and the Future of Yoga Therapy.' In L. Payne, T. Gold, and E. Goldman (eds) *Yoga Therapy and Integrative Medicine: Where Ancient Science Meets Modern Medicine*. Laguna Beach, CA: Basic Health Publications, Inc.

Kepner, J., Devi, N., Le Page, J., Le Page, L., Kraftsow, G., and Lee, M. (2014) 'The differences between yoga teacher training and yoga therapist training and the distinction between yoga teaching and yoga therapy.' *International Journal of Yoga Therapy 24*, 1, 7–21.

Kirby, A. C., Luber, K. M., and Menefee, S. A. (2013) 'An update on the current and future demand for care of pelvic floor disorders in the United States.' *American Journal of Obstetrics and Gynecology 209*, 6, 584.e1–584.e5845.

Koch, L. (2020) [Online course] *Hydrating Psoas and Resolving Scar Tissue Course.*

Koch, L. and Johnson, K. (2019) [Workshop] *Rewilding Psoas: WILD ~ A Collaboration with Kimberly Ann Johnson.* June 2, 2019. Encinitas, CA.

Lawrence, M. (2020) [Podcast: *This Is Yoga Therapy*] 'Yoga Therapy, Research and Eudaimonic Well-Being with Marlysa Sullivan.' Season 2, episode 3. Durango, CO: Inner Peace Yoga Therapy. Accessed on 23/08/21 at https://innerpeaceyogatherapy.com/yoga-therapy-research-and-eudaimonic-well-being-with-marlysa-sullivan.

Le Page, J. and Le Page, L. (2014) *Mudras for Healing and Transformation, 2nd edition.* Sebastopol, CA: Integrative Yoga Therapy.

Luber, K. M., Boero, S., and Choe, J. Y. (2001) 'The demographics of pelvic floor disorders: Current observations and future projections.' *American Journal of Obstetrics and Gynecology 184*, 7, 1496–1503.

Lyon, I. (2019) [Video] *What the Heck is Orienting? (And Why is it Important?!)* Accessed on 23/08/21 at https://youtu.be/XGYh1wPpOLA.

Lyons, M. (2019) [Podcast: *The Pelvic Health Podcast*] 'Menopause with physiotherapist Michelle Lyons.' Accessed on 23/08/21 at https://podcasts.apple.com/us/podcast/the-pelvic-health-podcast/id1022705760?i=1000456239509.

Maeda, T., Tomita, M., Nakazawa, A., Sakai, G., *et al.* (2017) 'Female functional constipation is associated with overactive bladder symptoms and urinary incontinence.' *BioMed Research International 2017*, 2138073.

Mandimika, C., Murk, W., Mcpencow, A., Lake, A., *et al.* (2015) 'Racial disparities in knowledge of pelvic floor disorders among community-dwelling women.' *Female Pelvic Medicine and Reconstructive Surgery 21*, 5, 287–292.

Markland, A., Richter, H., Fwu, C. W., Eggers, P., and Kusek, J. (2011) 'Prevalence and trends of urinary incontinence in adults in the United States, 2001 to 2008.' *The Journal of Urology 186*, 2, 589–593.

McCall, T. (2019) 'Foreword.' In N. Pearson, S. Prosko, and M. Sullivan (eds) *Yoga and Science in Pain Care: Treating the Person in Pain.* London and Philadelphia: Singing Dragon.

McCall, T., Satish, L., and Tiwari, S. (2016) 'History, Philosophy, and Practice of Yoga Therapy.' In S. Khalsa, L. Cohen, T. McCall, and S. Telles (eds) *The Principles and Practice of Yoga in Healthcare.* Edinburgh: Handspring.

McCool-Myers, M., Theurich, M., Zuelke, A., Knuettel, H., and Apfelbacher, C. (2018) 'Predictors of female sexual dysfunction: A systematic review and qualitative analysis through gender inequality paradigms.' *BMC Women's Health 18*, 1, 108.

McGonigal, K. (2021) *How to Create a Sankalpa.* Yoga International. Accessed on 23/08/21 at https://yogainternational.com/article/view/how-to-create-a-sankalpa.

Messelink, B., Benson, T., Berghmans, B., Bø, K., *et al.* (2005) 'Standardization of terminology of pelvic floor muscle function and dysfunction: Report from the pelvic floor clinical assessment group of the International Continence Society.' *Neurourology and Urodynamics 24*, 4, 374–380.

Meston, C. (n.d.) *The Sympathetic Nervous System and Women's Sexual Arousal.* Austin, TX: The Sexual Psychophysiology Laboratory at University of Texas, Austin. Accessed 23/08/21 at https://labs.la.utexas.edu/mestonlab/the-sympathetic-nervous-system-and-womens-sexual-arousal.

Miller, D. (2018) *Mindfulness and Interstitial Cystitis.* Herman and Wallace. Accessed on 23/08/21 at https://hermanwallace.com/blog/mindfulness-and-interstitial-cystitis.

Miller, J. (2019, first published 2015) *Jill Miller on The New Science of Self-Care: The Role of Myofascial Massage in Healing.* Yoga U. Accessed on 23/08/21 at www.yogauonline.com/yoga-anatomy/jill-miller-new-science-self-care-role-myofascial-massage-healing.

Myers, T. (2009, first published 2001) *Anatomy Trains: Myofascial Meridians for Manual and Movement Therapists.* Edinburgh and New York: Churchill Livingstone, Elsevier.

Nagoski, E. (2015) *Come As You Are: The Surprising New Science That Will Transform Your Sex Life.* New York: Simon and Schuster Paperbacks.

Neff, K. and Germer, C. (2013) 'A pilot study and randomized controlled trial of the mindful self-compassion program.' *Journal of Clinical Psychology 69*, 1, 28–44.

Nestor, J. (2020) [Audio: *Outside Podcast*] 'Changing how you breathe could change your life.' Outside podcast hosted by Keyes, C. and Roberts, M. Accessed on 23/08/21 at https://podcasts.apple.com/us/podcast/outside-podcast/id1090500561?i=1000493138580.

Ng, K. S., Sivakumaran, Y., Nassar, N., and Gladman, M. (2015) 'Fecal incontinence: Community prevalence and associated factors. Systematic review.' *Diseases of the Colon and Rectum 58*, 12, 1194–1209.

O'Connell, H. and DeLancey, J. (2005) 'Clitoral anatomy in nulliparous, healthy, premenopausal volunteers using unenhanced magnetic resonance imaging.' *The Journal of Urology 173*, 6, 2060–2063.

O'Dell, K., Morse, A., Crawford, S., and Howard, A. (2007) 'Vaginal pressure during lifting, floor exercises, jogging, and use of hydraulic exercise machines.' *International Urogynecology Journal and Pelvic Floor Dysfunction 18*, 12, 1481–1489.

O'Sullivan, P. (2015) [Video] *Prof. Peter O'Sullivan, Pelvic Pain: What are the Really Important Factors to Address in Management?* Accessed on 23/08/21 at https://youtu.be/HK7SiQtyqxw. [Comments at 2:06 that pelvic girdle pain (PGP) is not a feature of bones "out of place" or "unstable" and more likely due to sensitization, BPSS factors. At 9:35 states research does not show differences in mobility between people with PGP and those without.]

O'Sullivan, P., Beales, D., Beetham, J., Cripps, J., *et al.* (2002) 'Altered motor control strategies in subjects with sacroiliac joint pain during the active straight-leg-raise test.' *Spine 27*, 1, E1–E8.

Oates, J. (2017) 'The effect of yoga on menstrual disorders: A systematic review.' *Journal of Alternative and Complementary Medicine 23*, 6, 4017–4417.

Palsson, T., Gibson, W., Darlow, B., Bunzli, S., *et al.* (2019) 'Changing the narrative in diagnosis and management of pain in the sacroiliac joint area.' *Physical Therapy 99*, 11, 1511–1519.

Pearson, N., Prosko, S., and Sullivan, M. (2019) 'Yoga and Yoga Therapy.' In N. Pearson, S. Prosko, and M. Sullivan (eds) *Yoga and Science in Pain Care: Treating the Person in Pain.* London and Philadelphia: Singing Dragon.

PHRC (2019) *What is the Knack and Why Does it Work to Prevent Urine Leakage?* Pelvic Health and Rehabilitation Center. Accessed on 23/08/21 at https://pelvicpainrehab.com/urinary-incontinence/6711/what-is-the-knack-and-why-does -it-work-to-prevent-urine-leakage.

Porges, S. (1995) 'Orienting in a defensive world: Mammalian modifications of our evolutionary heritage. A Polyvagal Theory.' *Psychophysiology 32*, 4, 301–318.

Porges, S. (1998) 'Love: An emergent property of the mammalian autonomic nervous system.' *Psychoneuroendocrinology 23*, 8, 837–861.

Porges, S. (2004) *Neuroception: A Subconscious System for Detecting Threats and Safety.* Washington, DC: Zero to Three. Accessed on 23/08/21 at https://static1.squarespace.com/static/5c1d025fb27e390a78569537/t/5ccdff181905f41dbcb689e3/1557004058168/Neuroception.pdf.

Porges, S. (2015) 'Play as Neural Exercise: Insights from the Polyvagal Theory.' In D. Pearce-McCall (ed.) *The Power of Play for Mind Brain Health*, pp.3–7. Accessed on 23/08/21 at www.legeforeningen.no/contentassets/6df47feea03643c5a878ee7b87a467d2/sissel-oritsland-vedlegg-til-presentasjon-porges-play-as-neural-exercise.pdf.

Porges, S. (2017) *The Pocket Guide to Polyvagal Theory: The Transformative Power of Feeling Safe.* New York: W. W. Norton and Company, Inc.

Prosko, S. (2016) 'Optimizing pelvic floor health through yoga therapy.' International Association of Yoga Therapists. *Yoga Therapy Today 48*, 32–34. Accessed on 23/08/21 at https://secureservercdn.net/104.238.69.231/0gl.9c2.myftpupload.com/wp-content/uploads/2016/01/YTT_Winter2016_YTIP_PelvicFloor.pdf.

Prosko, S. (2017) [Online course: Embodia] *PhysioYoga and the Pelvic Floor.* Accessed on 23/08/21 at https://embodiaapp.com/courses/94-physioyoga-and-the-pelvic-floor-shelly-prosko.

Remski, M. (2019) *Practice and All Is Coming: Abuse, Cult Dynamics, and Healing in Yoga and Beyond.* Rangiora: Embodied Wisdom Publishing.

Rosenbaum, T. (2021) *Sexual Health in Women – Role of Physiotherapy.* Accessed on 23/08/21 at www.physiotimes.com/article/physio-speaks-sexual-health-in-women--role-of-physiotherapy---talli-y-rosenbaum.

Ross, A. and Michalsen, A. (2016) 'Yoga for Prevention and Wellness.' In S. Khalsa, L. Cohen, T. McCall, and S. Telles (eds) *The Principles and Practice of Yoga in Healthcare.* Edinburgh: Handspring.

Rudavsky, A. (2020) [Podcast: *The Pelvic Health Podcast*] 'The glottis and pelvic floor.' Accessed on 23/08/21 at https://podcasts.apple.com/us/podcast/the-pelvic-health-podcast/id1022705760?i=1000497416628.

Russell, N., Daniels, B., Smoot, B., and Allen, D. (2019) 'Effects of yoga on quality of life and pain in women with chronic pelvic pain.' Systematic Review and Meta-Analysis. *Journal of Women's Health Physical Therapy 43*, 3, 144–154.

Saad, M., de Medeiros, R., and Mosini, A. C. (2017) 'Are we ready for a true biopsychosocial-spiritual model? The many meanings of "spiritual".' *Medicines 4*, 4, 79.

Sapolsky, R. (2004, first published 1994, 1998 by Freeman, W. H.) *Why Zebras Don't Get Ulcers: The Acclaimed Guide to Stress, Stress-Related Diseases, and Coping, 3rd edition.* New York: Holt Paperbacks.

Sapsford, R., Richardson, C., Maher, C., and Hodges, P. (2008) 'Pelvic floor muscle activity in different sitting postures in continent and incontinent women.' *Archives of Physical Medicine and Rehabilitation 89*, 9, 1741–1747.

Satchidananda, S. (2008, first published 1978) *The Yoga Sutras of Patanjali.* Buckingham, VA: Integral Yoga Publications.

Saxena, R., Gupta, M., Shankar, N., Jain, S., and Saxena, A. (2017) 'Effects of yogic intervention on pain scores and quality of life in females with chronic pelvic pain.' *International Journal of Yoga 10*, 1, 9–15.

Schleip, R. (2015) *Fascia as an Organ of Communication.* Accessed on 23/08/21 at www.fascialfitness.net.au/articles/fascia-as-an-organ-of-communication.

Schrepf, A., Naliboff, B., Williams, D., Stephens-Shields, A., *et al.* (2018) 'Adverse Childhood Experiences and symptoms of urologic chronic pelvic pain syndrome: A multidisciplinary approach to the study of chronic pelvic pain research network study.' *Annals of Behavioral Medicine 52*, 865–877.

Sjödahl, J., Kvist, J., Gutke, A., and Oberg, B. (2009) 'The postural response of the pelvic floor muscles during limb movements: A methodological electromyography study in parous women without lumbopelvic pain.' *Clinical Biomechanics 24*, 2, 183–189.

Smith, M., Coppieters, M., and Hodges, P. (2007) 'Postural response of the pelvic floor and abdominal muscles in women with and without incontinence.' *Neurourology and Urodynamics 26*, 377–385.

Smith, M., Coppieters, M., and Hodges, P. (2008) 'Is balance different in women with and without stress urinary incontinence?' *Neurourology and Urodynamics 27*, 1, 71–78.

Smith, M., Russell, A., and Hodges, P. (2006) 'Disorders of breathing and continence have a stronger association with back pain than obesity and physical activity.' *Australian Journal of Physiotherapy 52*, 11–16.

Soljanik, I., Janssen, U., Lienemann, A., and Fritsch, H. (2007) 'The LFG-complex (levator ani muscle-fossa ischioanalis-gluteus maximus muscle) and its role for the functional integration of the pelvic floor.' *European Urology Supplements 6*, 2, 104.

Solomonova, E. (2015) 'First-person experience and yoga research: Studying neural correlates of an intentional practice.' *Frontiers in Human Neuroscience 9*, 85.

Sovik, R. (2021) *Finding Faith in the Spirit of Yoga.* Yoga International. Accessed on 23/08/21 at https://yogainternational.com/article/view/finding-faith-in-the-spirit-of-yoga.

Sovik, R. and Bhavanani, A.B. (2016) 'History, Philosophy, and Practice of Yoga.' In S. Khalsa, L. Cohen, T. McCall, and S. Telles (eds) *The Principles and Practice of Yoga in Healthcare.* Edinburgh: Handspring.

Stanton, A., Lorenz, T., Pulverman, C., and Meston, C. (2015) 'Heart rate variability: A risk factor for female sexual dysfunction.' *Applied Psychophysiology and Biofeedback 40*, 3, 229–237. Accessed on 23/08/21 at https://labs.la.utexas.edu/mestonlab/files/2016/05/2015-stanton-lorenz-pulverman-meston.pdf.

Sullivan, M., Erb, M., Schmalzl, L., Moonaz, S., Noggle Taylor, J., and Porges, S. (2018a) 'Yoga therapy and polyvagal theory: The convergence of traditional wisdom and contemporary neuroscience for self-regulation and resilience.' *Frontiers in Human Neuroscience 12*, 67.

Sullivan, M., Moonaz, S., Weber, K., Taylor, J. N., and Schmalzl, L. (2018b) 'Toward an explanatory framework for yoga therapy informed by philosophical and ethical perspectives.' *Alternative Therapies in Health and Medicine 24*, 1, 38–47.

Sweta, K., Godbole, A., Awasthi, H., and Pandey, U. (2018) 'Effect of mula bandha yoga in mild grade pelvic organ prolapse: A randomized controlled trial.' *International Journal of Yoga 11*, 2, 116–121.

Talasz, H., Kremser, C., Kofler, M., Kalchschmid, E., Lechleitner, M., and Rudisch, A. (2011) 'Phase-locked parallel movement of diaphragm and pelvic floor during breathing and coughing: A dynamic MRI investigation in healthy females.' *International Urogynecology Journal 22,* 1, 61–68.

Tanner, H. (2015) *Obturator Internus and Making Connections.* Herman and Wallace Pelvic Rehabilitation Institute. Accessed on 23/08/21 at https://hermanwallace.com/blog/obturator-internus-a-making-connections.

Tibbetts, V. and Peper, E. (1996) 'Effects of imagery and position on breathing patterns.' *The Proceedings of the 27th Annual Meeting of the Association for Applied Psychophysiology and Biofeedback 21.* [Small sample, but participants reported and sensors registered increased stress and bracing when imagining walking on concrete as compared to a soft meadow.]

Traditional Chinese Medicine World Foundation (n.d.) *Progression of Health Issues.* Accessed on 23/08/21 at www.tcmworld.org/what-is-tcm/progression-of-health-issues.

Tricycle (2021) *What are the Three Poisons? (Greed, Hatred and Delusion).* Accessed on 23/08/21 at https://tricycle.org/beginners/buddhism/three-poisons.

Tyagi, A. and Cohen, M. (2016) 'Yoga and heart rate variability: A comprehensive review of the literature.' *International Journal of Yoga 9,* 2, 97–113.

van der Kolk, B. (2014) *The Body Keeps the Score: Brain, Mind, and Body in the Healing of Trauma.* New York: Penguin Books.

Vandyken, B., Keizer, A., Vandyken, C., Macedo, L., Kuspinar, A., and Dufour, S. (2020) 'Pelvic floor muscle tenderness on digital palpation among women: Convergent validity with central sensitization.' *Brazilian Journal of Physical Therapy 25,* 3, 256–261.

Vandyken, C. (2021) Private email correspondence.

Vestal, L. (2019) [Online course] *Kegels That Work: A Workshop for Women Who Want to Stop Guessing + Start Taking Back Control.* Accessed on 23/08/21 at https://ot-pioneers.teachable.com/p/kegelsthatwork.

Vrijens, D., Drossaerts, J., van Koeveringe, G., Van Kerrebroeck, P., van Os, J., and Leue, C. (2015) 'Affective symptoms and the overactive bladder: A systematic review.' *Journal of Psychosomatic Research 78,* 2, 95–108.

Wade, D. T. and Halligan, P. W. (2017) 'The biopsychosocial model of illness: A model whose time has come.' *Clinical Rehabilitation 31,* 8, 995–1004.

Werntz, D., Bickford, R., Bloom, F., and Shannahoff-Khalsa, D. (1983) 'Alternating cerebral hemispheric activity and the lateralization of autonomic nervous function.' *Human Neurobiology 2,* 1, 39–43.

Wiebe, J. (2014) [Video] *Impact of Alignment on Diaphragm and Pelvic Floor Availability.* Accessed on 23/08/21 at https://youtu.be/FYOuh2-Hqmk.

Wiebe, J. (2015) *Training the Reflexive Response of the Pelvic Floor.* Accessed on 23/08/21 at www.juliewiebept.com/training-the-reflexive-response-of-the-pelvic-floor.

Wiebe, J. (2018) [Video] *How Breathing and the Core Influence the Pelvic Floor.* Kinetic Labs. Accessed on 23/08/21 at https://youtu.be/eRAaJN3FC6A.

Wiebe, J. and Clinton, S. (2018) [Online course] *From the Glottis to the Pelvic Floor: Making Clinical Connections.* Accessed on 23/08/21 at https://courses.juliewiebept.com/p/from-the-glottis-to-the-pelvic-floor-making-clinical-connections.

Wobser, A., Adkins, Z., and Wobser, R. (2020) 'Embryology section.' In *Anatomy, Abdomen and Pelvis, Bones (Ilium, Ischium, Pubis).* Accessed on 23/08/21 at www.ncbi.nlm.nih.gov/books/NBK519524.

Woon, J., Perumal, V., Maigne, J., and Stringer, M. (2013) 'CT morphology and morphometry of the normal adult coccyx.' *European Spine Journal: Official Publication of the European Spine Society, the European Spinal Deformity Society, and the European Section of the Cervical Spine Research Society* 22, 4, 863–870.

Yamasaki, Z. (2021) [Website and training program] *Transcending Sexual Trauma Through Yoga.* Accessed on 23/08/21 at www.zabieyamasaki.com/about/transcending-sexual-trauma-through-yoga [Includes trauma-informed yoga benefits and examples of invitational cues.]

Yogi Times (2021, first published 2016) *Demographics and Statistics of the Yoga Industry.* Accessed on 23/08/21 at www.yogitimes.com/article/unstoppable-trend-yoga-infographic-business.

Zomorodi, S., Abdi, S., and Rasulzadeh-Tabatabaee, S. (2014) 'Comparison of long-term effects of cognitive-behavioral therapy versus mindfulness-based therapy on reduction of symptoms among patients suffering from irritable bowel syndrome.' *Gastroenterology and Hepatology from Bed to Bench* 7, 2, 118–124.

APPENDIX A

Screening and Pelvic Self-Assessment Forms

To support implementation of the Pelvic Yoga Therapy Survey, please go to www.cheridostal.com to download the Pelvic Yoga Therapy Survey Pro Use Guide.

PELVIC YOGA THERAPY SURVEY

Pre: Collect and date the responses from this survey as part of a new client intake process.

Post: Repeat survey upon conclusion of your pelvic yoga-therapy program to compare data.

Client initials: _________ Date of survey completion: _______________

Pre or post: _________________________________

Please respond to each of the questions below using the following scale:

1 = Not at all true **3 = Neutral** **5 = A lot/very true**

1. My pelvic health concerns me or creates stress for me.

   1 2 3 4 5

2. I feel equipped to practice/exercise safely and effectively on my own.

   1 2 3 4 5

3. I experience incontinence (leaking of any kind with coughing, sneezing, etc.).

   1 **2** **3** **4** **5**

4. I experience frequency and/or urgency (indicate bladder, bowel, or both).

   1 **2** **3** **4** **5**

5. I experience pressure, fullness, or heaviness.

   1 **2** **3** **4** **5**

6. I'm able to feel and sense my pelvic-floor muscles during daily activities.

   1 **2** **3** **4** **5**

7. I feel informed and educated about my body.

   1 **2** **3** **4** **5**

8. I'm able to calm myself when needed.

   1 **2** **3** **4** **5**

9. I allow myself to relax and enjoy life.

   1 **2** **3** **4** **5**

10. I love my body.

   1 **2** **3** **4** **5**

Thank you for completing the survey!

PELVIC SELF-ASSESSMENT WORKSHEET

Gather supplies: Mirror, lube, journal and pen, pillows, any other comfort items desired.

Before you begin: Wash your hands thoroughly with soap and warm water.

Claim your space: Find a private place so you can relax and take your time.

Date: ______________

Time of day: ______________

Current day of cycle or date of last period, if relevant: ______________

Take a quiet minute and sense your body, observing sensations, breathing, energy, thoughts, and emotions. Record how you feel right now as a baseline before your pelvic self-assessment.

PELVIC-FLOOR AWARENESS – MAKING A CONNECTION

- Did you feel able to focus attention on your pelvic floor?
  Y / N / not sure
- Could you visualize and/or feel the PF coordination with breathing?
  Y / N / not sure

Notes on pelvic awareness: ______________________________

____

____

PELVIC-FLOOR ENGAGEMENT – OBSERVING THE WHOLE PERINEUM IN ACTION

- Clitoral nod?
  Y / N / not sure
- Vaginal close and lift?
  Y / N / not sure
- Anal "wink" or closing?
  Y / N / not sure

- Circle one word to best describe your engagement:
  absent / weak / normal / strong
- Did you feel muscles in other parts of your body want to engage instead?
  Y / N / not sure
  - If so, where in your body did you feel excess tension or effort?
- Did your pelvic-floor engagement feel complete and even side to side, front to back?

Notes on pelvic engagement: ______________________________

____

____

PELVIC-FLOOR RELAXATION – CHECK THE ONE THAT BEST DESCRIBES YOUR EXPERIENCE

- Fully relaxed and descended after engagement.
- Partially relaxed and/or descended after engagement.
- I did not feel or see my pelvic floor relax at all when attempted.
- I'm not sure.

Notes on pelvic relaxation: ______________________________

____

____

Did you choose visual assessment with mirror and/or internal self-touch for this session?

Rest and observe how you feel. Record how you feel now, making note of any changes that feel pleasant, concerning, or interesting. Thank yourself for completing this process.

COZEAN PELVIC DYSFUNCTION SCREENING PROTOCOL

INSTRUCTIONS: CHECK ALL THAT APPLY

☐ I sometimes have pelvic pain (in genitals, perineum, pubic or bladder area, or pain with urination) that exceeds a "3" on a 1–10 pain scale, with 10 being the worst pain imaginable

☐ I can remember falling onto my tailbone, lower back, or buttocks (even in childhood)

☐ I sometimes experience one or more of the following urinary symptoms

- Accidental loss of urine
- Feeling unable to completely empty my bladder
- Having to void within a few minutes of a previous void
- Pain or burning with urination
- Difficulty starting or frequent stopping/starting of urine stream

☐ I often or occasionally have to get up to urinate two or more times at night

☐ I sometimes have a feeling of increased pelvic pressure or the sensation of my pelvic organs slipping down or falling out

☐ I have a history of pain in my low back, hip, groin, or tailbone or have had sciatica

☐ I sometimes experience one or more of the following bowel symptoms

- Loss of bowel control
- Feeling unable to completely empty my bowels
- Straining or pain with a bowel movement
- Difficulty initiating a bowel movement

☐ I sometimes experience pain or discomfort with sexual activity or intercourse

☐ Sexual activity increases one or more of my other symptoms

☐ Prolonged sitting increases my symptoms

IF YOU CHECKED 3 OR MORE CIRCLES, PELVIC FLOOR DYSFUNCTION IS LIKELY. YOU MAY BENEFIT FROM AN ASSESSMENT FROM A PELVIC FLOOR PHYISCAL THERAPIST.

PELVIC SANITY

THE PRIMARY CARE PELVIC HEALTH SCREEN

Please read each statement to the subject and indicate a checkmark (√) beside each statement that is applicable.

	Do you urinate more than 8 times per day?
	Do you have difficulty initiating your urine stream and/or experience burning with urination?
	Do you experience very strong and/or uncontrollable urges to go to the bathroom?
	Do you experience any urine or fecal leakage (on the way to the bathroom, coughing/laughing/sneezing, exercising, etc.)?
	Do you have pain during or after a bowel movement?
	Do you struggle with having regular bowel movements or constipation?
	Do you ever experience painful intercourse?
	Do you experience pelvic pain and/or pelvic pressure, i.e. vaginal, rectal, penile, testicular, bladder, tailbone, or pelvic girdle?
	For women only, do you experience pain or cramping with menstruation that requires intervention (such as heat, medication, rest, etc.)?

This screening questionnaire is based on research that shows these symptoms are correlated to pelvic floor dysfunction. If you checked YES to at least one box on this list, consulting with a pelvic floor physiotherapist may be very helpful for your symptoms.

Keizer, A., Vandyken, B., Vandyken, C., Yardley, D., *et al.* (2019) 'Predictors of pelvic floor muscle dysfunction among women with lumbopelvic pain.' *Physical Therapy 99*, 12, 1703–1711.

APPENDIX B

Sample Practices

Yoga therapy does not prescribe protocols; we see each student holistically, distinctly. With that said, recognizing common themes can streamline practice development by seeing patterns of baseline PFM function and underlying ANS states.

These sequences focus primarily on physical practice to provide a framework within which you can layer personalized imagery and cues, meditation, pranayama, mantra, mudra, and so on as relevant to each student.

Sequence 1: Enhancing pelvic awareness

These exercises may help prevent pelvic-floor issues by enhancing awareness and understanding or as a starting point for new clients. Cultivate their ability to sense the PFM before adding more complex movements.

- Standing experiential anatomy, self-touch tour of pelvic bones (Chapter 4)
- Seated vulva cupping or gentle contact with props (Chapter 5)
- Constructive rest position (Chapter 6)

When the above practices seem integrated, consider progressing with:

- Pelvic tilt from supine (Chapter 9) or cat-cow initiated with pelvic awareness (Chapter 11)
- Table rocking (Chapter 11)
- Wall baby (Chapter 11), legs up the chair, or reclined bound angle restorative (Chapter 10) with hands in trimurti/yoni mudra over lower belly
- Savasana, personalized to client

Sequence 2: Soothing pelvic pain and overactive PFM (down-training focus)

Consider how we can build rapport to support relaxation and a feeling of safety, and how the practices chosen can down-train the ANS and PFM. You might layer in breath awareness, jaw massage, and more to enhance ease. Encourage contentment and an overall message to "do" less. This sequence may also be supportive for people with overactive bladder syndrome or interstitial cystitis.

- Prone savasana restorative to enhance relaxation and breath excursion (Chapter 10)
- Table rocking, emphasizing the expansion and widening on the way back, perhaps spending a few breaths there before coming forward (Chapter 11)
- Restorative supported child's pose (Chapter 11)
- Savasana with props filling negative spaces at ankles, knees, neck, and head (Chapter 11)

When the above practices seem integrated, consider progressing with:

- Constructive rest position (Chapter 6) moving into smooth, efficient pelvic tilts (Chapter 9)
- Single leg march (Chapter 9) focus on efficiency; potentially add knees to chest or happy baby
- Half dog at the wall (Chapter 9) or wide leg forward bend (Chapter 11)
- Wall baby (Chapter 11), legs up the chair, or reclined restorative (Chapter 10)
- Supported bridge (Chapter 5); if tolerated well, could extend legs up along the wall to enhance inversion's benefits
- Savasana; consider qualities of surrender, self-compassion, trust

Sequence 3: Building strength and balance for underactive PFM and asymmetry

Utilize the breath and sound strategies throughout these movements to enhance connection to and coherence in PFM activation (Chapter 5). Also, allow cues to support symmetrical PFM awareness and movement coordination according to what you observe in a student.

- Child's pose; consider using side bend to balance awareness between sides of PFM (Chapter 11)
- Cat-cow initiated with pelvic awareness (Chapter 11); trusting strength as dynamic, adaptive experience
- Table rocking; enjoy how push through balls of feet can activate deep core and PFM support; utilize femur rotation according to assessment (Chapter 11)
- Standing dynamic alignment explorations and/or inner earth and space, a standing flow (Chapter 6)

When these practices seem integrated, consider progressing with:

- Prone leg lift and/or bridge (Chapter 11)
- 90-90 barrel rolling and/or transverse plane butterfly from supine (Chapter 11); enhance adductor activation by holding a yoga block between knees during rolling
- Chair pose with block between knees (Chapter 11) or another active squat variation
- Ninja balance and front lunge repetitions or isometric holds (Chapter 11); once integrated could progress into additional narrow stance poses
- Heart womb mudra standing flow to integrate bilaterally (Chapter 11)
- Savasana; potential themes of security, strength, confidence, nonjudgment of asymmetry

Sequence 4: Practicing with prolapse

Remember, prolapse-like symptoms (pressure, bulging, heaviness) can be associated with either an underactive or overactive PFM tendency. First, focus on enhancing trusting awareness, efficient breath coordination, and "unloading" the PFM's role of supporting the pelvic organs. It's essential that we help people build skills to manage symptoms in everyday movements. Gradually help students learn how to practice relatively symptom-free, and then progress as indicated by the student's feedback.

- CRP into supported bridge (Chapter 5); elevate pelvis as much as needed to find comfort
- Bridge with block between knees to enhance awareness of PFM (Chapter 11); could also consider doing a wall bridge variation – from legs up the wall, press into heels to bridge dynamically; inversion further unloads pelvic organs
- Single leg march (Chapter 9) focused on learning effective IAP management
- Table rocking with focus on actively engaging from push of feet without increased pressure or bearing down sensations; consider this a prerequisite for squats (Chapter 11)
- Legs up the chair with strap around outer thighs and block between knees (Chapter 10)
- CRP or savasana with possible themes of acceptance, trust, compassionate boundaries

When these practices seem integrated, consider progressing with the following:

- Consider core cylinder and thoracic mobility: rib circumference feedback (Chapter 5), rib fanning (Chapter 6); consider side bending and twists
- Standing dynamic alignment and/or inner earth and space, a standing flow (Chapter 6)
- Sit to stand or chair pose with block between and strap around thighs for containment and connection (Chapter 11); if pressure exacerbated when working upright, first enhance skill from supine or table
- Rest in supported bridge; finish with supported savasana

APPENDIX C

Constipation Relief

Chronic constipation is no fun, and it's quite common in people with pelvic symptoms or conditions. The root causes of constipation can vary widely from lifestyle factors to more serious conditions like cancer, comorbidities that cause nerve damage, and more, so it's important that we ask our client to rule these out with their medical team.

Two potential causes of constipation that we can support with yoga therapy are slow transit and functional disorganization in the pelvic floor. Slow transit means the stool sits in the colon too long, allowing more water to be extracted than desired, hence the firm, dry quality. Maybe the students missed "the call" or perhaps their dietary habits perpetuate this sluggish pattern of poo. Educating the client about pelvic-floor function and elimination, and increasing their capacity to sense the PFM, may assist them in developing more efficient coordination for toileting, learning to let go with greater ease.

What's in a yoga therapist's scope for nutrition guidance?

Nutritional habits and perceived stressors can create an inflammatory environment that exacerbates pelvic pain, GI disorders, and incontinence symptoms. Nutrition, ayurvedic lifestyle management, and digestive health deserve their own books, and what works for one client nutritionally may not be wise for another.

As a yoga teacher and yoga therapist faculty trainer, one of the most common questions I hear is: "What type of support can we offer around nutrition and diet, since we're not licensed dieticians or nutritionists?" We refrain from offering specific macronutrient profiles or recommending supplements, as these lie outside the bounds of our scope. Creating a meal plan, prescribing a calorie range, or managing one's vitamin, mineral, and herbal supplement intake require advanced training. Please have trusted professionals waiting in the wings to support customized dietary changes.

We *can* support clients in becoming aware of their habits, like what environment they eat meals in and how, offering meals as a practice of slowing down, attuning their senses to what they're about to consume. One simple idea could be choosing to sit at the table with colleagues and chew slowly rather than eating quickly at their desk between meetings.

If we suggest, for example, a food journal, our role is first to help a student become aware of what they do daily and then help them identify patterns that may connect with the state of their stool. Compassion can be practiced in place of judgment as they work to build a more sustainable lifestyle. They take the lead, and we can gently steer them with general lifestyle and nutrition recommendations that are widely accepted as sound and beneficial.

We may suggest a warm beverage first thing in the morning and prior to meals, and increasing healthy fats like avocado and unctuous foods like steamed vegetables, juicy fruits, and broths. Even a slow, warmed oil massage can enhance circulation and movement as a student glides their hands over the contours of their body and may benefit the person's sense of wellbeing and calmness to facilitate positive digestive changes. Our goal here is to cultivate the opposite qualities of constipation – more lubrication, fluidity, and ease.

Save time for toileting

Our sigmoid colon stores stool until peristalsis (sometimes referred to as a "mass movement") makes it move down – which happens one to three times per day. This natural movement of the bowel that gives us "the urge" happens when we awaken from sleep and as a natural follow-up response to eating. What goes in must come out, folks.

I've noticed over the years that the simplest tip, and perhaps hardest to implement for many students, is to be body-aware enough to feel this subtle urge begin to cue an elimination event and *to make time for it* during their morning routine. Remember the story where my client high-fived me over the oranges because she finally eliminated? This pivot to make more space in her morning created more sustainable, easeful habits for her PFM and bowels. We could also implement an evening routine to drop into parasympathetic function, encouraging clients to get to bed earlier to make way for the morning movement.

You may be keen to know that Shelly Prosko (2015), a pelvic health physiotherapist and yoga therapist, created a beautiful toilet meditation which has been translated into many languages for your convenience.

Organize your pooping posture

Elevating your feet during bowel movements allows the puborectalis muscle to align the rectum as a more direct, vertical exit down into the toilet bowl. It's shaped like a lasso around your rectum; it conveniently alters the exit route to assist with retention or continence while standing, walking, and going about your day.

With your feet up on the tub, a stack of books, or a toileting stool, this muscle relaxes and "unkinks the hose," possibly making elimination more efficient. This can help folks learn to reduce the effort used to eliminate, lessening the strain on the pelvic tissues. For people with prolapse, constipation or a habit of straining could have been a contributing factor in the descent of their pelvic organs; this may provide an additional symptom-management strategy.

Restorative postures

When using a restorative sequence to support bowel movements, consider the region or location of this system and how we can influence it in multiple planes through asana. When we move our body in space or relative to gravity, our organs also move. Postures like prone savasana and supported child's pose where the trunk and abdomen are firmly supported can help facilitate deeper, more fluid breathing and bring relaxed awareness to the belly and its contents.

Moving into supported twists, sidelying postures that encourage lateral flexion of the trunk, and supported forward bends can all further enhance motility and mobility of the lower gastrointestinal tract, and may support apana vayu, the downward eliminating current of energy in the body. Keep in mind how the postures you select will influence the activity of the student's pelvic floor; investigate how your cues can facilitate relaxation in the PFM.

Restorative postures chosen for elimination may focus far less on creating musculoskeletal "stretch" or "opening" sensations and seek to provide a safe nest wherein the student can surrender, soften, and rest. Find ways to support your student in accessing the relaxation response through yoga-therapy practice and in the pace and rhythm of daily life.

Belly massage practice

Some students find great relief from a simple practice of self-touch that encourages relaxation and gentle mobilization of the colon's contents. Using broad, diffuse touch, invite students to trace the pathway of their large intestine from the lower right quadrant of the abdomen up toward the lower ribs, sweeping across the transverse colon to the left side, and then stroking down the left side toward the pelvic bowl.

At no point should belly massage trigger pain, distress, or disruptions to their breathing. We want to cue their self-touch belly massage in a way that helps them feel calm. They may even feel or hear their belly gurgling in response.

In cases of constipation, I use the analogy of a sold-out concert. The folks far away from the stage in the back row are nearest to the exit. They leave first when the show's over, everyone else must wait their turn. Similarly, when the descending colon is packed with firm, hard stool, we might consider gently massaging *only* down the lower left quadrant of the abdomen first. Once a successful bowel movement has occurred, and as a self-care and maintenance practice, the student could return to tracing lovingly along the entire pathway of this system from right to left.

In closing

We might think of constipation as a reflection of inactivity or sluggishness and suggest asana, walking, deep breathing, and restorative sequences to get things moving, literally. The opposite approach may be warranted for other kinds of digestive-symptom presentations. When our clients exhibit disturbances like IBS, cramping, spasms, reflux, or diarrhea, we may be working instead with a reactive quality in their system. Consider all presenting factors and plan asana selections accordingly so as not to exacerbate symptoms.

We can work with students to identify mental-emotional factors and help restore a sense of safety through nervous-system reeducation, pranayama, and restorative practices that instill peace and comfort. Every client is unique, and the suggestions in this appendix must be adapted accordingly.

Reference

Prosko, S. (2015) *The 6 Stages of Toilet Meditation.* Accessed on 23/08/21 at https://physioyoga.ca/the-6-stages-of-toilet-meditation.

Practices Index

Sample sequences are available in Appendix B for enhancing pelvic awareness, overactive/pain relief, underactive/strength building, and practicing with prolapse.

Subject Index

Note: page numbers given in *italics* refer to illustrations

Author Index